Injury & Trauma Sourcebook

Learning Disabilities Sourcebook, 4th Edition

Leukemia Sourcebook

Liver Disorders Sourcebook

Medical Tests Sourcebook, 4th Edition

Men's Health Concerns Sourcebook, 4th Edition

Mental Health Disorders Sourcebook, 5th Edition

Mental Retardation Sourcebook

Movement Disorders Sourcebook, 2nd Edition

Multiple Sclerosis Sourcebook

Muscular Dystrophy Sourcebook

Obesity Sourcebook

Osteoporosis Sourcebook

Pain Sourcebook, 3rd Edition

Pediatric Cancer Sourcebook

Physical & Mental Issues in Aging Sourcebook

Podiatry Sourcebook, 2nd Edition

Pregnancy & Birth Sourcebook, 3rd Edition

Prostate & Urological Disorders Sourcebook

Prostate Cancer Sourcebook

Rehabilitation Sourcebook

Respiratory Disorders Sourcebook, 2nd Edition

Sexually Transmitted Diseases Sourcebook, 5th Edition

Sleep Disorders Sourcebook, 3rd Edition

Smoking Concerns Sourcebook

Sports Injuries Sourcebook, 4th Edition

Stress-Related Disorders Sourcebook, 3rd Edition

Stroke Sourcebook, 2nd Edition

Surgery Sourcebook, 2nd Edition

Thyroid Disorders Sourcebook

Transplantation Sourcebook

Traveler's Health Sourcebook

Urinary Tract & Kidney Diseases & Disorders Sourcebook, 2nd Edition

Vegetarian Sourcebook

Women's Health Concerns Sourcebook, 3rd Edition

Workplace Health & Safety Sourcebook

Worldwide Health Sourcebook

Teen Health Series

Abuse & Violence Information for Teens

Accident & Safety Information for Teens

Alcohol Information for Teens, 2nd Edition

Allergy Information for Teens

Asthma Information for Teens, 2nd Edition

Body Information for Teens

Cancer Information for Teens, 2nd Edition

Complementary & Alternative Medicine Information for Teens

Diabetes Information for Teens, 2nd Edition

Diet Information for Teens, 3rd Edition

Drug Information for Teens, 3rd Edition

Eating Disorders Information for Teens, 2nd Edition

Fitness Information for Teens, 3rd Edition

Learning Disabilities Information for Teens

Mental Health Information for Teens, 3rd Edition

Pregnancy Information for Teens, 2nd Edition

Sexual Health Information for Teens, 3rd Edition

Skin Health Information for Teens, 2nd Edition

Sleep Information for Teens

Sports Injuries Information for Teens, 3rd Edition

Stress Information for Teens

Suicide Information for Teens, 2nd Edition

Tobacco Information for Teens, 2nd Edition

Childhood
Diseases and
Disorders
SOURCEBOOK

Third Edition

Health Reference Series

Third Edition

Childhood
Diseases and
Disorders
SOURCEBOOK

*Basic Consumer Health Information about the
Physical, Mental, and Developmental Health of Pre-
Adolescent Children, Including Facts about Infectious
Diseases, Asthma and Allergies, Cancer, Diabetes, Growth
Disorders, and Conditions Affecting the Blood, Heart,
Ear, Nose, Throat, Gastrointestinal Tract, Kidney, Liver,
Bones, Muscles, Brain, Lungs, Skin, and Eyes*

*Along with Information about Vaccines, Medications,
Wellness Promotion, a Glossary of Related Terms, and a List
of Resources for Parents and Caregivers*

**Edited by
Laura Larsen**

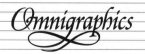

155 W. Congress, Suite 200, Detroit, MI 48226

Bibliographic Note
Because this page cannot legibly accommodate all the copyright notices, the Bibliographic Note portion of the Preface constitutes an extension of the copyright notice.

Edited by Laura Larsen

Health Reference Series

Karen Bellenir, *Managing Editor*
David A. Cooke, MD, FACP, *Medical Consultant*
Elizabeth Collins, *Research and Permissions Coordinator*
Cherry Edwards, *Permissions Assistant*
EdIndex, Services for Publishers, *Indexers*

* * *

Omnigraphics, Inc.
Matthew P. Barbour, *Senior Vice President*
Kevin M. Hayes, *Operations Manager*

* * *

Peter E. Ruffner, *Publisher*

Copyright © 2012 Omnigraphics, Inc.

ISBN 978-0-7808-1271-0

E-ISBN 978-0-7808-1272-7

Library of Congress Cataloging-in-Publication Data

Childhood diseases and disorders sourcebook : basic consumer health information about the physical, mental, and developmental health of pre-adolescent children ... / edited by Laura Larsen. -- 3rd ed.
   p. cm. -- (Health reference series)
   Summary: "Provides basic consumer health information about the physical and mental health of pre-adolescent children including common illnesses and injuries, disease prevention and screening, and wellness promotion. Includes index, glossary of related terms, and other resources"-- Provided by publisher.
   Includes bibliographical references and index.
   ISBN 978-0-7808-1271-0 (hardcover : alk. paper) 1. Pediatrics. 2. Children--Health and hygiene. 3. Children--Diseases. I. Larsen, Laura.
   RJ61.C5427 2012
   618.92--dc23
                                                      2012018883

Table of Contents

Visit www.healthreferenceseries.com to view *A Contents Guide to the Health Reference Series*, a listing of more than 16,000 topics and the volumes in which they are covered.

Part II: Childhood Infections and Related Concerns

Part III: Medical Conditions Appearing in Childhood

Part IV: Developmental and Pediatric Mental Health Concerns

Part V: Additional Help and Information

Preface

About This Book

According to the Centers for Disease Control and Prevention, in 2010, 82.1% of school-age children were reported in good or very good health. However, even healthy children often face illnesses and injuries. Other children sometimes suffer from chronic diseases that limit their daily activities or threaten future health. In addition, 20% of school-age children are currently considered obese. These matters, along with environmental hazards, lack of physical activity, poor diet, and other dangers, create concern for the well-being of our nation's children.

Childhood Diseases and Disorders Sourcebook, Third Edition, provides up-to-date information about common disorders that affect the physical, mental, and developmental health of school-age children. It discusses infectious diseases, asthma and allergies, cancer, diabetes, growth and developmental disorders, mental health and conduct disorders, and conditions affecting the blood, brain, muscles and bones, skin, and internal organs. Included are guidelines for promoting wellness and preventing injuries, along with a glossary of related terms and a list of organizations providing further information.

More in-depth information about disorders affecting infants, toddlers, and teenagers, and conditions not covered in detail, can be found in other *Health Reference Series* sourcebooks.

How to Use This Book

This book is divided into parts and chapters. Parts focus on broad areas of interest. Chapters are devoted to single topics within a part.

Part I: Introduction to Children's Health and Safety provides basic information on routine and emergency medical care for children, as well as guidelines for childhood wellness.

Part II: Childhood Infections and Related Concerns focuses on food-borne, bacterial, viral, and parasitic and fungal infections that can occur in childhood, as well as other diseases associated with infections.

Part III: Medical Conditions Appearing in Childhood describes conditions and disorders that are generally diagnosed during childhood. This part provides facts about allergies, cancer, diabetes, growth disorders, and disorders affecting the blood and heart, ear, nose, and throat, gastrointestinal tract, endocrine system, kidneys, liver, muscles and bones, brain, lungs, skin, and eyes.

Part IV: Developmental and Pediatric Mental Health Concerns details mental health disorders than can affect children as well as common developmental and learning disabilities.

Part V: Additional Help and Information provides a glossary of terms related to childhood diseases and disorders and concludes with a list of resources for parents and caregivers.

Bibliographic Note

This volume contains documents and excerpts from publications issued by the following U.S. government agencies: Centers for Disease Control and Prevention (CDC); Genetics Home Reference, U.S. National Library of Medicine; National Cancer Institute (NCI); National Dissemination Center for Children with Disabilities; National Eye Institute (NEI); National Diabetes Education Program (NDEP); National Digestive Diseases Information Clearinghouse (NDDIC); National Heart, Lung, and Blood Institute (NHLBI); National Institute of Allergy and Infectious Diseases (NIAID); National Institute of Arthritis and Musculoskeletal and Skin Diseases (NIAMS); National Institute of Child Health and Human Development (NICHD); National Institute of Diabetes and Digestive and Kidney Diseases (NIDDK); National Institute of Mental Health (NIMH); National Institute of Neurological Disorders and Stroke (NINDS); National Institute on

Deafness and Other Communication Disorders (NIDCD); Surgeon General; U.S. Department of Agriculture (USDA); U.S. Department of Health and Human Services (HHS); and U.S. Food and Drug Administration (FDA).

In addition, this volume contains copyrighted documents from the following organizations: A.D.A.M., Inc.; Akron Children's Hospital; American Academy of Orthopaedic Surgeons; American College of Emergency Physicians; American College of Gastroenterology; American Heart Association; American Liver Foundation; Ann & Robert H. Lurie Children's Hospital of Chicago; Asthma and Allergy Foundation of America; Child and Adolescent Services Research Center; Childhood Liver Disease Research and Education Network; Cleveland Clinic; Cure JM Foundation; International OCD Foundation; Lighthouse International; Magic Foundation; Massachusetts General Hospital, School Psychiatry Program and Mood and Anxiety Disorders Institute Resource Center; National Center for Learning Disabilities; Nemours Foundation; New York State Department of Health Bureau of Communicable Disease Control; Pediatric Otolaryngology Head and Neck Surgery Associates, P.A.; Safe Kids Worldwide; Seattle Children's Hospital, Research and Foundation; Southern Nevada Health District; and University of Michigan Health System.

Full citation information is provided on the first page of each chapter or section. Every effort has been made to secure all necessary rights to reprint the copyrighted material. If any omissions have been made, please contact Omnigraphics to make corrections for future editions.

Acknowledgements

Thanks go to the many organizations, agencies, and individuals who have contributed materials for this *Sourcebook* and to medical consultant Dr. David Cooke and prepress services provider WhimsyInk. Special thanks go to managing editor Karen Bellenir and research and permissions coordinator Liz Collins for their help and support.

About the Health Reference Series

The *Health Reference Series* is designed to provide basic medical information for patients, families, caregivers, and the general public. Each volume takes a particular topic and provides comprehensive coverage. This is especially important for people who may be dealing with a newly diagnosed disease or a chronic disorder in themselves or in a family member. People looking for preventive guidance, information about disease warning signs, medical statistics, and risk factors for health problems will also find answers to their questions in the *Health Reference Series*. The *Series*, however, is not intended to serve as a tool for diagnosing illness, in prescribing treatments, or as a substitute for the physician/patient relationship. All people concerned about medical symptoms or the possibility of disease are encouraged to seek professional care from an appropriate health care provider.

A Note about Spelling and Style

Health Reference Series editors use *Stedman's Medical Dictionary* as an authority for questions related to the spelling of medical terms and the *Chicago Manual of Style* for questions related to grammatical structures, punctuation, and other editorial concerns. Consistent adherence is not always possible, however, because the individual volumes within the *Series* include many documents from a wide variety of different producers and copyright holders, and the editor's primary goal is to present material from each source as accurately as is possible following the terms specified by each document's producer. This sometimes means that information in different chapters or sections may follow other guidelines and alternate spelling authorities. For example, occasionally a copyright holder may require that eponymous terms be shown in possessive forms (Crohn's disease *vs.* Crohn disease) or that British spelling norms be retained (leukaemia *vs.* leukemia).

Locating Information within the Health Reference Series

The *Health Reference Series* contains a wealth of information about a wide variety of medical topics. Ensuring easy access to all the fact sheets, research reports, in-depth discussions, and other material contained within the individual books of the *Series* remains one of our highest priorities. As the *Series* continues to grow in size and scope, however, locating the precise information needed by a reader may become more challenging.

A *Contents Guide to the Health Reference Series* was developed to direct readers to the specific volumes that address their concerns. It presents an extensive list of diseases, treatments, and other topics of general interest compiled from the Tables of Contents and major index headings. To access *A Contents Guide to the Health Reference Series*, visit www.healthreferenceseries.com.

Medical Consultant

Medical consultation services are provided to the *Health Reference Series* editors by David A. Cooke, MD, FACP. Dr. Cooke is a graduate of Brandeis University, and he received his M.D. degree from the University of Michigan. He completed residency training at the University of Wisconsin Hospital and Clinics. He is board-certified in Internal Medicine. Dr. Cooke currently works as part of the University of Michigan Health System and practices in Ann Arbor, MI. In his free time, he enjoys writing, science fiction, and spending time with his family.

Our Advisory Board

We would like to thank the following board members for providing guidance to the development of this *Series*:

- Dr. Lynda Baker, Associate Professor of Library and Information Science, Wayne State University, Detroit, MI

- Nancy Bulgarelli, William Beaumont Hospital Library, Royal Oak, MI

- Karen Imarisio, Bloomfield Township Public Library, Bloomfield Township, MI

- Karen Morgan, Mardigian Library, University of Michigan-Dearborn, Dearborn, MI

- Rosemary Orlando, St. Clair Shores Public Library, St. Clair Shores, MI

Health Reference Series *Update Policy*

The inaugural book in the *Health Reference Series* was the first edition of *Cancer Sourcebook* published in 1989. Since then, the *Series* has been enthusiastically received by librarians and in the medical community. In order to maintain the standard of providing high-quality health information for the layperson the editorial staff at Omnigraphics felt it was necessary to implement a policy of updating volumes when warranted.

Medical researchers have been making tremendous strides, and it is the purpose of the *Health Reference Series* to stay current with the most recent advances. Each decision to update a volume is made on an individual basis. Some of the considerations include how much new information is available and the feedback we receive from people who use the books. If there is a topic you would like to see added to the update list, or an area of medical concern you feel has not been adequately addressed, please write to:

Editor
Health Reference Series
Omnigraphics, Inc.
155 W. Congress, Suite 200
Detroit, MI 48226
E-mail: editorial@omnigraphics.com

Part One

Introduction to Children's Health and Safety

Chapter 1

Child Health Statistics

The National Survey of Children's Health (NSCH), conducted in 2007, contains many encouraging findings about the state of children's health in the United States. Overall, 84.4% of children in the United States are in excellent or very good health, and 88.5% receive an annual preventive health care checkup. Most children have access to a regular source of care when they are sick (93.1%) and have a personal doctor or nurse (92.2%), according to their parents.

The survey also presents information that can guide the nation in improving children's health and health care. Of children aged 1–17 years, only 78.4% receive an annual preventive dental visit, and 70.7% of children are reported to have excellent or very good oral health. Of children with family incomes below the federal poverty level (FPL), fewer than half are in excellent or very good oral health. In addition, many children with developmental, behavioral, or emotional conditions need mental health services, but only 60.0% of these children receive any mental health services, according to their parents. Only 57.5% receive their care through a "medical home," a regular source of medical care that meets the criteria of accessibility, continuity, comprehensiveness, coordination, compassion, and cultural sensitivity. This proportion varies substantially by the race and ethnicity of the child:

This chapter excerpted from "The Health and Well-Being of Children: A Portrait of States and the Nation 2007," U.S. Department of Health and Human Services, Health Resources and Services Administration, Maternal and Child Health Bureau (mchb.hrsa.gov), 2009.

68.0% of white children received care from a medical home, compared to 44.2% of black children, 63.0% of multiracial children, 38.5% of Hispanic children, and 48.6% of children of other races.

Health insurance is another area in need of systemic improvement. Nearly 10% of children lacked health insurance, and a total of 15.1% had at least one period in which they were uninsured during the year before the survey; both of these findings represent increases since the 2003 survey. Children in low-income households are more likely than children in higher-income households to have experienced a gap in health insurance in the past year: more than 24% of children in households whose income is less than 200% of the federal poverty level lacked consistent health insurance coverage. The survey also makes clear the risks associated with lack of health insurance for children. Uninsured children are more likely than those with insurance to go without preventive health and dental care and are less likely to receive needed mental health services than those with coverage.

Many aspects of children's home and family environment support their health and development. Of school-aged children, 84% read for pleasure on a typical day, a habit that can improve their school performance and support their intellectual development, and three-quarters of children eat meals with their families at least four days a week. The parents of 89.8% of children do not report usually or always feeling stress from their parenting roles. However, one major, preventable environmental threat to children is tobacco smoke in the household. Overall, 26.2% of children live in households where someone smokes, and this rate is higher for lower-income children. Of children with family incomes below the poverty level, 36.9% lived in a household with a smoker, as did 33.9% of children with household incomes between 100% and 199% of the poverty level.

Some groups of children are at higher risk of health problems and experience barriers to access to health care as well. Children in low-income households are less likely to be in excellent or very good physical or oral health, more likely to be diagnosed with asthma, more likely to display problem social behaviors, miss more days of school due to illness, and are more likely to have gaps in health care coverage than children in higher-income households. Low-income children are less likely to participate in activities outside of school, more likely to watch more than one hour of television a day in their early years, more likely to live in households where someone smokes, and more likely to live in neighborhoods that do not feel safe or supportive to their parents, and their parents are more likely to report parenting stress. These circumstances may combine to put children in low-income households at a health, developmental, and educational disadvantage.

Another population of children who may be especially vulnerable is children with special health care needs, defined as those who have a chronic physical, developmental, behavioral, or emotional condition and who also require health and related services of a type or amount beyond that required by children generally.

Compared to other children, children with special needs are more likely to have injuries that require medical care, are less likely to receive their care from a medical home, are less likely to be fully engaged in school, and miss more days of school each year. However, these children are also more likely to have health insurance and less likely to have a gap in coverage over the course of a year than are children without special health care needs.

Chapter 2

Doctor Visits and Your Child

When kids anticipate "going to the doctor," many become worried and apprehensive about the visit. Whether they're going to see their primary care doctor or a specialist—and whether for a routine exam, illness, or special problem—kids are likely to have fears, and some may even feel guilty.

Some fears and guilty feelings surface easily, so that kids can talk about them. Others are harbored secretly and remain unspoken. You can help your child express these fears and overcome them.

Common Fears and Concerns about Medical Exams

Things that often top kids' lists of concerns about going to the doctor include:

- **Separation:** Kids often fear that their parents may leave them in the exam room and wait in another room. The fear of separation from the parent during mysterious examinations is most common in kids under 7 years old, but can be frightening to older kids through ages 12 or 13.

- **Pain:** Kids may worry that a part of the exam or a medical procedure will hurt. They especially fear they may need an injection, particularly kids ages 6 through 12.

- **The doctor:** Some kids' concerns may be about the doctor's manner. A kid may misinterpret qualities such as speed, efficiency, or a detached attitude and view them as sternness, dislike, or rejection.

- **The unknown:** Apprehensive about the unknown, kids also worry that their problem may be much worse than their parents are telling them. Some who have simple problems suspect they may need surgery or hospitalization; some who are ill worry that they may die.

In addition, kids often harbor feelings of guilt: They may believe that their illness or condition is punishment for something they've done or neglected to do. Kids who feel guilty may also believe that examinations and medical procedures are part of their punishment.

How to Help

You can help by encouraging your kids to express their fears and by addressing them in words that they understand and aren't likely to misinterpret. Here are some practical ways to do this:

Explain the Purpose of the Visit

If the upcoming appointment is for a regular health checkup, explain that it's "a well-child visit. The doctor will check on how you're growing and developing, and also ask questions and examine you to make sure that your body is healthy. And you'll get a chance to ask any questions you want to about your body and your health." Also, stress that all healthy kids go to the doctor for such visits.

If the visit is to diagnose and treat an illness or other condition, explain—in very nonthreatening language—that the doctor "needs to examine you to find out how to fix this and help you get better."

It's a good idea to prepare kids by giving them advance notice of the visit and thus not a complete surprise. When explaining the purpose of the visit, talking about the doctor in a positive way also helps to promote the relationship between your child and the doctor.

Address Any Guilty Feelings

A child who is going to the doctor because of an illness or other condition might have unspoken feelings of guilt about it. Discuss the illness or condition in neutral language and reassure your child: "This isn't caused by anything you did or forgot to do. Illnesses like this happen to many kids. Aren't we lucky to have doctors who can find the causes and who know how to help us get well?"

If you, your spouse, other relatives, or friends had (or have) the same condition, share this information. Knowing that you and many others have been through the same thing may help relieve your child's guilt and fear.

If your child needs a doctor's attention because of a condition that resulted in ridicule or rejection by other kids (or even by adults), you'll need to double your efforts to relieve shame and blame. Head lice, embarrassing scratching caused by pinworm, and involuntary daytime wetting or bedwetting are examples of conditions that are often misunderstood by others.

Even if you've been very supportive, you should reassure your child again, before the visit to the doctor, that the condition is not his or her fault and that many kids have had it.

Of course, if your child has suffered an injury after disregarding safety rules, it's wise to point out (as matter-of-factly as possible) the cause-and-effect relationship between the action and the injury. However, you should still try to relieve guilt. You could say, "You probably didn't understand the danger involved in doing that, but I'm sure you understand now, and I know you won't do it that way again."

If your child repeatedly disobeys rules and becomes injured, speak to your doctor. This sort of worrisome behavior pattern needs a closer look.

In any of these cases, though, be sure to explain, especially to young kids, that going to the doctor for an examination is not a punishment. Be sure your kids understand that adults go to doctors just like kids do and that the doctor's job is to help people stay healthy and fix any problems.

Tell Kids What to Expect during a Routine Exam

Children learn best during play, and this may be a time when they feel most comfortable asking any questions regarding fears they may have. You can use a doll or teddy bear to show a young child how the nurse will measure height and weight or demonstrate parts of the routine exam.

Many children's books are available to help illustrate the doctor visit. You can offer opportunities for experiential play in simulated hospitals or doctor's offices at home, in the classroom at school, or at some children's museums.

It also helps to use role-playing to show how the doctor might:

- use a blood pressure cuff to "hug the arm";

- look in the mouth (and will need to hold the tongue down with a special stick for just a few seconds to see the throat);

- look at the eyes and into the ears;

- listen to the chest and back with a stethoscope;

- tap or press on the tummy to listen to or feel what's inside;

- look quickly to see that the "private areas" are healthy;

- tap on the knees;

- look at the feet.

It's important for parents to let their kids know that what they've taught them about the privacy of their bodies is still true, but that doctors, nurses, and parents must sometimes examine all parts of the body. Emphasize, though, that these people are the only exceptions. And reassure your child that you will be in the exam room with him or her.

Tell Kids What to Expect during Other Exams

If your child is going to the doctor because of an illness or medical condition or is going to visit a specialist, you may not even know what to expect during the examination.

When you're calling to make the appointment, you can ask to speak to the doctor or a nurse to find out, in a general way, what will take place during the office visit and exam. Then you can explain some of the procedures and their purpose in gentle language, appropriate to your child's age level. Your child will feel more secure understanding what's going to take place and why it's necessary.

Be honest, but not brutally honest. Let your child know if a procedure is going to be somewhat embarrassing, uncomfortable, or even painful, but don't go into alarming detail.

Reassure your child that you'll be there and that the procedure is truly necessary to fix—or find out how to fix—the problem. (Adolescents may prefer to be examined without a parent or with only a same-sex parent or same-sex chaperone present. That preference should be honored.)

Kids can cope with discomfort or pain more easily if they're forewarned, and they'll learn to trust you if you're honest with them.

If you don't know much about the illness or condition, admit that but reassure your child that you'll both be able to ask the doctor questions about it. Write down your child's questions.

If a blood sample will be taken during or after the examination, be careful how you explain this. Some young kids worry that "taking blood" means that *all* their blood will be taken. Let your child know that the body contains a great deal of blood and that only a very little bit of it (usually no more than 1 or 2 teaspoons [about 10 milliliters]) will be taken for testing.

Again, make certain that your child understands that the visit, with its embarrassing or uncomfortable procedures, is not a punishment for any misbehavior or disobedience.

Involve Your Child in the Process

- **Gathering information for the doctor:** If the situation isn't an emergency, allow your child to contribute to a list of symptoms that you create for the doctor. Include all symptoms you've observed, no matter how unrelated they may seem to the problem at hand. Also, before the visit, prepare a history (in the form of a list) of your child's previous illnesses and medical conditions and a history of illnesses and medical conditions among close members of the family (parents, siblings, grandparents, aunts, and uncles).

- **Writing down questions:** Ask your child to think of questions to ask the doctor. Write them down and give them to the doctor. Or, if kids are old enough, they can write down and ask the questions themselves. If the problem has occurred before, list the things that have worked and the things that haven't worked in previous treatment. Kids will be reassured by your active role in their medical care and will learn from your example. And you'll be prepared to give the doctor information vital to making an informed diagnosis.

Choose a Doctor Who Relates Well to Kids

Because your doctor is your best ally in helping your kids cope with health examinations, it's important to carefully select a doctor. Of course, you want one who's knowledgeable and competent. However, you also want a doctor who understands kids' needs and fears and who communicates easily with them, in a friendly manner and without talking down to them.

In the course of a physical exam, the doctor inspects, taps, and probes various parts of the body—procedures that may be embarrassing (or even physically uncomfortable) for kids. A good rapport between doctor and patient can minimize these feelings.

If your child's doctor seems critical, uncommunicative, disinterested, or unsympathetic, do not be afraid to change doctors. Ask for recommendations from other parents in your area or from other doctors whose opinions you trust.

If your child's illness or condition requires a specialist, ask your doctor to recommend someone who's knowledgeable, experienced, and friendly.

After all, adults want these characteristics in their own physicians, so as a parent you should serve as your child's advocate in seeking medical care.

Chapter 3

How to Give Medicine to Children

Giving Medication to Children

Are medications that are intended for children clinically tested on children?

If the product is to be used only for children, then it must be studied in the pediatric population. However, many therapies are developed for adults and then used in children without having been studied in children. Therefore, most marketed products that are mostly used in adults have not been studied in children—even though they may be used by doctors to treat children.

There has been improvement in this area in regard to prescription drugs. As of 2008, an estimated 50% to 60% of prescription drugs used to treat children have been studied in some part of the pediatric population.

How can parents find out if a medication has been tested for its effects on children?

With prescription medications, there is a "pediatric" section in the labeling that states whether the medication has been studied for its effects on children. The label will also tell you what ages have been studied.

This chapter excerpted from "Giving Medication to Children," June 9, 2009, and "Kids Aren't Just Small Adults—Medicines, Children, and the Care Every Child Deserves," June 7, 2011, U.S. Food and Drug Administration (www.fda.gov).

Most over-the-counter (OTC) products other than those for fever or pain have not actually been studied in children for effectiveness, safety, or dosing. They were approved for marketing many decades ago under a process where an expert panel looked at the evidence, including literature, and decided if a product should continue to be sold OTC.

Most of the time, these panels did not have pediatric studies and were mostly using information collected in adults to determine if the product could be used in children.

Should OTC medications be given to a child?

Parents need to weigh the benefit of treating the child's symptoms against the risk of any adverse affects of the drugs. For the common cold, for example, the symptoms will run their course. Remember, OTC cough and cold products do not treat the underlying cause of the problem. They treat the symptoms.

Read the labels to make sure the product is appropriate for your child's age. Just because a product's box says that it is intended for children does not mean it is intended for children of all ages.

Also, be sure that you understand the possible side effects so you can be aware that it may not be the disease that is causing a symptom.

What should parents keep in mind when giving medication to children?

Know that children can have different adverse reactions to a drug than adults. So for a product that has not been studied in children, it is possible for an adverse effect to occur that may not be listed on the drug's label.

Children are more sensitive than adults to many drugs. For example, antihistamines and alcohol—common ingredients in cold medications—can have adverse effects at lower doses on young patients, causing excitability or excessive drowsiness. Some drugs, like aspirin, can cause serious illness or even death in children with chickenpox or flu symptoms.

Also, realize that some diseases may be expressed differently in children than in adults, and some drugs don't work for kids even though they have been proven to work in adults.

All of these factors underscore the importance of speaking to your health care professionals and asking questions about the medicines that you are buying OTC or that are being prescribed for your child.

What are active ingredients, and why should parents be familiar with them?

A product is made up of many components. Some of these are "inactive" and just help make it taste better or dissolve better. Unless it is a combination product, usually there is only one "active" ingredient in a medication that makes it pharmaceutically active—that is, what causes the medicine to be effective against the disease or condition.

Many products, including products that treat different conditions, use the same active ingredients or the same class of active ingredients. So it is possible to overdose with a certain active ingredient if you are not careful.

You should not decide what OTC medications to take or to give a child based merely on what the large print on a product's box says. You must look for the active ingredient. Also, don't rely just on advertisements for information when it comes to giving medication to children.

How can parents make sure they give proper dosages of a medication to a child?

The main rule is: Use only as directed.

Use the measuring devices that come with the products, and use these devices as instructed. Never use home utensils such as spoons or other devices that have not been designed to measure medicine, and never have a child drink directly from a medicine bottle.

With measuring devices, pay attention to the small details. It can be easy to misread a measurement or a marking. You don't want to give your child a tablespoon when you're supposed to give him a teaspoon, or give her 5 milliliters (mL) when you're supposed to give her 0.5 mL. Mistakes like this can be deadly.

What has the U.S. Food and Drug Administration (FDA) recommended regarding OTC cough and cold medicines and children?

FDA recommends that OTC cough and cold medicines not be used to treat infants and children less than two years of age. Giving these products to these children can cause serious and potentially life-threatening side effects.

Many drug manufacturers have preemptively and voluntarily withdrawn cough and cold medicines that were being sold for use in this age group. That action was strongly supported by FDA.

If you are concerned about making your child feel more comfortable, talk with your doctor about what approaches to take. If your child's cold symptoms do not improve or get worse, contact your doctor. A persistent cough may signal a more serious condition such as bronchitis or asthma.

FDA knows of reports of serious side effects from OTC cough and cold medicines in children 2 to 11 years of age, but we haven't completed our review of information about the safety of these products in children of this age.

Kids Aren't Just Small Adults—Medicines, Children, and the Care Every Child Deserves

- Give the right medicine, in the right amount, to your child. Not all medicines are right for an infant or a child. Medicines with the same brand name can be sold in many different strengths, such as infant, children, and adult formulas. The amount and directions are also different for children of different ages or weights. Always use the right medicine and follow the directions exactly. Never use more medicine than directed, even if your child seems sicker than the last time.

- Talk to your doctor, pharmacist, or nurse to find out what mixes well and what doesn't. Medicines, vitamins, supplements, foods, and beverages don't always mix well with each other. Your health care professional can help.

- Know the difference between a tablespoon (tbsp) and a teaspoon (tsp). A tablespoon holds three times as much medicine as a teaspoon. On measuring tools, a teaspoon is equal to "5 cc" or "5 mL."

- Know your child's weight. Directions on some OTC medicines are based on weight. Never guess the amount of medicine to give to your child or try to figure it out from the adult dose instructions. If a dose is not listed for your child's age or weight, call your doctor or other members of your health care team.

- Prevent a poison emergency by always using a child-resistant cap. Relock the cap after each use. Be especially careful with any products that contain iron; they are the leading cause of poisoning deaths in young children.

- Store all medicines in a safe place. Today's medicines are tasty, colorful, and many can be chewed. Kids may think that these products are candy. To prevent an overdose or poisoning emergency, store all medicines and vitamins in a safe place out of your child's (and even your pet's) sight and reach. If your child takes too much, call the Poison Center Hotline at 800-222-1222 (open 24 hours every day, 7 days a week) or call 911.

- Check the medicine three times. First, check the outside packaging for such things as cuts, slices, or tears. Second, once you are at home, check the label on the inside package to be sure you have the right medicine. Make sure the lid and seal are not broken. Third, check the color, shape, size, and smell of the medicine. If you notice anything different or unusual, talk to a pharmacist or another health care professional.

Chapter 4

Recommended Childhood Vaccinations

Vaccines have contributed to a significant reduction in many childhood diseases, such as diphtheria, polio, measles, and whooping cough. It is now rare for American children to experience the devastating effects of these illnesses. Infant deaths due to childhood diseases have nearly disappeared in the United States and other countries with high vaccination coverage. But the germs that cause vaccine-preventable diseases and death still exist and can be passed on to people who are not protected by vaccines.

Like any medicine, vaccination has benefits and risks, and no vaccine is 100% effective in preventing disease. Most side effects of vaccines are usually minor and short-lived. A child may feel soreness at the injection site or experience a low-grade fever. Serious vaccine reactions are extremely rare, but they can happen. For example, signs of severe allergic reaction can include swelling, itching, weakness, dizziness, and difficulty breathing.

"But parents should also know that the risk of being harmed by a vaccine is much smaller than the risk of serious illness that comes with infectious diseases," says Norman Baylor, PhD, director of the Office of Vaccine Research and Review in the U.S. Food and Drug Administration (FDA)'s Center for Biologics Evaluation and Research (CBER).

This chapter excerpted from "A Parent's Guide to Kids' Vaccines," U.S. Food and Drug Administration (www.fda.gov), July 31, 2007, updated January 28, 2008. For more information, including currently recommended vaccine schedules, visit the Centers for Disease Control and Prevention (CDC)'s webpage on vaccines, available online at www.cdc.gov/vaccines/parents/index.html.

Vaccines may contain live, attenuated (but weakened), or killed (inactivated) forms of disease-causing bacteria or viruses, or components of these microorganisms. Vaccines stimulate the body to make antibodies—proteins that specifically recognize and target the disease-causing bacteria and viruses and help eliminate them from the body.

Steps to Take When You Vaccinate

Review the vaccine information sheets. These sheets explain both the benefits and risks of a vaccine. Health practitioners are required by law to provide them.

Talk to your doctor about the benefits and risks of vaccines, along with the potential consequences of not vaccinating against certain diseases. Some parents are surprised to learn that children can die of measles, chicken pox, and other vaccine-preventable diseases.

Before your child receives a vaccine, tell your doctor if you, your child, or a sibling has ever had a bad reaction to a vaccine. If your child or a sibling has had an allergic reaction or other severe reaction to a dose of vaccine, talk with your health care provider about whether that vaccine should be taken again.

Ask about conditions under which your child should not be vaccinated. This might include being sick or having a history of certain allergic or other adverse reactions to previous vaccinations or their components. For example, eggs are used to grow influenza (flu) vaccines, so a child who is allergic to eggs should not get a flu vaccine.

Adverse reactions and other problems related to vaccines should be reported to the Vaccine Adverse Event Reporting System, which is maintained by FDA and the Centers for Disease Control and Prevention. For a copy of the vaccine reporting form, call 800-822-7967 or report online to www.vaers.hhs.gov

Commonly Used Vaccines

Diphtheria, Tetanus, Pertussis (DTaP) Vaccine

- What it's for: Protects against the bacterial infections diphtheria, tetanus (lockjaw), and pertussis (whooping cough). Tripedia, Infanrix and DAPTACEL are licensed for children six weeks to seven years old. Diphtheria can infect the throat, causing a thick covering that can lead to problems with breathing, paralysis, or heart failure. Tetanus can cause painful tightening of the muscles, seizures, and paralysis. Whooping cough causes severe coughing spells and can lead to pneumonia, seizures, brain damage, and death.

- Common side effects: Mild fever, redness, soreness or swelling at the injection site, fussiness or crying more than usual.

- Tell your health care provider beforehand if your child is moderately or severely ill, has had a severe reaction to a previous shot, or has a known sensitivity to ingredients of the vaccine, including latex.

Tetanus, Diphtheria, Pertussis (Tdap) Vaccine

- What it's for: Boostrix is licensed for use for people ages 10 to 18 years. Adacel is licensed for people ages 11 years and older, up to age 64. Protects against the bacterial infections diphtheria, tetanus (lockjaw), and pertussis (whooping cough).

- Common side effects: Mild fever, pain and redness at injection site, headache, tiredness.

- Tell your health care provider beforehand if your child has had any allergic reaction to any vaccine that protects against diphtheria, tetanus, or pertussis diseases; any ingredient contained in the vaccine; or to latex.

Haemophilus Influenzae Type B (Hib) Vaccine

- What it's for: Protects against Hib disease, which can cause meningitis (an infection of the covering of the brain and spinal cord), pneumonia (lung infection), severe swelling of the throat, and infections of the blood, joints, bones, and covering of the heart. Approved for children who are at least two months old.

- Common side effects: Redness, warmth or swelling at site of injection, fever.

- Tell your health care provider beforehand if your child is moderately or severely ill or has ever had a life-threatening allergic reaction to a previous dose of Hib vaccine.

Hepatitis A Vaccine

- What it's for: Protects against liver disease caused by the hepatitis A virus. Hepatitis A can cause mild "flu-like" illness, jaundice (yellow skin or eyes), severe stomach pains, and diarrhea. A person who has hepatitis A can easily pass the disease to others within the same household. Havrix and VAQTA are licensed for use in children ages 12 months and up.

- Common side effects: Soreness at the injection site, headache, loss of appetite, tiredness.

- Tell your health care provider beforehand if your child has ever had a severe allergic reaction to a previous dose of the vaccine.

Hepatitis B Vaccine

- What it's for: Protects against liver disease caused by the hepatitis B virus. Hepatitis B can lead to liver damage, liver cancer, and death. Recombivax HB and Engerix-B are licensed for use in babies at birth.

- Common side effects: Soreness at injection site and fever.

- Tell your health care provider beforehand if your child is moderately or severely ill or has ever had a life-threatening allergic reaction to baker's yeast used for making bread or to a previous dose of the vaccine.

Human Papillomavirus (HPV) Vaccine

- What it's for: Gardasil is licensed for the prevention of cervical cancer, abnormal and precancerous cervical lesions, abnormal and precancerous vaginal and vulvar lesions, and genital warts in females ages 9 to 26.

- Common side effects: Pain, redness or swelling, itching at the site of injection, dizziness, fainting.

- Tell your health care provider beforehand if your child has had an allergic reaction to yeast or another component of HPV vaccine or to a previous dose of the vaccine.

Influenza (Flu) Vaccine—Inactivated Shot

- What it's for: Protects children six months and older against the influenza virus strains contained in the vaccine. Influenza is a contagious respiratory illness caused by the influenza virus. It can cause mild to severe illness and at times can lead to death. The influenza viruses that cause disease in people may change every year, so yearly vaccination is needed to reduce the chances of getting sick.

- Common side effects: Soreness at the injection site, low-grade fever, and aches. The influenza vaccine is made from killed or inactivated influenza viruses, so you can't get the flu from the flu shot.

- Tell your health care provider beforehand if your child is moderately or severely ill, has ever had an allergic reaction to eggs or to a previous dose of the flu vaccine, or has ever had Guillain-Barré syndrome (GBS), a serious neurological disorder that can occur either spontaneously or after certain infections. The disorder typically involves weakness in the legs and arms that can be severe.

Influenza (Flu) Vaccine—Live Intranasal

- What it's for: FluMist is sprayed into both nostrils and protects against flu in healthy children and adolescents ages 5 to 17. In September 2007, FDA approved FluMist for use in children between the ages of 2 and 5.

- Common side effects: Runny nose, headache, vomiting, muscle aches, low-grade fever. This vaccine, which contains weakened viruses, usually doesn't cause illness because the viruses have lost their disease-causing properties.

- Tell your health care provider beforehand if your child is pregnant; is moderately or severely ill; has a weakened immune system; has ever had an allergic reaction to eggs or to a previous dose of the flu vaccine; has a history of asthma or any other history of coughing, wheezing, or shortness of breath; or has a history of Guillain-Barré syndrome.

Measles, Mumps, Rubella (MMR) Vaccine

- What it's for: Protects against measles, mumps, and rubella in children ages 12 months and up. Measles is a respiratory infection that causes skin rash and flu-like symptoms. It can cause severe disease leading to ear infection, pneumonia, seizures, and brain damage. Mumps causes fever, headache, and swollen glands, especially salivary glands. It can also lead to deafness, meningitis (infection of the brain and spinal cord covering), painful swelling of the testicles or ovaries. Rubella, also called German measles, is an infection of the skin and lymph nodes and can cause arthritis. Rubella infection during pregnancy can lead to birth defects.

- Common side effects: Fever and mild rash. In rare cases, swelling of the glands in the cheeks or neck.

- Tell your health care provider beforehand if your child is ill or has ever had an allergic reaction to gelatin, the antibiotic neomycin, or a previous dose of the MMR vaccine.

Meningococcal Disease Vaccine

- What it's for: Menactra is licensed for use in people ages 11 years and older, up to age 55. In October 2007, FDA approved expanding the age range for Menactra to include children ages 2 to 10 years. Menomune is licensed for use in children 2 years and older. These vaccines protect against meningococcal disease, a serious illness caused by a bacteria. It is a leading cause of bacterial meningitis in children 2–18 years old in the United States. Meningitis is an infection of fluid surrounding the brain and the spinal cord.

- Common side effects: Sore arm, headache, fatigue.

- Tell your health care provider beforehand if your child has had a severe allergic reaction to a previous dose of meningococcal vaccine; has a known sensitivity to vaccine components or latex, which is used in the vial stopper; or has bleeding disorders or a history of Guillain-Barré syndrome, a serious neurological disorder that can occur either spontaneously or after certain infections. The disorder typically involves weakness in the legs and arms that can be severe.

Pneumococcal Conjugate Vaccine

- What it's for: Prevnar (Pneumococcal 7-valent Conjugate Vaccine) protects infants and toddlers against serious pneumococcal disease, such as meningitis and blood infections, and some ear infections.

- Common side effects: Redness, tenderness, swelling at injection site, fever, fussiness, drowsiness, loss of appetite.

- Tell your health care provider beforehand if your child is moderately or severely ill or has ever had an allergic reaction to a previous dose.

Pneumococcal Vaccine Polyvalent

- What it's for: Pneumovax 23 is licensed for use in children with certain health conditions who are two years or older for the prevention of the 23 most prevalent types of pneumococcal bacteria. Pneumococcal disease can lead to serious infections of the blood; the lungs, such as pneumonia; and the covering of the brain (meningitis).

- Common side effects: Soreness, warmth, redness, swelling at the site of injection.

- Tell your health care provider beforehand if your child is allergic to any component of the vaccine, has a respiratory illness or other active infection, or has severely compromised cardiovascular and/or pulmonary function.

Polio Vaccine

- What it's for: The inactivated poliovirus vaccine (IPV) protects against the virus that causes polio, an illness that can cause paralysis or death. For children at least two months old.

- Common side effects: Soreness at injection site, muscle aches, low-grade fever.

- Tell your health care provider beforehand if your child has ever had a severe allergic reaction to a previous shot or an allergic reaction to the antibiotics neomycin, streptomycin, or polymyxin B.

Rotavirus Vaccine

- What it's for: RotaTeq is a live vaccine given by mouth to prevent rotavirus gastroenteritis in infants. This viral infection of the stomach and intestines can cause severe diarrhea, vomiting, and fever, which may lead to serious dehydration. For children who are at least 6 weeks old, but younger than 32 weeks.

- Common side effects: Mild, temporary diarrhea or vomiting.

- Tell your health care provider beforehand if your child has a known or weakened immune system, is allergic to any of the ingredients of the vaccine, or has ever had an allergic reaction after getting a dose of the vaccine.

Varicella (Chicken Pox) Vaccine

- What it's for: Varivax (varicella virus vaccine live) protects against chicken pox in people one year and older. Chicken pox, which is caused by the varicella-zoster virus, causes itchy blisters and fever. Complications of chicken pox can include skin infection, scarring, brain swelling, and pneumonia.

- Common side effects: Soreness or swelling at the injection site, fever, mild rash.

- Tell your health care provider beforehand if your child is moderately or severely ill or has ever had a life-threatening allergic reaction to gelatin, the antibiotic neomycin, or a previous dose of chicken pox vaccine.

Chapter 5

Promoting Wellness

Chapter Contents

Section 5.1

Nutrition for Children

"Dietary Guidelines," "Choose MyPlate: 10 Tips to a Great Plate," and "Be a Healthy Role Model for Children: 10 Tips for Setting Good Examples," U.S. Department of Agriculture Center for Nutrition Policy and Promotion (www.choosemyplate.gov), June 2011.

Dietary Guidelines

The *Dietary Guidelines for Americans* are jointly issued and updated every five years by the Department of Agriculture (USDA) and the Department of Health and Human Services (HHS). They provide authoritative advice for Americans ages two and older about consuming fewer calories, making informed food choices, and being physically active to attain and maintain a healthy weight, reduce risk of chronic disease, and promote overall health.

The *Dietary Guidelines for Americans* describe a healthy diet as one that follows these characteristics:

- Emphasizes fruits, vegetables, whole grains, and fat-free or low-fat milk and milk products

- Includes lean meats, poultry, fish, beans, eggs, and nuts

- Is low in saturated fats, trans fats, cholesterol, salt (sodium), and added sugars

The recommendations in the *Dietary Guidelines* and in MyPlate are for the general public over two years of age. MyPlate is not a therapeutic diet for any specific health condition. Individuals with a chronic health condition should consult with a health care provider to determine what dietary pattern is appropriate for them.

MyPlate helps individuals use the *Dietary Guidelines* to do the following:

- Make smart choices from every food group

- Find balance between food and physical activity

- Get the most nutrition out of calories
- Stay within daily calorie needs

Choose MyPlate: 10 Tips to a Great Plate

Making food choices for a healthy lifestyle can be as simple as using these 10 tips. Use the ideas in this section to balance your calories, to choose foods to eat more often, and to cut back on foods to eat less often.

1. **Balance calories:** Find out how many calories you need for a day as a first step in managing your weight. Go to www.Choose MyPlate.gov to find your calorie level. Being physically active also helps you balance calories.

2. **Enjoy your food, but eat less:** Take the time to fully enjoy your food as you eat it. Eating too fast or when your attention is elsewhere may lead to eating too many calories. Pay attention to hunger and fullness cues before, during, and after meals. Use them to recognize when to eat and when you've had enough.

3. **Avoid oversized portions:** Use a smaller plate, bowl, and glass. Portion out foods before you eat. When eating out, choose a smaller size option, share a dish, or take home part of your meal.

4. **Foods to eat more often:** Eat more vegetables, fruits, whole grains, and fat-free or 1% milk and dairy products. These foods have the nutrients you need for health—including potassium, calcium, vitamin D, and fiber. Make them the basis for meals and snacks.

5. **Make half your plate fruits and vegetables:** Choose red, orange, and dark-green vegetables like tomatoes, sweet pota-toes, and broccoli, along with other vegetables for your meals. Add fruit to meals as part of main or side dishes or as dessert.

6. **Switch to fat-free or low-fat (1%) milk:** They have the same amount of calcium and other essential nutrients as whole milk, but fewer calories and less saturated fat.

7. **Make half your grains whole grains:** To eat more whole grains, substitute a whole-grain product for a refined product— such as eating whole wheat bread instead of white bread or brown rice instead of white rice.

8. **Foods to eat less often:** Cut back on foods high in solid fats, added sugars, and salt. They include cakes, cookies, ice cream, candies, sweetened drinks, pizza, and fatty meats like ribs, sausages, bacon, and hot dogs. Use these foods as occasional treats, not everyday foods.

9. **Compare sodium in foods:** Use the Nutrition Facts label to choose lower sodium versions of foods like soup, bread, and frozen meals. Select canned foods labeled "low sodium," "reduced sodium," or "no salt added."

10. **Drink water instead of sugary drinks:** Cut calories by drinking water or unsweetened beverages. Soda, energy drinks, and sports drinks are a major source of added sugar, and calories, in American diets.

Be a Healthy Role Model for Children: 10 Tips for Setting Good Examples

You are the most important influence on your child. You can do many things to help your children develop healthy eating habits for life. Offering a variety of foods helps children get the nutrients they need from every food group. They will also be more likely to try new foods and to like more foods. When children develop a taste for many types of foods, it's easier to plan family meals. Cook together, eat together, talk together, and make mealtime a family time!

1. **Show by example:** Eat vegetables, fruits, and whole grains with meals or as snacks. Let your child see that you like to munch on raw vegetables.

2. **Go food shopping together:** Grocery shopping can teach your child about food and nutrition. Discuss where vegetables, fruits, grains, dairy, and protein foods come from. Let your children make healthy choices.

3. **Get creative in the kitchen:** Cut food into fun and easy shapes with cookie cutters. Name a food your child helps make. Serve "Janie's Salad" or "Jackie's Sweet Potatoes" for dinner. Encourage your child to invent new snacks. Make your own trail mixes from dry whole-grain, low-sugar cereal and dried fruit.

4. **Offer the same foods for everyone:** Stop being a "short-order cook" by making different dishes to please children. It's easier to plan family meals when everyone eats the same foods.

5. **Reward with attention, not food:** Show your love with hugs and kisses. Comfort with hugs and talks. Choose not to offer sweets as rewards. It lets your child think sweets or dessert foods are better than other foods. When meals are not eaten, kids do not need "extras"—such as candy or cookies—as replacement foods.

6. **Focus on each other at the table:** Talk about fun and happy things at mealtime. Turn off the television. Take phone calls later. Try to make eating meals a stress-free time.

7. **Listen to your child:** If your child says he or she is hungry, offer a small, healthy snack—even if it is not a scheduled time to eat. Offer choices. Ask "Which would you like for dinner: broccoli or cauliflower?" instead of "Do you want broccoli for dinner?"

8. **Limit screen time:** Allow no more than two hours a day of screen time like TV and computer games. Get up and move during commercials to get some physical activity.

9. **Encourage physical activity:** Make physical activity fun for the whole family. Involve your children in the planning. Walk, run, and play with your child—instead of sitting on the sidelines. Set an example by being physically active and using safety gear, like bike helmets.

10. **Be a good food role model:** Try new foods yourself. Describe its taste, texture, and smell. Offer one new food at a time. Serve something your child likes along with the new food. Offer new foods at the beginning of a meal, when your child is very hungry. Avoid lecturing or forcing your child to eat.

Section 5.2

Physical Fitness and Health

This section excerpted from "How Much Physical Activity Do Children Need?" March 30, 2011, and "Physical Activity for Everyone: Making Physical Activity Part of a Child's Life," February 16, 2011, Centers for Disease Control and Prevention (www.cdc.gov).

Physical Activity Guidelines for Children

How much physical activity do children need?

Children and adolescents should do 60 minutes (one hour) or more of physical activity each day.

This may sound like a lot, but don't worry! Your child may already be meeting the *Physical Activity Guidelines for Americans*. Encourage your child to participate in activities that are age appropriate, enjoyable, and offer variety! Just make sure your child or adolescent is doing three types of physical activity:

1. **Aerobic activity:** Aerobic activity should make up most of your child's 60 or more minutes of physical activity each day. This can include either moderate-intensity aerobic activity, such as brisk walking, or vigorous-intensity activity, such as running. Be sure to include vigorous-intensity aerobic activity on at least three days per week.

2. **Muscle strengthening:** Include muscle strengthening activities, such as gymnastics or push-ups, at least three days per week as part of your child's 60 or more minutes.

3. **Bone strengthening:** Include bone strengthening activities, such as jumping rope or running, at least three days per week as part of your child's 60 or more minutes.

How do I know if my child's aerobic activity is moderate or vigorous intensity?

1. As a rule of thumb, on a scale of 0 to 10, where sitting is a 0 and the highest level of activity is a 10, moderate-intensity

activity is a 5 or 6. When your son does moderate-intensity activity, his heart will beat faster than normal and he will breathe harder than normal. Vigorous-intensity activity is a level 7 or 8. When your son does vigorous-intensity activity, his heart will beat much faster than normal and he will breathe much harder than normal.

2. Another way to judge intensity is to think about the activity your child is doing and compare it to the average child. What amount of intensity would the average child use? For example, when your daughter walks to school with friends each morning, she's probably doing moderate-intensity aerobic activity. But while she is at school, when she runs or chases others by playing tag during recess, she's probably doing vigorous-intensity activity.

What do you mean by "age-appropriate" activities?

Some physical activity is better suited for children than adolescents. For example, children do not usually need formal muscle-strengthening programs, such as lifting weights. Younger children usually strengthen their muscles when they do gymnastics, play on a jungle gym, or climb trees. As children grow older and become adolescents, they may start structured weight programs. For example, they may do these types of programs along with their football or basketball team practice.

Making Physical Activity a Part of a Child's Life

How is it possible for my child to meet the Guidelines?

Many physical activities fall under more than one type of activity. This makes it possible for your child to do two or even three types of physical activity in one day! For example, if your daughter is on a basketball team and practices with her teammates every day, she is not only doing vigorous-intensity aerobic activity but also bone-strengthening. Or, if your daughter takes gymnastics lessons, she is not only doing vigorous-intensity aerobic activity but also muscle- and bone-strengthening! It's easy to fit each type of activity into your child's schedule—all it takes is being familiar with the *Guidelines* and finding activities that your child enjoys.

What can I do to get—and keep—my child active?

As a parent, you can help shape your child's attitudes and behaviors toward physical activity, and knowing these guidelines is a great place to start. Throughout their lives, encourage young people to be physically active for one hour or more each day, with activities ranging from informal, active play to organized sports. Here are some ways you can do this:

- Set a positive example by leading an active lifestyle yourself.

- Make physical activity part of your family's daily routine by taking family walks or playing active games together.

- Give your children equipment that encourages physical activity.

- Take young people to places where they can be active, such as public parks, community baseball fields, or basketball courts.

- Be positive about the physical activities in which your child participates and encourage new activities.

- Make physical activity fun. Fun activities can be anything your child enjoys, either structured or nonstructured. Activities can range from team sports or individual sports to recreational activities such as walking, running, skating, bicycling, swimming, playground activities, or free-time play.

- Instead of watching television after dinner, encourage your child to find fun activities to do individually or with friends and family, such as walking, playing chase, or riding bikes.

- Be safe! Always provide protective equipment such as helmets, wrist pads, or kneepads, and ensure that activity is age appropriate.

Section 5.3

Obesity in Children

This section excerpted from "Basics about Childhood Obesity," April 26, 2011, "Data and Statistics," April 21, 2011, and "A Growing Problem," November 28, 2011, Centers for Disease Control and Prevention (www.cdc.gov).

How is childhood overweight and obesity measured?

Body mass index (BMI) is a measure used to determine childhood overweight and obesity. It is calculated using a child's weight and height. BMI does not measure body fat directly, but it is a reasonable indicator of body fatness for most children and teens.

A child's weight status is determined using an age- and sex-specific percentile for BMI rather than the BMI categories used for adults because children's body composition varies as they age and varies between boys and girls.

Centers for Disease Control and Prevention (CDC) growth charts (at http://www.cdc.gov/growthcharts/cdc_charts.htm) are used to determine the corresponding BMI-for-age and sex percentile for children and adolescents (aged 2–19 years):

- Overweight is defined as a BMI at or above the 85th percentile and lower than the 95th percentile for children of the same age and sex.

- Obesity is defined as a BMI at or above the 95th percentile for children of the same age and sex.

What are the consequences of childhood obesity?

Childhood obesity can have a harmful effect on the body in a variety of ways. Obese children are more likely to have the following symptoms:

- High blood pressure and high cholesterol, which are risk factors for cardiovascular disease (CVD)

- Increased risk of impaired glucose tolerance, insulin resistance, and type 2 diabetes

- Breathing problems, such as sleep apnea, and asthma

- Joint problems and musculoskeletal discomfort

- Fatty liver disease, gallstones, and gastro-esophageal reflux (i.e., heartburn)

- A greater risk of social and psychological problems, such as discrimination and poor self-esteem, which can continue into adulthood

Childhood obesity can lead to health risks later in life as well.

- Obese children are more likely to become obese adults. Adult obesity is associated with a number of serious health conditions including heart disease, diabetes, and some cancers.

- If children are overweight, obesity in adulthood is likely to be more severe.

What are obesity rates among all children in the United States?

- Approximately 17% (or 12.5 million) of children and adolescents aged 2–19 years are obese.

- Since 1980, obesity prevalence among children and adolescents has almost tripled.

- There are significant racial and ethnic disparities in obesity prevalence among U.S. children and adolescents. In 2007–2008, Hispanic boys, aged 2 to 19 years, were significantly more likely to be obese than non-Hispanic white boys, and non-Hispanic black girls were significantly more likely to be obese than non-Hispanic white girls.

What causes childhood obesity?

Childhood obesity is the result of eating too many calories and not getting enough physical activity.

Why focus on food and physical activity environments?

There are a variety of environmental factors that determine whether or not the healthy choice is the easy choice for children and their parents. American society has become characterized by environments that promote increased consumption of less healthy food and physical inactivity. It can be difficult for children to make healthy food choices and get enough physical activity when they are exposed to environments in their home, child care center, school, or community that are influenced by the following unhealthy choices:

- **Sugar drinks and less healthy foods on school campuses:** About 55 million school-aged children are enrolled in schools across the United States, and many eat and drink meals and snacks there. Yet, more than half of U.S. middle and high schools still offer sugar drinks and less healthy foods for purchase.

- **Advertising of less healthy foods:** Nearly half of U.S. middle and high schools allow advertising of less healthy foods, which impacts students' ability to make healthy food choices. In addition, foods high in total calories, sugars, salt, and fat, and low in nutrients, are highly advertised and marketed through media targeted to children and adolescents, while advertising for healthier foods is almost nonexistent in comparison.

- **Variation in licensure regulations among child care centers:** More than 12 million children regularly spend time in child care arrangements outside the home. However, not all states use licensing regulations to ensure that child care facilities encourage more healthful eating and physical activity.

- **Lack of daily, quality physical activity in all schools:** Most adolescents fall short of the *2008 Physical Activity Guidelines for Americans* recommendation of at least 60 minutes of aerobic physical activity each day, as only 18% of students in grades 9–12 met this recommendation in 2007.

- **No safe and appealing place, in many communities, to play or be active:** Many communities are built in ways that make it difficult or unsafe to be physically active. For some families, getting to parks and recreation centers may be difficult, and public transportation may not be available. Half of the children in the United States do not have a park, community center, and sidewalk in their neighborhood.

- **Limited access to healthy affordable foods**: Some people have less access to stores and supermarkets that sell healthy, affordable food such as fruits and vegetables, especially in rural, minority, and lower-income neighborhoods.

- **Greater availability of high-energy-dense foods and sugar drinks:** High-energy-dense foods are ones that have a lot of calories in each bite. A recent study among children showed that a high-energy-dense diet is associated with a higher risk for excess body fat during childhood. Sugar drinks are the largest source of added sugar and an important contributor of calories in the diets of children in the United States.

- **Increasing portion sizes:** Portion sizes of less healthy foods and beverages have increased over time in restaurants, grocery stores, and vending machines. Research shows that children eat more without realizing it if they are served larger portions.

- **Lack of breastfeeding support:** Breastfeeding protects against childhood overweight and obesity. However, in the United States, while 75% of mothers start out breastfeeding, only 13% of babies are exclusively breastfed at the end of six months.

- **Television and media:** Children 8–18 years of age spend an average of 7.5 hours a day using entertainment media, including TV, computers, video games, cell phones, and movies. TV viewing is a contributing factor to childhood obesity because it may take away from the time children spend in physical activities; lead to increased energy intake through snacking and eating meals in front of the TV; and influence children to make unhealthy food choices through exposure to food advertisements.

Section 5.4

Healthy Sleep Habits

Everyone needs sleep; our bodies require it to survive. Following a sleep routine when your children are young can help your entire family develop healthy sleeping habits. Sounds simple enough, but parents with young children know that a child who doesn't sleep well can turn a family's life into a bad dream.

Not enough sleep can result in daytime sleepiness, irritability, frustration, attention problems, and difficulty controlling impulses and emotions. Children who don't get enough sleep may not appear sleepy, but instead seem to be hyperactive or disobedient.

Sleep Problems

A parent's natural instinct is to comfort young children when they can't fall asleep. However, making a habit of feeding, rocking, holding, or lying in the bed with your son can create problems.

He may learn to associate falling asleep with these activities and will be unable to sleep without them. In addition, everyone wakes up briefly several times each night. Most people aren't even aware of it and return to sleep quickly. However, a young child who associates sleep with the habits mentioned here will not be able to fall asleep again until that same activity occurs. This is known as sleep-onset association disorder.

To prevent this in an infant, always put your baby to bed drowsy, but awake; in a toddler, help him not to associate falling asleep with your presence. Since your son probably will cry until he learns to fall asleep without you, try gradually increasing the time before responding to him and decreasing the time you are in his room.

Also, make sure he has his security friend or object if he takes one to bed. If you must enter your daughter's room, do not turn on the lights or remove her from bed unless it's necessary for her safety or comfort. By following these guidelines, children will usually learn to fall asleep by themselves within a week.

Older children may have trouble sleeping because of fear. If you lie down with your child at naps and bedtime, now is the time to teach him to fall asleep on his own. Begin by sitting on a chair near the bed until he falls asleep. After several nights, move closer to the door. Eventually move the chair out of the room. Leave the door open if he doesn't get out of bed, but close it if he does.

This process can take one to three weeks to learn. Use rewards, such as star charts or small prizes and lots of verbal praise, to speed the process. Be consistent—by letting your child backslide just once, she may think she can get away with it again.

Sleep problems tend to occur at predictable ages. Infants less than three months old normally wake and sleep for short periods throughout the day and night, including waking for feedings. Sleep-onset association disorder also occurs in older infants and toddlers, causing frequent waking and feeding at night

Delaying bedtime by needing to use the bathroom or wanting a drink can occur in children over two years into the early school-age years. Sleep terrors, fear of the dark, or nightmares often begin in children ages two to four.

Sleepwalking usually begins in children over six. Teenagers often have a sleep problem called delayed phase sleep disorder, which causes trouble falling asleep before midnight and difficulty being fully awake until after 9 or 10 a.m. This problem is made worse by high schools having early start times.

Other sleep problems in teens are caused by caffeine; nicotine or illegal drug use; psychiatric disorders, such as depression; or medical conditions like narcolepsy or insomnia.

Most common sleep problems can be corrected with a little guidance and some common sense.

Signs of Sleep Problems

Signs that your child may have a sleep problem include:

- snoring;

- apnea or pauses when breathing during sleep;

- can't fall asleep at night or stay awake during the day;

- school performance suffers;

- needs help from a parent to fall asleep;
- wakes up repeatedly throughout the night;
- behavior problems and mood swings.

Consequences of Lack of Sleep

Lack of sleep affects both children and adults. People who get less sleep than they need, even if it's only an hour less, develop sleep debt, which can interfere with daily routines and activities.

Even when you don't feel sleepy, sleep debt can negatively affect how you function throughout the day. It can cause you to fall asleep at dangerous times, like when driving. Sleepiness can increase the risk of accidents and injuries in both children and adults.

Lack of sleep also can impact how your child performs in school or sports. Studies indicate that people who don't get enough sleep die sooner than those who sleep normally.

How Much Sleep Is Enough?

While the development of the brain plays a role in establishing sleep-wake cycles and how much sleep a person needs, learning and conditioning also have an effect. This is good news for parents, who can help their children develop healthy sleep habits.

When establishing sleep routines, keep the following in mind:

- Newborns up to 3 months will sleep between 16 to 20 hours in a 24-hour period, sleeping for 1 to 4 hours and waking for 1 to 2 hours.

- Depending on the baby, newborns will begin to tell the difference between day and night between 6 weeks and 3 months of age.

- A 4- to 5-month-old will sleep 14 or 15 hours each day with up to 6 to 8 hours of continuous sleep.

- A 6- to 12-month-old will sleep 13 to 14 hours a day with two naps.

- Between 70% and 80% of 9-month-olds will sleep through the night.

- Toddlers sleep about 12 hours a day with usually one nap.

- Preschoolers, ages three to six, sleep 10 or 11 hours each day. Naps decrease during this time and usually end around age five (or sooner in some children).

- School-age children need up to 10 hours of sleep.

- Teens should get 9 hours of sleep each night.

- Most adults should sleep 8 hours.

Healthy Sleep Tips

It's much easier to prevent a sleep problem than to treat one, so here are some tips to help your child establish life-long patterns of good sleep:

- Set a regular bedtime and stick to it.

- Create a consistent bedtime routine, typically around 30 minutes long. This may include giving your child a warm bath or reading a story.

- Make after-dinner playtime a relaxing time. Too much activity close to bedtime can keep children awake.

- Avoid big meals within four hours of bedtime.

- Avoid giving children caffeinated products including cocoa less than six hours before bedtime.

- Set a comfortable bedroom temperature—not too warm or cold.

- Keep the bedroom dark. If necessary, use a small nightlight. Expose your child to natural sunlight soon after awakening in the morning.

- Keep the noise level low.

- Don't give in to requests for one more kiss or a tissue.

- A firm and consistent approach to a stall tactic will help avoid reinforcing the behavior. If your son needs to use the bathroom, send him by himself. This limits more contact with you.

- Except for younger children who need naps, avoid naps during the day.

- Exercise can promote good sleep, but not within two hours of bedtime.

- Avoid emotional conversations, watching TV that is exciting or scary, or playing electronic or computer games before bedtime.

- Keep the TV out of your child's bedroom.

- Talk with your pediatrician about medications that may affect your child's sleep. Ask for alternative medications if necessary.

- If your older child is having sleep problems, encourage her to keep a sleep diary to record how much time she slept the night before and how she feels the next day. After one week, review the diary with her and look for potential influences on the quality and quantity of her sleep, such as watching TV, drinking something caffeinated, or arguing with a sibling before bed.

- Teenagers should not alter their bedtime and waking time by more than one hour on weekends or while on vacation.

Section 5.5

The Importance of Handwashing

Why is hand washing important?

Proper hand washing is the most effective way to prevent the spread of infectious diseases.

Is there a right way to wash your hands?

There is more to hand washing than you think!

- Rub your hands together vigorously with warm, soapy water to remove dirt, oils, and germs from the skin.

- The soapy lather traps the dirt, oil, and germs, making them easier to wash away.

Follow these five simple steps:

- Turn on the faucet to start the warm running water. Wet your hands.

- Apply soap and lather well, scrubbing between fingers, wrists, backs of hands, and under nails for at least 30 seconds.

- Rinse with warm water running from your wrist down to your fingertips, then into the sink.

- With the water still running, dry your hands well. Disposable towels or air hand dryers are required in public restrooms.

- Using the disposable towel, turn off the sink faucet and then dispose. Keep washed hands covered to prevent recontamination.

Once you have properly washed your hands, an alcohol-based hand sanitizer may be used. Use hand lotion if dry skin becomes a problem.

What type of soap should I use?

Liquid soap is required at all public hand washing areas; however, bar soap may be used in your home. A self-draining holder that is cleaned frequently is recommended for bar soap.

When family members are sick, use liquid soap and disposable towels. Avoid bar soap and shared cloth towels as they may spread germs.

What should we teach children about hand washing?

It is important to teach children how to wash their hands using the same steps listed here. Teach them to sing "Row, Row, Row Your Boat," or the "Happy Birthday" song twice while washing their hands to ensure they wash them for the proper length of time.

Adults and children should wash their hands:

- after touching bare human body parts other than clean hands and clean, exposed portions of arms;

- before and after eating or drinking;

- after playing outdoors;

- after playing with pets;

- after using the bathroom;

- after coughing, sneezing, or blowing their noses;

- after handling soiled equipment or utensils;

- after food preparation, as often as necessary to remove soil and contamination and to prevent cross-contamination when changing tasks;

- after switching between working with raw food and working with ready-to-eat food;

- after using tobacco;

- after engaging in other activities that contaminate the hands.

Even though hands may appear to be clean, they may carry germs that cause disease.

Don't assume that children know how to wash their hands properly. Supervision, especially in a child care setting, is essential to forming good hand washing habits in children.

Finally, children learn by example. Let them see good hand washing habits from adults who care for them.

Section 5.6

The Effects of Secondhand Smoke on Children

This section excerpted from "The Health Consequences of Involuntary Exposure to Tobacco Smoke," Office of the Surgeon General, U.S. Department of Health and Human Services (www.surgeongeneral.gov), January 4, 2007, reviewed by David A. Cooke, MD, FACP, April 2012, and "Health Effects of Secondhand Smoke," Centers for Disease Control and Prevention (www.cdc.gov), March 21, 2011.

The Health Consequences of Involuntary Exposure to Tobacco Smoke

- Secondhand smoke contains more than 250 chemicals known to be toxic or carcinogenic (cancer causing), including formaldehyde, benzene, vinyl chloride, arsenic, ammonia, and hydrogen cyanide. Children who are exposed to secondhand smoke are inhaling many of the same cancer-causing substances and poisons as smokers.

Health Effects of Secondhand Smoke in Children

- Because their bodies are developing, infants and young children are especially vulnerable to the poisons in secondhand smoke.

- Both babies whose mothers smoke while pregnant and babies who are exposed to secondhand smoke after birth are more likely to die from sudden infant death syndrome (SIDS) than babies who are not exposed to cigarette smoke.

- Mothers who are exposed to secondhand smoke while pregnant are more likely to have lower birth weight babies, which makes babies weaker and increases the risk for many health problems.

- Babies whose mothers smoke while pregnant or who are exposed to secondhand smoke after birth have weaker lungs than other babies, which increases the risk for many health problems.

- Secondhand smoke exposure causes acute lower respiratory infections such as bronchitis and pneumonia in infants and young children.

- Secondhand smoke exposure causes children who already have asthma to experience more frequent and severe attacks.

- Secondhand smoke exposure causes respiratory symptoms, including cough, phlegm, wheeze, and breathlessness, among school-aged children.

- Children exposed to secondhand smoke are at increased risk for ear infections and are more likely to need an operation to insert ear tubes for drainage.

Exposure to Secondhand Smoke among Children

- The Surgeon General has concluded that there is no risk-free level of secondhand smoke exposure. Even brief exposures can be harmful.

- On average, children are exposed to more secondhand smoke than nonsmoking adults.

- Based on levels of cotinine (a biological marker of secondhand smoke exposure), an estimated 22 million children aged 3–11 years and 18 million youth aged 12–19 years were exposed to secondhand smoke in the United States in 2000.

- Children aged 3–11 years and youth aged 12–19 years are significantly more likely than adults to live in a household with at least one smoker.

- Children aged 3–11 years have cotinine levels more than twice as high as nonsmoking adults.

- Children who live in homes where smoking is allowed have higher cotinine levels than children who live in homes where smoking is not allowed.

Health Effects of Secondhand Smoke

- Studies show that older children whose parents smoke get sick more often. Their lungs grow less than children who do not breathe secondhand smoke, and they get more bronchitis and pneumonia.

- Wheezing and coughing are more common in children who breathe secondhand smoke.

- Secondhand smoke can trigger an asthma attack in a child. Children with asthma who are around secondhand smoke have more severe and frequent asthma attacks. A severe asthma attack can put a child's life in danger.

- Children whose parents smoke around them get more ear infections. They also have fluid in their ears more often and have more operations to put in ear tubes for drainage.

Parents can help protect their children from secondhand smoke by taking the following actions:

- Do not allow anyone to smoke near your child.

- Do not smoke or allow others to smoke in your home or car. Opening a window does not protect your children from smoke.

- Use a smoke-free day care center.

- Do not take your child to restaurants or other indoor public places that allow smoking.

- Teach children to stay away from secondhand smoke.

Section 5.7

Skin Cancer Prevention

This section excerpted from "Protecting Children from the Sun," Centers for Disease Control and Prevention (www.cdc.gov), June 14, 2011.

Just a few serious sunburns can increase your child's risk of skin cancer later in life. Kids don't have to be at the pool, beach, or on vacation to get too much sun. Their skin needs protection from the sun's harmful ultraviolet (UV) rays whenever they're outdoors.

- **Seek shade.** UV rays are strongest and most harmful during midday, so it's best to plan indoor activities then. If this is not possible, seek shade under a tree, an umbrella, or a pop-up tent. Use these options to prevent sunburn, not to seek relief after it's happened.

- **Cover up.** Clothing that covers your child's skin helps protect against UV rays. Although a long-sleeved shirt and long pants with a tight weave are best, they aren't always practical. A T-shirt, long shorts, or a beach cover-up are good choices, too—but it's wise to double up on protection by applying sunscreen or keeping your child in the shade when possible.

- **Get a hat.** Hats that shade the face, scalp, ears, and neck are easy to use and give great protection. Baseball caps are popular among kids, but they don't protect their ears and neck. If your child chooses a cap, be sure to protect exposed areas with sunscreen.

- **Wear sunglasses.** They protect your child's eyes from UV rays, which can lead to cataracts later in life. Look for sunglasses that wrap around and block as close to 100% of both UVA and UVB rays as possible.

- **Apply sunscreen.** Use sunscreen with at least SPF 15 and UVA and UVB protection every time your child goes outside. For the best protection, apply sunscreen generously 30 minutes before going outdoors. Don't forget to protect ears, noses, lips, and the tops of feet.

Take sunscreen with you to reapply during the day, especially after your child swims or exercises. This applies to waterproof and water-resistant products as well.

Follow the directions on the package for using a sunscreen product on babies less than six months old. All products do not have the same ingredients; if your or your child's skin reacts badly to one product, try another one or call a doctor. Your baby's best defense against sunburn is avoiding the sun or staying in the shade.

The U.S. Food and Drug Administration has announced significant changes to sunscreen product labels that will help consumers decide how to buy and use sunscreen and allow them to protect themselves and their families from sun-induced damage more effectively.

Keep in mind, sunscreen is not meant to allow kids to spend more time in the sun than they would otherwise. Try combining sunscreen with other options to prevent UV damage.

Too Much Sun Hurts

Turning pink? Unprotected skin can be damaged by the sun's UV rays in as little as 15 minutes. Yet it can take up to 12 hours for skin to show the full effect of sun exposure. So, if your child's skin looks "a little pink" today, it may be burned tomorrow morning. To prevent further burning, get your child out of the sun.

Tan? There's no other way to say it—tanned skin is damaged skin. Any change in the color of your child's skin after time outside—whether sunburn or suntan—indicates damage from UV rays.

Cool and cloudy? Children still need protection. UV rays, not the temperature, do the damage. Clouds do not block UV rays, they filter them—and sometimes only slightly.

Oops! Kids often get sunburned when they are outdoors unprotected for longer than expected. Remember to plan ahead, and keep sun protection handy—in your car, bag, or child's backpack.

Chapter 6

Preventing Childhood Injuries

Chapter Contents

Section 6.1

Preventing Burns

Burn Prevention for Big Kids At Home

Flame burns (caused by direct contact with fire) are more common among older children. Because young children have thinner skin than older children and adults, their skin burns at lower temperatures and more deeply. There are several precautions parents and caregivers can take to keep children safe from burns.

Top Tips

In the kitchen:

- Do not allow children to use a microwave until they are both tall enough to reach in safely and able to understand that steam can cause burns.
- Place hot foods and liquids on the center of the table.
- Always supervise young children in the kitchen and around electrical appliances and outlets.

Around the house:

- Set your water heater to 120 degrees or lower to avoid burns.
- Keep matches, gasoline, lighters, and all other flammable materials locked away and out of children's reach.
- Cover unused electrical outlets.

Fire Prevention for Big Kids At Home

Big kids are curious about fire. Teaching your children about the hazards of playing with matches and other flammable materials, as well as practicing a fire escape route with your family, can help prevent accidents and injuries. Fires resulting from children's play are the leading cause of residential fire-related death and injury among children ages nine and under.

Also, many children are scared by fire, and they may hide or act irrationally, making escape unlikely. Planning and practicing a fire escape route with your family and talking to your children about what to expect in a fire are simple steps anyone can take. A prepared child is more likely to escape unharmed.

Top Tips

In the kitchen:

- Don't wear loose-fitting clothing in the kitchen.
- Never leave the kitchen unattended while cooking, and never leave a child alone while cooking.
- Keep anything that can catch fire (like dish towels or wooden spoons) away from your stovetop.

In the bedroom:

- Install smoke alarms in and outside of every sleeping area and test smoke alarms monthly.
- Teach children what to do when they hear the sound of the smoke alarm.
  - Crawl low under smoke.
  - Touch doors before opening them; if the door is hot, use another exit.
  - Never go back into a burning building; children should be reminded not to stop or return for anything, such as a toy or to call 911.
  - Upon leaving the burning building, children whose clothes have caught fire should immediately stop, drop to the ground, and roll back and forth quickly to extinguish the flames.

Around the house:

- Practice an escape plan with your child.
- Teach young children not to play with matches or lighters. Lock up matches and lighters out of their sight and reach.
- Keep all portable heaters out of children's reach and at least three feet away from flammable objects.

- Avoid plugging several appliance cords into the same electrical socket.

- Keep children away from candles and other open flames.

Section 6.2

Preventing Drowning

This section excerpted from "Unintentional Drowning: Fact Sheet," Centers for Disease Control and Prevention (www.cdc.gov), May 16, 2011.

Every day, about 10 people die from unintentional drowning. Of these, 2 are children aged 14 or younger. Drowning is the sixth leading cause of unintentional injury death for people of all ages, and the second leading cause of death for children ages 1 to 14 years.

More than one in five people who die from drowning are children 14 and younger. For every child who dies from drowning, another four received emergency department care for nonfatal submersion injuries.

More than 55% of drowning victims treated in emergency departments require hospitalization or transfer for higher levels of care (compared to a hospitalization rate of 3%–5% for all unintentional injuries). These injuries can be severe.

Nonfatal drownings can cause brain damage that may result in long-term disabilities including memory problems, learning disabilities, and permanent loss of basic functioning (e.g., permanent vegetative state).

What factors influence drowning risk?

- **Lack of supervision and barriers:** Supervision by a lifeguard or designated water-watcher is important to protect young children when they are in the water, whether a pool or bathtub. But when children are not supposed to be in the water, supervision alone isn't enough to keep them safe.

  Barriers such as pool fencing should be used to help prevent young children from gaining access to the pool area without caregivers' awareness. There is an 83% reduction in the risk of childhood drowning with a four-sided isolation pool fence, compared to three-sided property-line fencing.

Among children ages one to four years, most drownings occur in residential swimming pools. Most young children who drowned in pools were last seen in the home, had been out of sight less than five minutes, and were in the care of one or both parents at the time.

- **Natural water settings (such as lakes, rivers, or the ocean):** The percent of drownings in natural water settings increases with age. When a location was known, 65% of drownings among those 15 years and older occurred in natural water settings.

- **Lack of life jacket use in recreational boating:** In 2009, the U.S. Coast Guard received reports for 4,730 boating incidents; 3,358 boaters were reported injured, and 736 died. Among those who drowned, 9 out of 10 were not wearing life jackets.

- **Alcohol use:** Alcohol use is involved in up to half of adolescent and adult deaths associated with water recreation and about one in five reported boating fatalities.

- **Seizure disorders:** For persons with seizure disorders, drowning is the most common cause of unintentional injury death, with the bathtub as the site of highest drowning risk.

What has research found?

- Participation in formal swimming lessons can reduce the risk of drowning by 88% among children aged one to four years.

- Seconds count. Cardiopulmonary resuscitation (CPR) performed by bystanders has been shown to improve outcomes in drowning victims. The more quickly intervention occurs, the better chance of improved outcomes.

How can drowning be prevented?

Take the following steps to help prevent water-related injuries:

- **Supervision when in or around the water:** Designate a responsible adult to watch young children while in the bath and all children swimming or playing in or around water. Supervisors of preschool children should provide "touch supervision" and be close enough to reach the child at all times. Adults should not be involved in any other distracting activity (such as reading, playing cards, talking on the phone, or mowing the lawn) while supervising children.

- **Buddy system:** Always swim with a buddy. Select swimming sites that have lifeguards whenever possible.

- **Seizure disorder safety:** If you or a family member has a seizure disorder, provide one-on-one supervision around water, including swimming pools. Consider taking showers rather than using a bathtub for bathing.

- **Learn to swim:** Formal swimming lessons can protect young children from drowning. However, even when children have had formal swimming lessons, constant, careful supervision when children are in the water, and barriers, such as pool fencing, to prevent unsupervised access are necessary.

- **Learn CPR:** In the time it might take for paramedics to arrive, your CPR skills could make a difference in someone's life.

- **Do not use air-filled or foam toys:** Do not use air-filled or foam toys, such as "water wings," "noodles," or inner tubes, in place of life jackets (personal flotation devices). These toys are not designed to keep swimmers safe.

- **Avoid alcohol:** Avoid drinking alcohol before or during swimming, boating, or water skiing. Do not drink alcohol while supervising children.

Take these precautions if you have a swimming pool at home:

- **Four-sided fencing:** Install a four-sided pool fence that completely separates the house and play area of the yard from the pool area. The fence should be at least four feet high. Use self-closing and self-latching gates that open outward with latches that are out of reach of children. Also, consider additional barriers such as automatic door locks or alarms to prevent access or notify you if someone enters the pool area.

- **Clear the pool and deck of toys:** Remove floats, balls, and other toys from the pool and surrounding area immediately after use so children are not tempted to enter the pool area unsupervised.

Take these steps if you are in or around natural bodies of water:

- Know the local weather conditions and forecast before swimming or boating. Strong winds and thunderstorms with lightning strikes are dangerous.

- Use U.S. Coast Guard–approved life jackets when boating, regardless of distance to be traveled, size of boat, or swimming ability of boaters.

- Know the meaning of and obey warnings represented by colored beach flags, which may vary from one beach to another.

- Watch for dangerous waves and signs of rip currents (e.g., water that is discolored and choppy, foamy, or filled with debris and moving in a channel away from shore). If you are caught in a rip current, swim parallel to shore; once free of the current, swim toward shore.

Section 6.3

Preventing Falls

Excerpted from "Falls Prevention Tips," © 2012 Safe Kids Worldwide (www.safekids.org). All rights reserved. Reprinted with permission.

Prevent window falls.

- Install window guards to prevent children from falling out of windows. For windows above the first floor, install window guards with an emergency release device in case of fire.

- Install window stops so that windows open no more than four inches.

- Keep windows locked and closed when they are not being used.

- Keep furniture away from windows so kids cannot climb to the ledge.

- If you have double-hung windows—the kind that can open down from the top as well as up from the bottom—it is generally safer to open the top pane, but growing kids may have enough strength, dexterity, and curiosity to open the bottom pane.

- Do not rely on window screens to prevent falls.

- Keep windows locked when they are closed.

- Supervise children at all times, especially around open windows.

- Never try to move a child who appears to be seriously injured after a fall—call 911 and let trained medical personnel move the child with proper precautions.

Playground equipment should be kept in good repair and securely anchored above a soft surface.

- Recommended surface materials include sand, pea gravel, wood chips, mulch, and shredded rubber. Rubber mats, synthetic turf, and other artificial materials are also safe surfaces and require less maintenance.

- Avoid playgrounds with asphalt, concrete, grass, dirt, and soil surfaces under the equipment. A fall onto a shock-absorbing surface is less likely to cause a serious injury than a fall onto a hard surface.

- Surfacing should be at least 12 inches deep and extend at least six feet in all directions around stationary equipment. Depending on the height of the equipment, surfacing may need to extend farther than six feet.

- For swings, make sure that the surfacing extends, in the back and front, twice the height of the suspending bar, so if the top of the swing set is 10 feet high, the surfacing should extend 20 feet.

Use of appropriate safety equipment is essential.

- Children should always wear activity-specific, properly fitting safety gear when participating in recreational activities.

- See *Bike and Wheels Safety for Big Kids at Play* tip sheet for more information [at www.safekids.org/safety-basics/big-kids/ at-play/bike-and-wheels-safety.html].

Prevent furniture tip overs.

- If a piece of furniture is unstable or top-heavy, secure it to a stud in the wall using brackets, braces, anchors, or wall straps. Large items such as TVs, microwaves, fish tanks, bookcases, heavy furniture, and appliances can topple off stands and fall on children.

- If possible, use a stand specifically designed for your TV as recommended by the manufacturer or place your TV on sturdy furniture appropriate for its size. Make sure both the stand and

TV are properly secured to the wall and push your TV as far back on the stand as possible, out of your child's reach.

- If you have a newer, flat screen TV, make sure it is properly anchored to the wall.

- Read the manufacturer's instructions for tips or warnings regarding placement of your TV or furniture.

- Keep heavier items on lower shelves or in lower drawers.

- Tie up loose cords, as a child pulling on an electrical cord, or tripping on one, could pull an appliance off a stand.

- Do not keep remote controls, candy, toys, or other items that attract children on top of furniture, as your child might be enticed to reach for these items.

When taking your children to the grocery store, take these steps to prevent shopping cart falls.

- Put your child in a stroller, wagon, or front pack instead of in a shopping cart.

- Ask your older child to walk and praise him or her for behaving and staying near you.

- Use the shopping carts that have a wheeled child carrier that is permanently attached and made part of the shopping cart. Some of these models look like cars or benches attached to the shopping cart.

- If you are placing your child in the shopping cart seat, always use a harness or safety belt to restrain your child. If the belt is missing or broken, select another cart and tell the store manager so a replacement can be installed.

- Never leave your child alone or unattended in a shopping cart and stay close to the cart at all times.

- Do not let your child ride in the cart basket, under the basket, on the sides, or on the front of the cart. Do not let an older child push the cart with another younger child in it.

Take these basic precautions to help prevent falls around the home.

- Use nonslip rugs on the floor and mats or decals in the bathtub or shower.

- Keep hallways and stairs well-lit and clear of clutter.

- Never let children play on high porches, decks, stairs, or balconies.

- Safety gates at the tops of stairs must be attached to the wall, as these are more secure than the kind held in place by outward pressure. Use safety gates that meet current safety standards to avoid entrapment and other hazards.

Section 6.4

Preventing Poisoning

"Poison Prevention for Big Kids at Home,"
© 2012 Safe Kids Worldwide (www.safekids.org). All rights reserved.
Reprinted with permission.

Big kids may spend more time without adult supervision. You can best protect your children by keeping harmful substances out of their sight and reach, and by testing for lead and carbon monoxide.

Although household cleaners are a frequent cause of poisoning, kids can also be fatally poisoned by iron, alcohol, and carbon monoxide. Because no prevention method is 100% effective, learn how to keep poison exposure from turning into tragedy for you and your family.

Top Tips

In the kitchen:

- Keep cleaning products in their original containers. Never put a potentially poisonous product in something other than its original container (like a plastic soda bottle), where it could be mistaken for something harmless.

- Know which household products are poisonous.

- Lock up poisons out of children's sight and reach.

In the bathroom:

- Always read labels and follow the exact directions. Give children medicines based on their weights and ages, and only use the dispensers that come packaged with children's medications.

- Never refer to medicine or vitamins as "candy."

- Do not have children help you take medication.

Around the house:

- Be aware of medications that may be in your handbag. Store handbags out of the reach of young children.

- Install carbon monoxide (CO) detectors in your home.

- Prevent CO buildup in the first place—make sure heating appliances are in good working order and used only in well-ventilated areas.

- Don't run a car engine in the garage, even to warm it up; move the car outside first.

Section 6.5

Preventing Motor Vehicle Injuries

Regardless of age, all passengers need to be buckled in. Follow specific guidelines for your child's height, age, and weight to determine the best child safety restraint. For children ages five to nine, who are under 4 feet 9 inches tall and less than 80 to 100 pounds, a car seat or booster seat is a must for the best protection.

Top Tips

- Use a car seat with a harness or booster seat with the vehicle lap *and* shoulder safety belts until your child passes the Safety Belt Fit Test.

- Vehicle seat belts are designed to fit an average-sized adult. To get the best protection from a seat belt, children usually need a booster until they are about 4 feet 9 inches tall and weigh between 80 and 100 pounds. Many children will be between 8 and 12 years of age before they meet these height and weight requirements.

- Use a booster seat correctly in a back seat every time your child rides in a car.

- Older kids get weighed and measured less often than babies, so check your child's growth a few times a year.

- Be sure to correctly install your car seat or booster seat. Booster seats are not installed the same way car seats are. Booster seats sit on the vehicle seat and are used to properly position the adult seat belt for an older child.

- A booster seat uses no harness. It uses the vehicle's lap *and* shoulder belts only. Be sure the seat belt is properly buckled.

- For children who are riding in booster seats, never place the shoulder belt under the child's arm or behind the child's back.

- Be sure all occupants wear safety belts correctly every time. Children learn from adult role models.

- Tell all drivers who transport your child that a car seat or booster seat use is a must when your child is in their vehicles.

- Treat seat belts as you would any cord or rope. Do not allow children to play with them at any time.

When your child reaches 4 feet 9 inches and between 80 to 100 pounds, use the Safety Belt Fit Test to determine if the child is big enough to use the adult seat belt without a booster. Use the Safety Belt Fit Test on every child under 13.

The Safety Belt Fit Test

- Have your child sit in a back seat with his or her bottom and back against the vehicle's seat back. Do the child's knees bend at the seat's edge?

  - If yes, go on.

  - If not, the child must stay in a booster seat.

- Buckle the seat belt. Does the lap belt stay low on the hips or high on the thigh?

  - If yes, go on.

  - If it rests on the soft part of the stomach, the child must stay in a booster seat.

- Look at the shoulder belt. Does it lie on the collarbone and shoulder?

  - If yes, go on. If it is on the face or neck, the child must remain in a booster seat.

  - Never put the shoulder belt under the child's arm or behind the child's back. Do not allow children to play with the shoulder portion of a seat belt. Treat it like any cord.

- Can the child maintain the correct seating position with the shoulder belt on the shoulder and the lap belt low across the hips, or high on the thighs?

  - If yes, the child has passed the Safety Belt Fit Test.

  - If no, the child should return to a booster seat and re-test in a month.

Chapter 7

Fevers and Febrile Seizures in Children

Chapter Contents

Section 7.1

Fevers in Children

"Children and Fever: What Parents Should Know,"
© American College of Emergency Physicians, 2011.
Used with permission.

The more a parent knows about a child's special health needs, the more effective he or she will be when responding to an illness or emergency. To help you prepare for a fever, here's some information from the American College of Emergency Physicians.

What is a fever?

Believe it or not, fever in itself is not an illness, but a symptom for a wide range of childhood conditions. In fact, elevated body temperature plays a role in the body's normal response to fighting infection. For children, fever is defined as a rectal temperature of 100.4 degrees Fahrenheit (38 degrees Celsius) or an oral temperature above 99.5 degrees Fahrenheit (37.5 degrees Celsius).

How common are fevers in children?

Fever is one of the most common reasons for parents to visit an emergency department with their child or infant. Children tend to have an average of nine upper respiratory tract infections a year that include fevers, and children in day care or preschool tend to have more.

"Fever itself is rarely a problem," said Dr. Sharon Mace of the American College of Emergency Physicians. "However, it is a sign that infection may be present. Therefore, when a child has a fever, the focus should be on the child, and the possible infection, and not the reading on the thermometer."

Contact a physician for any child with a fever who:

- is under two months of age, because infants don't have well-developed immune systems and could have serious infections;

- has a body temperature higher than 102 degrees Fahrenheit;

- looks very sick, is poorly responsive and uninterested in his or her surroundings, is sluggish, and won't suck on breast or bottle;

- cries constantly, continuously, or without relief;

- is difficult to awaken;

- has a stiff neck;

- has purple spots on the skin;

- has difficulty breathing;

- is drooling excessively or having great difficulty swallowing;

- has symptoms of earache or sore throat;

- has a limp or will not use an arm or leg;

- has significant abdominal pain;

- has painful urination or difficulty urinating;

- has any amount of redness or swelling on his or her body; or

- has a seizure (fit or convulsion).

If the illness does not appear sufficiently serious, you can help children by not over-dressing them and by encouraging them to drink small amounts of clear fluids frequently.

Also keep in mind that children's normal body temperature varies considerably, from 97.5 degrees Fahrenheit to 99 degrees Fahrenheit. It will probably be lowest in the early morning and tend to rise as the day progresses and during active play.

"Don't rely on touch to judge a fever," said Dr. Mace. "If a child is extremely ill or dehydrated, he or she could have decreased circulation to the skin and feel cool despite having a fever. Also, when a child's temperature starts to drop, circulation to the skin may increase, allowing heat to escape, but the child may appear flushed or feel hot, despite a decreasing temperature."

Do not give children under age 19 aspirin to treat a fever, because it has been linked to Reye's Syndrome, a disease that can be fatal. Acetaminophen is effective treatment; use one 80-mg (children's chewable) tablet for each 12 pounds of body weight.

Section 7.2

Febrile Seizures

This section excerpted from "Febrile Seizures Fact Sheet,"
National Institute of Neurological Disorders and Stroke
(www.ninds.nih.gov), January 10, 2012.

What are febrile seizures?

Febrile seizures are convulsions brought on by a fever in infants or small children. During a febrile seizure, a child often loses consciousness and shakes, moving limbs on both sides of the body. Less commonly, the child becomes rigid or has twitches in only a portion of the body, such as an arm or a leg, or on the right or the left side only. Most febrile seizures last a minute or two, although some can be as brief as a few seconds while others last for more than 15 minutes.

The majority of children with febrile seizures have rectal temperatures greater than 102 degrees Fahrenheit. Most febrile seizures occur during the first day of a child's fever. Children prone to febrile seizures are not considered to have epilepsy, since epilepsy is characterized by recurrent seizures that are not triggered by fever.

How common are febrile seizures?

Approximately one in every 25 children will have at least one febrile seizure, and more than one-third of these children will have additional febrile seizures before they outgrow the tendency to have them. Febrile seizures usually occur in children between the ages of six months and five years and are particularly common in toddlers. Children rarely develop their first febrile seizure before the age of six months or after three years of age. The older a child is when the first febrile seizure occurs, the less likely that child is to have more.

What makes a child prone to recurrent febrile seizures?

A few factors appear to boost a child's risk of having recurrent febrile seizures, including young age (less than 15 months) during the first seizure, frequent fevers, and having immediate family members with a history of febrile seizures. If the seizure occurs soon after a fever has begun or when the temperature is relatively low, the risk of recurrence is higher. A long initial febrile seizure does not substantially boost the risk of recurrent febrile seizures, either brief or long.

Are febrile seizures harmful?

Although they can be frightening to parents, the vast majority of febrile seizures are short and harmless. During a seizure, there is a small chance that the child may be injured by falling or may choke from food or saliva in the mouth. Using proper first aid for seizures can help avoid these hazards.

There is no evidence that short febrile seizures cause brain damage. Large studies have found that children with febrile seizures have normal school achievement and perform as well on intellectual tests as their siblings who don't have seizures. Even when seizures are very long (more than one hour), most children recover completely, but a few might be at risk of subsequent seizures without fever (epilepsy).

In other words, between 95% and 98% of children who experience febrile seizures do not go on to develop epilepsy. However, although the absolute risk remains small, some groups of children—including those with cerebral palsy, delayed development, or other neurological abnormalities—have an increased risk of developing epilepsy. The type of febrile seizure also matters; children who have prolonged febrile seizures (particularly lasting more than an hour) or seizures that affect only part of the body, or that recur within 24 hours, are at a somewhat higher risk. Among children who don't have any of these risk factors, only one in 100 develops epilepsy after a febrile seizure.

What should be done for a child having a febrile seizure?

Seizures are frightening, but it is important that parents and caregivers stay calm and carefully observe the child. To prevent accidental injury, the child should be placed on a protected surface such as the floor or ground. The child should not be held or restrained during a convulsion. To prevent choking, the child should be placed on his or her side or stomach. When possible, gently remove any objects from the child's mouth. Never place anything in the child's mouth during a convulsion. Objects placed in the mouth can be broken and obstruct the child's airway. Look at your watch when the seizure starts. If the seizure lasts 10 minutes, the child should be taken immediately to the nearest medical facility. Once the seizure has ended, the child should be taken to his or her doctor to check for the source of the fever. This is especially urgent if the child shows symptoms of stiff neck, extreme lethargy, or abundant vomiting.

How are febrile seizures diagnosed and treated?

Before diagnosing febrile seizures in infants and children, doctors sometimes perform tests to be sure that seizures are not caused by something other than simply the fever itself. For example, if a doctor suspects the child has meningitis (an infection of the membranes surrounding the brain), a spinal tap may be needed to check for signs of the infection in the cerebrospinal fluid (fluid that bathes the brain and spinal cord). If there has been severe diarrhea or vomiting, dehydration could be responsible for seizures. Also, doctors often perform other tests such as examining the blood and urine to pinpoint the cause of the child's fever.

A child who has a febrile seizure usually doesn't need to be hospitalized. If the seizure is prolonged or is accompanied by a serious infection, or if the source of the infection cannot be determined, a doctor may recommend that the child be hospitalized for observation.

How are febrile seizures prevented?

If a child has a fever most parents will use fever-lowering drugs such as acetaminophen or ibuprofen to make the child more comfortable, although there are no studies that prove that this will reduce the risk of a seizure.

Prolonged daily use of oral anticonvulsants, such as phenobarbital or valproate, to prevent febrile seizures is usually not recommended because of their potential for side effects and questionable effectiveness for preventing such seizures.

Children especially prone to febrile seizures may be treated with the drug diazepam orally or rectally, whenever they have a fever. The majority of children with febrile seizures do not need to be treated with medication, but in some cases a doctor may decide that medicine given only while the child has a fever may be the best alternative. This medication may lower the risk of having another febrile seizure.

In addition, some children are prone to having very long (lasting an hour or more) febrile seizures. When a child has had a long febrile seizure, subsequent ones might also be long. Because very long febrile convulsions are associated with increased risk of developing epilepsy, some doctors will suggest the child be treated with a rectal form of the drug diazepam to stop the seizure and prevent it from becoming long.

Chapter 8

Responding to Medical Emergencies

Is It an Emergency?: When Your Child Has an Emergency

Nothing is more terrifying to parents than when their child has a medical emergency. Unintentional injuries are the leading cause of death in children and teens ages 1 to 21 in the U.S. The most common injuries are related to motor vehicle crashes, drowning, fires and burns, suffocation, choking, unintentional firearm injuries, falls, and poisoning. However, parents can take an active role in protecting their children by providing good care and practicing injury prevention.

To prepare for a childhood medical emergency, become familiar with the signs and symptoms of childhood emergencies, work with your pediatrician to complete a medical history form for your child, and develop a plan in case of a medical emergency. Ask when you should go directly to an emergency department, when you should call an ambulance, and what to do when the pediatrician's office is closed. In addition, become familiar with the policies of emergency departments in your community—for example, some allow parents to be with their children during invasive medical procedures, and some do not.

If you take your child to an emergency department, bring your child's medications in their original containers, as well as his or her medical history form. If you suspect your child has swallowed poison

"Is It an Emergency?" and "Warning Signs of a Childhood Medical Emergency," © American College of Emergency Physicians, 2011. Used with permission.

or any potentially harmful medications, call poison control first (800-222-1222), and then bring the suspected poisons or medications with your child to the emergency department.

In a medical emergency, go to the nearest emergency department, unless directed to another nearby hospital by the child's physician or emergency services personnel. An ambulance may transport the child to the nearest emergency department or to a nearby specialty center, if appropriate. If necessary, after stabilization, your child may be transferred to a hospital with advanced pediatric capabilities.

Since hospitals can be frightening places for children, try to bring along a favorite toy, blanket, or book to help make your child less anxious.

When a child experiences a medical emergency, it's important to stay calm and to call for help. Although this may be difficult, it is the responsibility of the parent or caretaker to do so—and remaining calm can help save the child's life.

- If you need immediate help, call 911 (or your local emergency services number).

- If needed and you know how, start rescue breathing or CPR (cardiopulmonary resuscitation).

- If you have learned first aid, apply the techniques to stop serious bleeding, manage shock, handle fractures, and control a fever until help arrives. In addition, if needed and you know how, perform basic choking-rescue procedures for infants and children.

- If the child is having a seizure, place him or her on a carpeted floor with the child's head turned to the side. Stay with your child until help arrives. Check to make sure that nothing is in the mouth or interfering with the child's ability to breathe. Do not place anything in the child's mouth when he or she is actively seizing. Placing your finger in the child's mouth could place you at risk of being bitten and cause the child to vomit and aspirate (breathe in vomit).

If you take a child to the emergency department, help calm him or her by explaining what to expect once you arrive:

- Listen. Give permission to ask questions, cry, and talk about feelings. Let the child know it's okay to be afraid and to say something hurts.

- Be comforting, but honest, including when giving information about procedures that may be painful.

- Share your feelings but remain calm; children sense when adults are anxious. Staying calm under stressful circumstances can save the child's life.

Warning Signs of a Childhood Medical Emergency: Call 911 or Seek Immediate Medical Attention

- Confusion, delirium, severe headache, unconsciousness, or vomiting, especially following a head injury

- Strange or withdrawn behavior, or any significant change from normal behavior

- Abnormal or difficult breathing

- Inability to stand up or unsteady walking

- Decreasing responsiveness or alertness

- Excessive sleepiness

- Irritability

- Skin or lips that look purple or blue (gray for darker-skinned children)

- Uncontrolled bleeding

- Increasing or severe, persistent pain

- Fever accompanied by changes in behavior (especially with a severe, sudden headache accompanied by mental changes, back/ neck stiffness, or rashes)

- Severe or persistent vomiting or diarrhea

Part Two

Childhood Infections and Related Concerns

Chapter 9

Foodborne Illness

What are foodborne illnesses?

Foodborne illnesses are caused by eating food or drinking beverages contaminated with bacteria, parasites, or viruses. Harmful chemicals can also cause foodborne illnesses if they have contaminated food during harvesting or processing. Foodborne illnesses can cause symptoms that range from an upset stomach to more serious symptoms. Most foodborne infections are undiagnosed and unreported, though the Centers for Disease Control and Prevention estimates that every year about 76 million people in the United States become ill from pathogens, or disease-causing substances, in food. Of these people, about 5,000 die.

What are the causes of foodborne illnesses?

Harmful bacteria are the most common cause of foodborne illnesses. Some bacteria may be present on foods when you purchase them. Raw foods are the most common source of foodborne illnesses because they are not sterile; examples include raw meat and poultry that may have become contaminated during slaughter. Seafood may become contaminated during harvest or through processing. One in 10,000 eggs

This chapter excerpted from "Bacteria and Foodborne Illness," National Digestive Diseases Information Clearinghouse, National Institute of Diabetes and Digestive and Kidney Diseases (digestive.niddk.nih.gov), May 2007. Reviewed by David A. Cooke, MD, FACP, April 2012.

may be contaminated with *Salmonella* inside the egg shell. Produce such as spinach, lettuce, tomatoes, sprouts, and melons can become contaminated with *Salmonella*, *Shigella*, or *Escherichia coli* (*E. coli*) O157:H7. Contamination can occur during growing, harvesting, processing, storing, shipping, or final preparation. Contamination may also occur during food preparation in a restaurant or a home kitchen. The most common form of contamination from handled foods is the calicivirus, also called the Norwalk-like virus.

When food is cooked and left out for more than two hours at room temperature, bacteria can multiply quickly. Most bacteria grow undetected because they don't produce a bad odor or change the color or texture of the food. Freezing food slows or stops bacteria's growth but does not destroy the bacteria. The microbes can become reactivated when the food is thawed. Refrigeration also can slow the growth of some bacteria. Thorough cooking is needed to destroy the bacteria.

What are the symptoms of foodborne illnesses?

In most cases of foodborne illnesses, symptoms resemble intestinal flu and may last a few hours or even several days. Symptoms can range from mild to serious and include the following:

- Abdominal cramps
- Nausea
- Vomiting
- Diarrhea, which is sometimes bloody
- Fever
- Dehydration

What are the risk factors of foodborne illnesses?

Some people are at greater risk for bacterial infections because of their age or an unhealthy immune system. Young children, pregnant women and their fetuses, and older adults are at greatest risk.

What are the complications of foodborne illnesses?

Some microorganisms, such as *Listeria monocytogenes* and *Clostridium botulinum*, cause far more serious symptoms than vomiting and diarrhea. They can cause spontaneous abortion or death.

In some people, especially children, hemolytic uremic syndrome (HUS) can result from infection by a particular strain of bacteria,

E. coli O157:H7, and can lead to kidney failure and death. HUS is a rare disorder that affects primarily children between the ages of 1 and 10 years and is the leading cause of acute renal failure in previously healthy children. A child may become infected after consuming contaminated food or beverages, such as meat, especially undercooked ground beef; unpasteurized juices; contaminated water; or through contact with an infected person.

The most common symptoms of HUS infection are vomiting, abdominal pain, and diarrhea, which may be bloody. In 5% to 10% of cases, HUS develops about 5 to 10 days after the onset of illness. This disease may last from 1 to 15 days and is fatal in 3% to 5% of cases. Other symptoms of HUS include fever, lethargy or sluggishness, irritability, and paleness or pallor. In about half the cases, the disease progresses until it causes acute renal failure, which means the kidneys are unable to remove waste products from the blood and excrete them into the urine. A decrease in circulating red blood cells and blood platelets and reduced blood flow to organs may lead to multiple organ failure. Seizures, heart failure, inflammation of the pancreas, and diabetes can also result. However, most children recover completely.

See a doctor right away if you or your child has any of the following symptoms with diarrhea:

- High fever—temperature over 101.5° F, measured orally

- Blood in the stools

- Diarrhea that lasts more than three days

- Prolonged vomiting that prevents keeping liquid down and can lead to dehydration

- Signs of severe dehydration, such as dry mouth, sticky saliva, decreased urination, dizziness, fatigue, sunken eyes, low blood pressure, or increased heart rate and breathing rate

- Signs of shock, such as weak or rapid pulse or shallow breathing

- Confusion or difficulty reasoning

How are foodborne illnesses diagnosed?

Your doctor may be able to diagnose foodborne illnesses from a list of what you've eaten recently and from results of appropriate laboratory tests. Diagnostic tests for foodborne illnesses should include examination of the feces. A sample of the suspected food, if available, can also be tested for bacterial toxins, viruses, and parasites.

How are foodborne illnesses treated?

Most cases of foodborne illnesses are mild and can be treated by increasing fluid intake, either orally or intravenously, to replace lost fluids and electrolytes. People who experience gastrointestinal or neurologic symptoms should seek medical attention.

In the most severe situations, such as HUS, hospitalization may be needed to receive supportive nutritional and medical therapy. Maintaining adequate fluid and electrolyte balance and controlling blood pressure are important. Doctors will try to minimize the impact of reduced kidney function. Dialysis may be needed until the kidneys can function normally. Blood transfusions also may be needed.

How are foodborne illnesses prevented?

Most cases of foodborne illnesses can be prevented through proper cooking or processing of food, which kills bacteria. In addition, because bacteria multiply rapidly between 40° F and 140° F, food must be kept out of this temperature range.

Follow these tips to prevent harmful bacteria from growing in food:

- Refrigerate foods promptly. If prepared food stands at room temperature for more than two hours, it may not be safe to eat. Set your refrigerator at 40° F or lower and your freezer at 0° F.

- Cook food to the appropriate internal temperature—145° F for roasts, steaks, and chops of beef, veal, and lamb; 160° F for pork, ground veal, and ground beef; 165° F for ground poultry; and 180° F for whole poultry. Use a meat thermometer to be sure. Foods are properly cooked only when they are heated long enough and at a high enough temperature to kill the harmful bacteria that cause illnesses.

- Prevent cross-contamination. Bacteria can spread from one food product to another throughout the kitchen and can get onto cutting boards, knives, sponges, and countertops. Keep raw meat, poultry, seafood, and their juices away from all ready-to-eat foods.

- Handle food properly. Always wash your hands for at least 20 seconds with warm, soapy water before and after handling raw meat, poultry, fish, shellfish, produce, or eggs. Wash your hands after using the bathroom, changing diapers, or touching animals.

- Wash utensils and surfaces before and after use with hot, soapy water. Better still, sanitize them with diluted bleach—one teaspoon of bleach to one quart of hot water.

- Wash sponges and dish towels weekly in hot water in the washing machine.
- Keep cold food cold and hot food hot.
- Maintain hot cooked food at 140° F or higher.
- Reheat cooked food to at least 165° F.
- Refrigerate or freeze perishables, produce, prepared food, and leftovers within two hours.
- Never defrost food on the kitchen counter. Use the refrigerator, cold running water, or the microwave oven.
- Never let food marinate at room temperature—refrigerate it.
- Divide large amounts of leftovers into small, shallow containers for quick cooling in the refrigerator.
- Remove the stuffing from poultry and other meats immediately and refrigerate it in a separate container.
- Wash all unpackaged fruits and vegetables, and those packaged and not marked "prewashed," under running water just before eating, cutting, or cooking. Scrub firm produce such as melons and cucumbers with a clean produce brush. Dry all produce with a paper towel to further reduce any possible bacteria.
- Do not pack the refrigerator. Cool air must circulate to keep food safe.

What are other disorders related to foodborne illnesses?

Scientists suspect that foodborne pathogens are linked to chronic disorders and can even cause permanent tissue or organ destruction. Research suggests that when some people are infected by foodborne pathogens, the activation of their immune system can trigger an inappropriate autoimmune response, which means the immune system attacks the body's own cells. In some people, an autoimmune response leads to a chronic health condition. Chronic disorders that may be triggered by foodborne pathogens are the following:

- Arthritis
- Inflammatory bowel disease
- Kidney failure
- Guillain-Barré syndrome
- Autoimmune disorders

What are common sources of foodborne illness?

- **Sources of illness:** Raw and undercooked meat and poultry
  - **Symptoms:** Abdominal pain, diarrhea, nausea, and vomiting
  - **Bacteria:** *Campylobacter jejuni*, *E. coli* O157:H7, *L. monocytogenes*, *Salmonella*

- **Sources of illness:** Raw foods; unpasteurized milk and dairy products, such as soft cheeses
  - **Symptoms:** Nausea, vomiting, fever, abdominal cramps, and diarrhea
  - **Bacteria:** *L. monocytogenes*, *Salmonella*, *Shigella*, *Staphylococcus aureus*, *C. jejuni*

- **Sources of illness:** Raw and undercooked eggs (raw eggs are often used in foods such as homemade hollandaise sauce, Caesar and other salad dressings, tiramisu, homemade ice cream, home-made mayonnaise, cookie dough, and frostings)
  - **Symptoms:** Nausea, vomiting, fever, abdominal cramps, and diarrhea
  - **Bacterium:** *Salmonella enteritidis*

- **Sources of illness:** Raw and undercooked shellfish
  - **Symptoms:** Chills, fever, and collapse
  - **Bacteria:** *Vibrio vulnificus*, *Vibrio parahaemolyticus*

- **Sources of illness:** Improperly canned goods; smoked or salted fish
  - **Symptoms:** Double vision, inability to swallow, difficulty speaking, and inability to breathe; seek medical help right away if you experience any of these symptoms
  - **Bacterium:** *C. botulinum*

- **Sources of illness:** Fresh or minimally processed produce; con-taminated water
  - **Symptoms:** Bloody diarrhea, nausea, and vomiting
  - **Bacteria:** *E. coli* O157:H7, *L. monocytogenes*, *Salmonella*, *Shigella*, *Yersinia enterocolitica*, viruses, and parasites

Chapter 10

Streptococcal Bacterial Infections

Chapter Contents

Section 10.1

Group A Streptococcal Infections

This section excerpted from "Group A Streptococcal (GAS) Disease,"
Centers for Disease Control and Prevention (www.cdc.gov), April 3, 2008.

What is group A **Streptococcus *(GAS)?***

Group A *Streptococcus* is a bacterium often found in the throat and
on the skin. People may carry group A streptococci in the throat or on
the skin and have no symptoms of illness. Most GAS infections are
relatively mild illnesses such as strep throat or impetigo. Occasionally
these bacteria can cause severe and even life-threatening diseases.

Severe, sometimes life-threatening, GAS disease may occur when
bacteria get into parts of the body where bacteria usually are not found,
such as the blood, muscle, or the lungs. These infections are termed "invasive GAS disease." Two of the most severe, but least common, forms
of invasive GAS disease are necrotizing fasciitis and streptococcal toxic
shock syndrome. Necrotizing fasciitis (occasionally described by the
media as "the flesh-eating bacteria") is a rapidly progressive disease
that destroys muscles, fat, and skin tissue. Streptococcal toxic shock
syndrome (STSS) results in a rapid drop in blood pressure and causes
organs (e.g., kidney, liver, lungs) to fail. STSS is not the same as the
"toxic shock syndrome" due to the bacteria *Staphylococcus aureus* that
has been associated with tampon usage. While 10%–15% of patients
with invasive group A streptococcal disease die from their infection,
approximately 25% of patients with necrotizing fasciitis and more
than 35% with STSS die.

How are group A streptococci spread?

These bacteria are spread through direct contact with mucus from
the nose or throat of persons who are infected or through contact
with infected wounds or sores on the skin. Ill persons, such as those
who have strep throat or skin infections, are most likely to spread the
infection. Persons who carry the bacteria but have no symptoms are
much less contagious. Treating an infected person with an antibiotic
for 24 hours or longer generally eliminates their ability to spread the

bacteria. However, it is important to complete the entire course of anti-biotics as prescribed. It is not likely that household items like plates, cups, or toys spread these bacteria.

How common is invasive group A streptococcal disease?

About 9,000–11,500 cases of invasive GAS disease occur each year in the United States, resulting in 1,000–1,800 deaths annually. STSS and necrotizing fasciitis each comprise an average of about 6%–7% of these invasive cases. In contrast, there are several million cases of strep throat and impetigo each year.

Why does invasive group A streptococcal disease occur?

Invasive GAS infections occur when the bacteria get past the de-fenses of the person who is infected. This may occur when a person has sores or other breaks in the skin that allow the bacteria to get into the tissue, or when the person's ability to fight off the infection is decreased because of chronic illness or an illness that affects the immune system. Also, some virulent strains of GAS are more likely to cause severe disease than others.

Who is most at risk of getting invasive group A streptococcal disease?

Few people who come in contact with GAS will develop invasive GAS disease. Most people will have a throat or skin infection, and some may have no symptoms at all. Although healthy people can get invasive GAS disease, people with chronic illnesses like cancer, diabe-tes, and chronic heart or lung disease, and those who use medications such as steroids, have a higher risk. Persons with skin lesions (such as cuts, chicken pox, and surgical wounds), the elderly, and adults with a history of alcohol abuse or injection drug use also have a higher risk for disease.

What are the early signs and symptoms of necrotizing fasciitis and streptococcal toxic shock syndrome?

The following are early signs and symptoms of necrotizing fasciitis:

- Severe pain and swelling, often rapidly increasing
- Fever
- Redness at a wound site

The following are early signs and symptoms of STSS:

- Fever

- Abrupt onset of generalized or localized severe pain, often in an arm or leg

- Dizziness

- Influenza-like syndrome

- Confusion

- A flat red rash over large areas of the body (only occurs in 10% of cases)

How is invasive group A streptococcal disease treated?

GAS infections can be treated with many different antibiotics. For STSS and necrotizing fasciitis, high dose penicillin and clindamycin are recommended. For those with very severe illness, supportive care in an intensive care unit may also be needed. For persons with necrotizing fasciitis, early and aggressive surgery is often needed to remove damaged tissue and stop disease spread. Early treatment may reduce the risk of death from invasive group A streptococcal disease. However, even the best medical care does not prevent death in every case.

What can be done to help prevent group A streptococcal infections?

The spread of all types of GAS infection can be reduced by good hand washing, especially after coughing and sneezing and before preparing foods or eating. Persons with sore throats should be seen by a doctor who can perform tests to find out whether the illness is strep throat. If the test result shows strep throat, the person should stay home from work, school, or day care until 24 hours after taking an antibiotic. All wounds should be kept clean and watched for possible signs of infection such as redness, swelling, drainage, and pain at the wound site. A person with signs of an infected wound, especially if fever occurs, should immediately seek medical care. It is not necessary for all persons exposed to someone with an invasive group A strep infection to receive antibiotic therapy to prevent infection. However, in certain circumstances, antibiotic therapy may be appropriate. That decision should be made after consulting with your doctor.

Section 10.2

Pneumococcal Disease

This section excerpted from "Pneumococcal Disease - Q&A,"
Centers for Disease Control and Prevention (www.cdc.gov), April 1, 2011.

What is pneumococcal disease?

Pneumococcal disease is defined as infections that are caused by the bacterium *Streptococcus pneumoniae*, also known as pneumococcus. The most common types of pneumococcal infections include middle ear infections, sinus infections, lung infections (pneumonia), blood stream infections (bacteremia), and meningitis. Some of these infections are considered to be "invasive." Invasive disease means that germs invade parts of the body that are normally free from germs. For example, pneumococcal bacteria can invade the bloodstream, causing bacteremia, and/or the tissues and fluids surrounding the brain and spinal cord, causing meningitis. When this happens, disease is usually very severe, causing hospitalization or even death.

Which children are most likely to get pneumococcal disease?

Young children are much more likely than older children and young adults to get pneumococcal disease. Children younger than two years of age, children in group child care, and children who have certain illnesses (for example, sickle cell disease, HIV infection, and chronic heart or lung conditions) are at higher risk than other children to get pneumococcal disease. Children with cochlear implants or cerebrospinal (CSF) fluid leaks are more likely to get pneumococcal meningitis. In addition, pneumococcal disease is more common among children of certain racial or ethnic groups, such as Alaska Natives, American Indians living in certain communities, and African Americans, than among other groups.

How common is pneumococcal disease?

Each year in the United States pneumococcus causes more than 4,800 cases of blood stream infections (bacteremia), meningitis, or other invasive disease in children younger than five years of age. Children under two years of age average more than one middle ear infection each year, many of which are caused by pneumococcus. Pneumococcus is the most common cause of bacteremia, pneumonia, meningitis and otitis media (middle ear infections) in young children.

What are the symptoms of pneumococcal disease?

- **Meningitis:** High fever, headache, and stiff neck are common symptoms of meningitis in anyone over the age of two years. These symptoms can develop over several hours, or they may take one to two days. Other symptoms may include nausea, vomiting, discomfort looking into bright lights, confusion, and sleepiness. In newborns and young infants, the classic symptoms of fever, headache, and neck stiffness may be absent or difficult to detect; infants may only appear slow or inactive, or be irritable, have vomiting, or be feeding poorly.

- **Pneumonia:** In adults, pneumococcal pneumonia is often characterized by sudden onset of illness with symptoms including shaking chills, fever, shortness of breath or rapid breathing, pain in the chest that is worsened by breathing deeply, and a productive cough. In infants and young children, signs and symptoms may not be specific, and may include fever, cough, rapid breathing or grunting.

- **Otitis media:** Children who have otitis media (middle ear infection) typically have a painful ear, and the eardrum is often red and swollen. Other symptoms that may accompany otitis media include sleeplessness, fever, and irritability.

- **Blood stream infections:** Infants and young children with blood stream infections—also known as bacteremia—typically have nonspecific symptoms including fevers and irritability.

How serious is pneumococcal disease?

Invasive pneumococcal disease may be a very serious illness in young children. Meningitis is the most severe type of pneumococcal disease. Of children younger than five years of age with pneumococcal meningitis, about 5% will die of their infection and others may have long-term problems such as blindness or hearing loss. Many children with pneumococcal pneumonia or blood stream infections will be ill enough to be hospitalized. About 1% of children with blood stream infections or pneumonia with a blood stream infection will die of their illness. Sinus infections and ear infections are usually mild and are much more common than serious forms of pneumococcal disease. Some children, however, develop recurrent ear infections and may need tympanostomy tubes (ear tubes).

How is pneumococcal disease spread?

The bacteria that cause pneumococcal disease are spread through contact with persons who are ill or healthy persons who carry the bacteria in the back of the nose. Transmission is mostly through the spread of respiratory droplets from the nose or mouth of a person with a pneumococcal infection. It is common for people, especially children, to carry the bacteria in their throats without being ill from it.

How is pneumococcal disease treated/cured?

Pneumococcal disease is treated with antibiotics. Before the introduction of pneumococcal conjugate vaccine (PCV) to prevent infection, many types of pneumococcal bacteria were becoming resistant to some of the antibiotics used to treat pneumococcal infections. Antibiotic-resistant pneumococcal infections have significantly declined but remain a concern in some populations. Appropriate use of antibiotics may also slow or reverse emerging drug resistance found among pneumococcal infections.

Who needs to be vaccinated with pneumococcal vaccines?

The pneumococcal conjugate vaccine (PCV13 or Prevnar 13) protects against 13 types of pneumococci (the bacteria that cause pneumococcal disease). It is recommended for use in infants and young children. The vaccine should be given to all infants at 2, 4, and 6 months of age, followed by a booster dose at 12 through 15 months of age. Previously unvaccinated, healthy children 24 months through four years of age only need to receive one dose of this vaccine. Additional doses of PCV13 may be recommended, depending on the child's age and health status. For more information, please consult your child's health care provider.

The pneumococcal polysaccharide vaccine (PPSV), Pneumovax, is a 23-valent polysaccharide vaccine that is currently recommended for use in all adults who are 65 years and older and for persons who are 2 years and older and at high risk for disease such as persons with sickle cell disease, HIV infection, or other immunocompromising conditions. It is also recommended for use in adults 19 through 64 years of age who smoke cigarettes or who have asthma and adults living in nursing homes or long-term-care facilities.

Section 10.3

Rheumatic Fever

Anyone can get rheumatic fever, but those who do are often 5 to 15 years old.

What is rheumatic fever and what causes it?

It's an inflammatory reaction that can occur after a streptococcal infection of the throat ("strep throat"). Most strep throats don't lead to rheumatic fever. When they do, the time between the strep throat and rheumatic fever is about two to four weeks. Rheumatic fever is not contagious; however, the strep infection that comes before it is catching. If a strep throat is treated, rheumatic fever can almost always be prevented.

How does rheumatic fever affect the body?

It may affect many parts of the body. It can cause painful, swollen joints; skin rash, especially on the chest or abdomen; abnormal movements; or bumps under the skin. It can also affect the heart and produce inflamed or scarred heart valves.

What are the common symptoms of rheumatic fever?

- Sudden onset of a sore throat, especially with painful swallowing
- Fever
- Tender, swollen glands under the jaw angle

The symptoms may be mild in some children. If your child has a sore throat, you can't know for sure if it's strep throat unless you take him or her to a doctor.

Does rheumatic fever always affect the heart?

No. When it does, the damage may either disappear or remain. When rheumatic fever causes permanent heart damage, it's called rheumatic heart disease.

Is there a cure for rheumatic fever?

There's no "miracle drug" to cure it. An attack of rheumatic fever usually subsides within a few weeks to a few months, but heart damage may last for life. That's why prevention is so important.

If my child has had rheumatic fever, must I restrict his or her activities?

Most children don't need to have their activities restricted after the acute stage of this illness. But talk to your doctor because the answer varies from child to child.

Can you get rheumatic fever more than once?

Yes. Your child is much more likely than others to have another "attack." Taking an antibiotic (usually penicillin) regularly for many years can prevent most recurrences. The antibiotic prevents strep throat and protects the patient from getting rheumatic fever again.

If my child has rheumatic heart disease, how can I protect him or her from more problems?

People with rheumatic heart disease are at risk of developing an infection on their damaged heart valves. This infection is called "bacterial endocarditis" or "infective endocarditis." You can help prevent this problem by keeping teeth clean and cavities filled. In the past, the American Heart Association recommended that people with rheumatic heart disease take a dose of antibiotics before certain dental or surgical procedures. However, our association does not suggest this type of preventive treatment any longer for people with rheumatic heart disease unless they have already had a bout of endocarditis or have an artificial heart valve.

Section 10.4

Scarlet Fever

"Scarlet Fever: A Group A Streptococcal Infection," Centers for Disease Control and Prevention (www.cdc.gov), June 24, 2011.

Scarlet fever results from group A strep infection. If your child has a sore throat and rash, your health care provider can test for strep. Prompt treatment with antibiotics can protect your child from possible complications.

Not as common as it once was, scarlet fever—scarlatina—is a bacterial infection caused by group A *Streptococcus* or "group A strep." This illness affects a small percentage of people who have strep throat or, less commonly, streptococcal (type of bacterial) skin infections. Scarlet fever is treatable with antibiotics and usually is a mild illness, but it needs to be treated to prevent rare but serious complications.

Although anyone can get scarlet fever, it usually affects children between 5 and 18 years of age. The classic symptom of the disease is not the fever, but a certain type of red rash that feels rough, like sandpaper.

How Do You Get Scarlet Fever?

Common symptoms of scarlet fever include the following:

- A very red, sore throat
- A fever (101° F or above)
- A red rash with a sandpaper feel
- Bright red underarm, elbow, and groin skin creases
- A whitish coating on the tongue or back of the throat
- A "strawberry" tongue
- Headache
- Nausea and/or vomiting
- Swollen glands
- Body aches

Group A strep bacteria live in a person's nose and throat. The bacteria are spread through contact with droplets from an infected person's cough or sneeze. If you touch your mouth, nose, or eyes after touching something that has these droplets on it, you may become ill. If you drink from the same glass or eat from the same plate as the sick person, you could also become ill. It is possible to get scarlet fever from contact with sores from group A strep skin infections.

Scarlet Fever: What to Expect

Illness usually begins with a fever and sore throat. There also may be chills, vomiting, and abdominal pain. The tongue may have a whitish coating and appear swollen. It may also have a strawberry-like (red and bumpy) appearance. The throat and tonsils may be very red and sore, and swallowing may be painful.

One or two days after the illness begins, the characteristic red rash appears (although the rash can appear before illness to as many as seven days later). Certain strep bacteria produce a toxin (poison) that causes some people to break out in the rash—the "scarlet" of scarlet fever. The rash may first appear on the neck and chest, then spread over the body. Typically, the rash begins as small, flat red blotches that gradually become fine bumps and feel like sandpaper.

Although the cheeks might have a flushed appearance, there may be a pale area around the mouth. Underarm, elbow, and groin skin creases may become brighter red than the rest of the rash. These are called Pastia's lines. The scarlet fever rash generally fades in about seven days. As the rash fades, the skin may peel around the finger tips, toes, and groin area. This peeling can last up to several weeks.

Scarlet fever is treatable with antibiotics. Since either viruses or other bacteria can also cause sore throats, it's important to ask the doctor about a strep test (a simple swab of the throat) if your child complains of having a sore throat. If the test is positive, meaning your child is infected with group A strep bacteria, your child's doctor will prescribe antibiotics to avoid possible, although rare, complications.

Complications from Scarlet Fever

Complications from scarlet fever can be prevented by treatment with antibiotics. These complications may include the following:

- Rheumatic fever
- Kidney disease (inflammation of the kidneys, called post-streptococcal glomerulonephritis)

- Ear infections (otitis media)

- Skin infections

- Abscesses of the throat

- Pneumonia

- Arthritis

Preventing Infection: Wash Those Hands

The best way to keep from getting infected is to wash your hands often and avoid sharing eating utensils, linens, towels, or other personal items. It is especially important for anyone with a sore throat to wash his or her hands often. There is no vaccine to prevent strep throat or scarlet fever.

Section 10.5

Strep Throat

"Strep Throat," National Institute of Allergy and Infectious Diseases (www.niaid.nih.gov), August 20, 2008.

Strep throat is the most common throat infection caused by bacteria.

It is found most often in children between the ages of 5 and 15, although it can occur in younger children and adults. Children younger than 3 years old can get strep infections, but these usually don't affect the throat.

Strep throat infections usually occur in the late fall, winter, and early spring.

Cause

Strep throat is usually caused by group A *Streptococcus* bacteria. Your health care provider may call the infection "acute streptococcal pharyngitis."

Transmission

You can get strep throat by direct contact with saliva or fluids from the nose from an infected person. Most people do not get group A strep infections from casual contact with others. A crowded environment like a dormitory, school, or nursing home, however, can make it easier for the bacteria to spread. There have also been reports of contaminated food, especially milk and milk products, causing infection.

Symptoms

If you have strep throat infection, you will have a red and painful sore throat and may have white patches on your tonsils. You also may have swollen lymph nodes in your neck, run a fever, and have a headache. Nausea, vomiting, and abdominal pain can occur but are more common in children than in adults.

You can get sick within three days after being exposed to the germ. Once infected, you can pass the infection to others for up to two to three weeks even if you don't have symptoms. After 24 hours of taking antibiotics, you will no longer spread the bacteria to others.

Diagnosis

Your health care provider will take a throat swab to find out if you have strep throat infection. If the result of the rapid test is negative, you may get a follow-up culture, which takes 24 to 48 hours, to confirm the results. If the culture test is also negative, your health care provider may suspect you do not have strep, but rather another type of infection.

The results of these throat cultures will help your health care provider decide on the best treatment. Most sore throats are caused by viruses, and antibiotics are useless against viruses.

Treatment

If you have strep throat, your health care provider will prescribe an antibiotic. This will help lessen symptoms. After 24 hours of taking the medicine, you will no longer be able to spread the infection to others. Treatment will also reduce the chance of complications.

Current guidelines by expert groups recommend penicillin as the medicine of choice for treating strep throat because penicillin has been proven to be effective, safe, and inexpensive. If you are allergic to penicillin there are other antibiotics your health care provider can give you to clear up the illness.

During treatment, you may start to feel better within four days. This can happen even without treatment. Still, it is very important to finish all your medicine to prevent complications.

Section 10.6

Impetigo

This section excerpted from "Impetigo,"
© 2012 A.D.A.M, Inc. Reprinted with permission.

Impetigo is a common skin infection.

Causes

Impetigo is caused by *Streptococcus* (strep) or *Staphylococcus* (staph) bacteria. Methicillin-resistant *Staphylococcus aureus* (MRSA) is becoming a common cause.

The skin normally has many types of bacteria on it, but intact skin is an effective barrier that keeps bacteria from entering and growing in the body. When there is a break in the skin, bacteria can enter the body and grow there, causing inflammation and infection. Breaks in the skin may occur with:

- animal bites;
- injury or trauma to the skin;
- human bites;
- insect bites.

Impetigo may also occur on skin where there is no visible break.

It is most common in children, particularly those in unhealthy living conditions.

In adults, it may follow other skin disorders or a recent upper respiratory infection such as a cold or other virus. It is similar to cellulitis, but it only involves the top layers of the skin.

Impetigo is contagious, meaning it can spread to others. You can catch this infection if the fluid that oozes from the blisters touches an open area on your skin.

Symptoms

- A single or possibly many blisters filled with pus; easy to pop and—when broken—leave a reddish raw-looking base (in infants)
- Itching blister
  - Filled with yellow or honey-colored fluid
  - Oozing and crusting over
- Rash—may begin as a single spot, but if person scratches, it may spread to other areas
- Skin lesions on the face, lips, arms, or legs that spread to other areas
- Swollen lymph nodes near the infection (lymphadenopathy)

Exams and Tests

Diagnosis is based mainly on the appearance of the skin lesion.

A culture of the skin or lesion usually grows the bacteria *Streptococcus* or *Staphylococcus*. The culture can help determine if MRSA is the cause, because specific antibiotics are used to treat this infection.

Treatment

The goal is to cure the infection and relieve the symptoms.

A mild infection may be treated with a prescription antibacterial cream. More severe cases may require antibiotics, taken by mouth.

Wash (do not scrub) the skin several times a day, preferably with an antibacterial soap, to remove crusts and drainage.

Outlook (Prognosis)

The sores of impetigo heal slowly and seldom scar. The cure rate is extremely high, but the condition often comes back in young children.

Possible Complications

- Kidney failure (post-streptococcal glomerulonephritis) (rare)
- Many patches of impetigo (in children)
- Permanent skin damage and scarring (very rare)
- Spread of the infection to other parts of the body (common)

Prevention

Prevent the spread of infection.

- If you have impetigo, always use a clean washcloth and towel each time.
- Do not share towels, clothing, razors, and other personal care products with other family members.
- Wash your hands thoroughly after touching the skin lesions.

Good general health and hygiene help to prevent infection. Thoroughly clean minor cuts and scrapes with soap and clean water. You can also use a mild antibacterial soap.

Impetigo is contagious, so avoid touching the draining (oozing) lesions.

Chapter 11

Other Bacterial Infections

Chapter Contents

Section 11.1

Cat Scratch Disease

This section excerpted from "Cat Scratch Disease," Centers for Disease Control and Prevention (www.cdc.gov), June 23, 2011.

What is cat scratch disease?

Cat scratch disease (CSD) is a bacterial disease caused by *Bartonella henselae*. Most people with CSD have been bitten or scratched by a cat and developed a mild infection at the point of injury. Lymph nodes, especially those around the head, neck, and upper limbs, become swollen. Additionally, a person with CSD may experience fever, headache, fatigue, and a poor appetite. Rare complications of *B. henselae* infection are bacillary angiomatosis and Parinaud oculoglandular syndrome.

Can my cat transmit **Bartonella henselae** *to me?*

Sometimes, yes, cats can spread *B. henselae* to people. Most people get CSD from cat bites and scratches. Kittens are more likely to be infected and to pass the bacterium to people. About 40% of cats carry *B. henselae* at some time in their lives. Cats that carry *B. henselae* do not show any signs of illness; therefore, you cannot tell which cats can spread the disease to you. People with immunocompromised conditions, such as those undergoing immunosuppressive treatments for cancer, organ transplant patients, and people with HIV/AIDS, are more likely than others to have complications of CSD. Although *B. henselae* has been found in fleas, so far there is no evidence that a bite from an infected flea can give you CSD.

How can I reduce my risk of getting cat scratch disease from my cat?

- Avoid "rough play" with cats, especially kittens. This includes any activity that may lead to cat scratches and bites.

- Wash cat bites and scratches immediately and thoroughly with running water and soap.

- Do not allow cats to lick open wounds that you may have.

- Control fleas.

- If you develop an infection (with pus and pronounced swelling) where you were scratched or bitten by a cat or develop symptoms, including fever, headache, swollen lymph nodes, and fatigue, contact your physician.

Section 11.2

Diphtheria

"Diphtheria," New York State Department of Health Bureau of Communicable Disease Control (http://www.health.ny.gov/diseases/communicable/control), 2012. Reprinted with permission.

What is diphtheria?

Diphtheria is a highly contagious and potentially life-threatening bacterial disease caused by *Corynebacterium diphtheriae*. There are two types of diphtheria: respiratory and cutaneous. Respiratory diphtheria involves the nose, throat and tonsils, and cutaneous diphtheria involves the skin. Cutaneous diphtheria is discussed here.

What is respiratory diphtheria?

Respiratory diphtheria presents as a sore throat with low-grade fever and a membrane attached to the tonsils, pharynx, or nose. Neck swelling is usually present in severe disease. Respiratory diphtheria can lead to severe breathing problems, heart failure, blood disorders, paralysis, coma, and even death.

Who gets respiratory diphtheria?

Respiratory diphtheria is extremely rare in the United States because of widespread immunization. Most of the infrequent cases of diphtheria in the U.S. are among unvaccinated or inadequately vaccinated persons, particularly those who travel to areas where diphtheria is common and those who come into close contact with travelers from such areas.

How is diphtheria spread?

Diphtheria is transmitted from person to person through close contact with the discharge from an infected person's eyes, nose, throat, or skin.

What are the symptoms of respiratory diphtheria?

Symptoms include sore throat, low-grade fever, muscle weakness, loss of appetite, and enlarged lymph nodes located in the neck. A grayish colored membrane may form over the nose, throat, and tonsils, blocking the airway and making it difficult to swallow. Persons may develop a barking cough and hoarseness with extensive involvement of the throat.

How soon do symptoms appear?

Symptoms usually appear 2 to 5 days after infection, with a range of 1 to 10 days.

What are the complications of untreated respiratory diphtheria?

Death occurs in approximately 5% to 10% of all respiratory cases with higher death rates (of up to 20%) among persons younger than 5 and older than 40 years of age.

What is the treatment for respiratory diphtheria?

Diphtheria demands immediate medical attention; any delay in treatment can result in death. A person with diphtheria should be hospitalized, isolated, and treated with diphtheria antitoxin and antibiotics, such as penicillin and erythromycin.

When and for how long is a person able to spread respiratory diphtheria?

Untreated patients who are infected with the diphtheria germ may be contagious for up to four weeks. If the patient is treated appropriately, the contagious period can be limited to less than four days.

Does past infection with diphtheria make a person immune?

Recovery from diphtheria is not always followed by lasting immunity.

Is there a vaccine for diphtheria?

Diphtheria vaccine for children is combined with tetanus and acellular pertussis to form a triple vaccine known as DTaP (diphtheria, tetanus, acellular pertussis). In 2005, a new vaccine was approved as a single booster vaccination for adolescents and adults called Tdap (tetanus, diphtheria, and acellular pertussis). Td (tetanus and diphtheria) is also a vaccine used as a booster vaccination in adolescents and adults; however, it does not contain the pertussis vaccine.

DTaP should be given at 2, 4, 6, 15 to 18 months of age, and between 4 and 6 years of age.

The preferred age for Tdap vaccination is 11 to 12 years. However, all adolescents aged 11 to 18 years should receive a single dose of Tdap instead of the Td for booster immunization if they have completed the recommended childhood DTaP vaccination series and have not received Td or Tdap. An interval of 5 years between Td and Tdap is encouraged; however, an interval of less than 5 years between Td and Tdap administration can be used. Thereafter, Td should be given every 10 years to maintain immunity.

Adults aged 19 to 64 years should receive a single dose of Tdap to replace a single dose of Td for active booster vaccination if they received their last dose of Td greater than 10 years earlier. Thereafter, Td should be given every 10 years to maintain immunity.

What can be done to prevent diphtheria?

The single most effective control measure is maintaining the highest possible level of immunization in the community. Other methods of control include prompt treatment of cases and a community surveillance program.

What is cutaneous (skin) diphtheria?

In the United States, cutaneous diphtheria, although rare, is most often seen among persons with poor hygiene who live in crowded conditions. Skin infections with diphtheria are still common in tropical countries and are even more contagious than respiratory diphtheria.

Skin wounds are characterized by a scaling rash, sores, or by blisters which can occur anywhere on the body. Skin wounds may be painful, swollen, and reddened. The skin infection is treated by thorough cleansing with soap and water and appropriate antibiotics.

Section 11.3

H. Pylori *Bacteria and Peptic Ulcers*

"Peptic Ulcers," July 2009, reprinted with permission from www.kidshealth .org. Copyright © 2009 The Nemours Foundation. This information was provided by KidsHealth, one of the largest resources online for medically reviewed health information written for parents, kids, and teens. For more articles like this one, visit www.KidsHealth.org, or www.TeensHealth.org.

Many people think that spicy foods cause peptic ulcers, but the truth is that bacteria called *Helicobacter pylori* (or *H. pylori*) are the main culprit. And while many believe that adults in high-stress jobs are the only ones affected, people of any age—even children—can develop ulcers.

About Peptic Ulcers

An ulcer is a sore, which means it's an open, painful wound. Peptic ulcers are ulcers that form in the stomach or the upper part of the small intestine, called the duodenum. An ulcer in the stomach is called a gastric ulcer and an ulcer in the duodenum is called a duodenal ulcer.

Both a gastric ulcer and a duodenal ulcer result when *H. pylori* or a drug weakens the protective mucous coating of the stomach and duodenum, allowing acid to get through to the sensitive lining beneath. Both the acid and the bacteria can irritate the lining and cause an ulcer to form.

H. pylori infection is usually contracted in childhood, perhaps through food, water, or close contact with an infected individual. Infections are more common in adults older than age 60 and in developing countries. And most people with *H. pylori* don't display any symptoms until they're older. In fact, they may go through life unaware that they're infected.

Although *H. pylori* infection usually doesn't cause problems in childhood, if left untreated it can cause gastritis (the irritation and inflammation of the lining of the stomach), peptic ulcer disease, and even stomach cancer later in life.

In the past, having peptic ulcers meant living with a chronic condition for several years or even a lifetime. But today, a better understanding of the cause of peptic ulcers and how to treat them means that most people can be cured.

Causes of Peptic Ulcers in Kids

Although stress and certain foods may aggravate an ulcer, most ulcers are caused by an *H. pylori* infection or the use of common nonsteroidal anti-inflammatory drugs (NSAIDs) such as ibuprofen.

However, whereas most experts agree that *H. pylori* infection is a primary cause of peptic ulcers in adults, not everyone thinks that the bacteria are a major culprit in childhood ulcers. Some doctors make the distinction between duodenal ulcers, which are commonly associated with *H. pylori* infection, and gastric ulcers, which may stem from other causes.

It's recognized that certain medical conditions can contribute to the development of ulcers. For instance, children with severe burns can develop ulcers secondary to the stress of their injuries. This is also true for infants who become septic, or very ill with a bacterial infection. In otherwise healthy kids, peptic ulcers are very unusual.

Some doctors believe that more kids get drug-related gastric ulcers than other types of peptic ulcers. Even moderate use of NSAIDs can cause gastrointestinal problems and bleeding in some children. Acetaminophen does not cause stomach ulcers and is a good alternative to NSAIDs for most childhood conditions.

Signs and Symptoms

Although peptic ulcers are rare in kids, if your child has any of the following signs and symptoms, call your doctor:

- Burning pain in the abdomen between the breastbone and the belly button (the most common ulcer symptom)

- Nausea

- Vomiting

- Chest pain (usually dull and achy)

- Loss of appetite

- Frequent burping or hiccupping

- Weight loss

- Feeding difficulties

- Blood in vomit or bowel movements, which may appear dark red or black

These signs and symptoms are common in many childhood illnesses and don't necessarily indicate an ulcer, but they should be reported to your doctor. Based on your child's medical history and symptoms, the doctor may refer your child to a pediatric gastroenterologist (a doctor who specializes in disorders of the stomach, intestines, and associated organs) for further evaluation.

Diagnosis

The doctor may do an upper gastrointestinal (GI) series to get a close look at your child's gastrointestinal tract. An upper GI series is a set of X-rays of the esophagus, stomach, and duodenum.

The doctor may also order an upper endoscopy, especially if an ulcer is suspected. This procedure, performed under sedation, involves inserting an endoscope—a small, flexible tube with a tiny camera on the end—down the throat and into the stomach and duodenum. It lets the doctor see the lining of the esophagus, stomach, and duodenum to check for possible ulcers, inflammation, or food allergies. It also can be used to perform tissue tests to check for *H. pylori*.

The endoscopy is sometimes used with a test called a pH probe in which a small wire is inserted into the lower part of the esophagus to measure the amount of acid going into that area.

If there's any evidence of inflammation, the doctor will test for *H. pylori*. This test is important because treatment for an ulcer caused by *H. pylori* is different from the treatment for an ulcer caused by NSAIDs.

H. pylori may be diagnosed through:

- tissue tests (performed during an endoscopy);

- blood tests (which can detect the presence of *H. pylori* antibodies; blood tests are easy to perform, although a positive test may indicate exposure to *H. pylori* in the past and not an active infection);

- stool tests (which can detect the presence of *H. pylori* antigens; stool tests are becoming more common for detecting *H. pylori*, and some doctors think they're more accurate than blood tests);

- breath tests (which can detect carbon broken down by *H. pylori* after the patient drinks a solution; breath tests are also used mostly in adults).

Treatment

The good news is that most *H. pylori*–related ulcers are curable with treatment that combines two different kinds of antibiotics and an acid suppressor. The antibiotics are taken over a one- to two-week period and the antacid is given for two months or longer. The ulcer may take eight weeks to heal, but the pain usually goes away after a few days or a week.

To be sure the treatment has worked, doctors may order a stool test to verify the absence of *H. pylori*. If symptoms persist or worsen, doctors might do a follow-up endoscopy 6 to 12 months later to check for *H. pylori*.

Likewise, ulcers related to NSAIDs rarely require surgery and usually improve with an acid suppressor and stopping or changing the NSAID. No antibiotics are needed to treat this type of ulcer.

Caring for Your Child

If your child is diagnosed with an *H. pylori*–related ulcer, make sure he or she takes all of the antibiotics as directed by the doctor. Even if the symptoms disappear, the infection may not be gone until all of the medication has been taken.

If your child has a medication-related ulcer, the doctor will tell you to avoid NSAIDs, including any medication containing ibuprofen or aspirin. Also, be sure to give your child the prescribed acid-reducing medication.

Unless a particular food is bothersome, most doctors don't recommend dietary restrictions for kids with ulcers. A good diet with a variety of foods is essential to all kids' growth and development.

Alcohol and smoking can aggravate an ulcer. Also make sure that your child avoids coffee, tea, sodas, and foods that contain caffeine, which can stimulate the secretion of acid in the stomach and may make an ulcer worse.

When to Call the Doctor

Call your child's doctor immediately if your child has any of these symptoms:

• Sudden, sharp, persistent belly pain

• Bloody or black bowel movements

• Bloody vomit or vomit that looks like coffee grounds

If your child has peptic ulcer disease, these signs and symptoms could indicate a serious problem, such as:

• perforation (when the ulcer becomes too deep and breaks through the stomach or duodenal wall);

• bleeding (when acid or the ulcer breaks a blood vessel);

• obstruction (when the ulcer blocks the path of food from going through the intestines).

If your child is taking NSAIDs and shows symptoms of peptic ulcer disease, seek prompt medical attention. Delaying diagnosis and treatment can lead to complications and possibly the need for surgery. But with timely treatment, almost all peptic ulcers can be cured.

Section 11.4

Haemophilus Influenza *Type B*

This section excerpted from "Hib Disease," Centers for Disease Control and Prevention (www.cdc.gov), July 2011.

What is Hib disease?

Hib disease is a serious illness caused by the bacteria *Haemophilus influenzae* type b. Babies and children younger than five years old are most at risk for Hib disease. It can cause lifelong disability and be deadly. The Hib vaccine prevents Hib disease.

What are the symptoms of Hib disease?

Hib disease causes different symptoms depending on which part of the body it affects.

The most common type of Hib disease is meningitis. This is an infection of the covering of the brain and spinal cord. It causes the following:

- Fever
- Loss of alertness
- Stiff neck

Hib disease can also cause the following:

- Throat swelling that makes it hard to breathe
- Joint infection
- Skin infection
- Pneumonia (lung infection)
- Bone infection

How serious is Hib disease?

Hib disease is very dangerous. Most children with Hib disease need care in the hospital. Even with treatment, as many as 1 out of 20 children with Hib meningitis dies. As many as 1 out of 5 children who survive Hib meningitis will have brain damage or become deaf.

How does Hib spread?

Hib spreads when an infected person coughs or sneezes. Usually, the Hib bacteria stay in a person's nose and throat and do not cause illness. But if the bacteria spread into the lungs or blood, the person will get very sick. Spread of Hib is common among family members and in child care centers.

What is the Hib vaccine?

The Hib vaccine is a shot that protects against Hib disease. The vaccine protects children by preparing their bodies to fight the bacteria. Almost all children (at least 95 children out of 100) who get all doses of the vaccine will be protected from Hib disease.

Vaccines, like any medicine, can have side effects. But severe side effects from the Hib vaccine are very rare.

When should my child get the Hib vaccine?

Children should get three or four doses of the Hib vaccine at the following ages for best protection:

- One dose at 2 months

- A second dose at 4 months

- For some brands, one dose at 6 months

- A final dose at 12 through 15 months of age

If my child does not get the Hib vaccine, will he get Hib disease?

Without the vaccine, your child has a much greater chance of getting Hib disease. Most cases of Hib disease in the U.S. today are in children who have not had the Hib vaccine.

Before the Hib vaccine, Hib disease was the most common cause of meningitis in children younger than five years in the U.S. About 20,000 children got severe Hib disease each year, and about 1,000 died. Today, with the vaccine, cases of severe Hib disease have dropped by more than 99%. Many more children would get sick from Hib if people stopped vaccinating.

Section 11.5

Lyme Disease

This section excerpted from "Lyme Disease," National Institute of Allergy and Infectious Diseases (www.niaid.nih.gov), March 29, 2011.

A History of Lyme Disease

In the early 1970s, a mysterious group of rheumatoid arthritis cases occurred among children in Lyme, Connecticut, and two neighboring towns. Puzzled, researchers looked at several possible causes, such as contact with germs (microbes) in water or air. Realizing that most of the children with arthritis lived and played near wooded areas, they then focused their attention on deer ticks.

By the mid-1970s, researchers began describing the signs and symptoms of this new disease, now termed Lyme disease, to help physicians diagnose patients. However, it was not until 1981 that researchers identified the cause of Lyme disease and discovered the connection between the deer tick and the disease.

Symptoms

Typically, the first symptom of Lyme disease is a rash known as erythema migrans, which starts as a small red spot at the site of the tick bite and gets larger over a period of days or weeks, forming a circular or oval-shaped red rash. The rash may look like a bull's eye, appearing as a red ring around a clear area with a red center. It appears within a few weeks of a tick bite and usually occurs at the place of the bite. The rash can range in size from that of a small coin to the width of a person's back. As infection spreads, rashes can appear at different sites on the body. The rash is often accompanied by other symptoms, such as fever, headache, stiff neck, body aches, and fatigue. Although these symptoms may be like those of common viral infections, such as the flu, Lyme disease symptoms tend to last longer or may come and go over time.

Some people who have Lyme disease may develop arthritis or nervous system problems and, more rarely, heart problems. Lyme disease may also cause eye inflammation, hepatitis (liver disease), and severe fatigue. However, these problems usually only appear in conjunction with other symptoms of the disease.

Diagnosis

Health care providers may have difficulty diagnosing Lyme disease because many of its symptoms are similar to those of other illnesses, such as the flu. The bull's eye rash is the only symptom that is unique to Lyme disease, but not everyone infected with Lyme bacteria develops the rash. An infected tick must be attached to the skin for at least 36 hours to transmit Lyme bacteria. Although transmission cannot occur without the tick bite, many people may not remember being bitten because the deer tick is tiny and its bite is usually painless.

If a person has symptoms of Lyme disease but does not have the distinctive rash, health care providers will rely on a detailed medical history, along with a careful physical exam and laboratory tests to check for the presence of antibodies to *B. burgdorferi* to help provide a diagnosis.

It takes a few weeks for someone infected with *B. burgdorferi* to produce antibodies against the bacteria. Health care providers frequently use one of two antibody tests as a first-level screening. The screening tests are designed to be very "sensitive," meaning that almost everyone who has Lyme disease and some people who do not will test positive. If the screening test is positive or indeterminate, a second, different test known as a Western blot test should be performed. Used appropriately, this test is designed to be "specific," meaning that it will usually be positive only if a person is truly infected. If the Western blot is negative, it suggests that the first test was a false positive.

The Centers for Disease Control and Prevention (CDC) does not recommend a Western blot test without conducting the first-level blood screening. Using the Western blot alone increases the potential for false positive results, which may cause individuals to be treated for Lyme disease when they do not have it and, subsequently, not receive treatment for the true cause of their illness.

Treatment

Antibiotics are prescribed to effectively treat Lyme disease. These medicines can help speed healing of the erythema migrans rash and keep symptoms, such as arthritis and nervous system problems, from developing. In general, the sooner treatment begins after infection, the quicker and more complete the recovery.

After receiving treatment for Lyme disease, patients may still experience muscle or joint aches and nervous system symptoms, such as trouble with memory and concentration. To help combat these problems, researchers are trying to find out how long a person should take antibiotics for the various symptoms that may follow a bout with Lyme disease. Individuals who have previously had Lyme disease can be infected again if bitten by an infected tick.

Prevention

The best way to prevent Lyme disease is to avoid contact with deer ticks, especially during the summer months when infections are most common. Other useful tips are as follows:

- Wear long pants, long sleeves, and long socks to keep ticks off the skin. Tuck shirts into pants, and pant legs into socks or shoes, to keep ticks on the surface of your clothing. If outside for a long period of time, tape the area where pants and socks meet to prevent ticks from crawling under clothing.

- Wear light-colored clothing to make it easier to spot ticks.

- Spray clothing with the repellant permethrin, found in lawn and garden stores. Do not apply permethrin directly to the skin.

- Spray exposed clothing and skin with repellant containing 20% to 30% DEET to prevent tick bites. Carefully read and understand manufacturer instructions when using repellant, especially when using the products on infants and children.

- Pregnant women in particular should avoid ticks in Lyme disease areas as infection may be transmitted to the fetus.

- Avoid wooded areas and nearby shady grasslands. Deer ticks are common in these areas and particularly common where the two areas merge.

- Maintain a clear backyard by removing yard litter and excess brush that could attract deer and rodents.

- Once indoors after being outside, check for ticks, especially in the hairy areas of the body, and wash all clothing.

- Before letting pets indoors, check them for ticks. Ticks may fall off and then attach to humans. Pets can also develop Lyme disease.

Risk of infection can be decreased by promptly removing ticks. After finding a tick, remove it using fine-tipped tweezers; do not use petroleum jelly, a hot match, nail polish, or other products. Grab the tick close to the skin and pull up gently so that all parts of the tick are removed. Wash hands afterward with soap and water or waterless alcohol-based hand rub, and clean the area with an antiseptic, such as rubbing alcohol, or soap and water. Place the tick in a tightly closed container for examination by the local health department or health care provider.

Section 11.6

Methicillin-Resistant Staphylococcus Aureus *(MRSA)*

This section excerpted from "MRSA Infections," Centers for Disease Control and Prevention (www.cdc.gov), August 9, 2010.

Definition of MRSA

Methicillin-resistant *Staphylococcus aureus* (MRSA) is a type of staph bacteria that is resistant to certain antibiotics called beta-lactams. These antibiotics include methicillin and other more common antibiotics such as oxacillin, penicillin, and amoxicillin. In the community, most MRSA infections are skin infections. More severe or potentially life-threatening MRSA infections occur most frequently among patients in health care settings. While 25% to 30% of people are colonized* in the nose with staph, less than 2% are colonized with MRSA.

*Colonized: When a person carries the organism/bacteria but shows no clinical signs or symptoms of infection. For *Staph aureus* the most common body site colonized is the nose.

Symptoms of MRSA

As with all regular staph infections, recognizing the signs and receiving treatment for MRSA skin infections in the early stages reduces the chances of the infection becoming severe.

Severe Infections

MRSA in health care settings usually causes more severe and potentially life-threatening infections, such as bloodstream infections, surgical site infections, or pneumonia. The signs and symptoms will vary by the type and stage of the infection.

Skin Infections

In the community, most MRSA infections are skin infections that may appear as pustules or boils that often are red, swollen, painful, or have pus or other drainage. They often first look like spider bites or bumps that are red, swollen, and painful. These skin infections commonly occur at sites of visible skin trauma, such as cuts and abrasions, and areas of the body covered by hair (e.g., back of neck, groin, buttock, armpit, beard area of men).

Personal Prevention of MRSA Skin Infections

The key to preventing MRSA infections is for everyone to practice good hygiene:

1. Keep your hands clean by washing thoroughly with soap and water or using an alcohol-based hand rub.

2. Keep cuts and scrapes clean and covered with a bandage until healed.

3. Avoid contact with other people's wounds or bandages.

4. Avoid sharing personal items such as towels or razors.

If you have it, prevent spreading MRSA skin infections to others by following these steps:

Cover your wound: Keep wounds that are draining, or have pus, covered with clean, dry bandages until healed. Follow your health care provider's instructions on proper care of the wound. Pus from infected wounds can contain staph, including MRSA, so keeping the infection covered will help prevent the spread to others.

Clean your hands: You, your family, and others in close contact should wash their hands frequently with soap and water or use an alcohol-based hand rub, especially after changing the bandage or touching the infected wound.

Do not share personal items: Avoid sharing personal items, such as towels, washcloths, razors, clothing, or uniforms, that may have had contact with the infected wound or bandage. Wash sheets, towels, and clothes that become soiled with water and laundry detergent.

Maintain a clean environment: Establish cleaning procedures for frequently touched surfaces and surfaces that come into direct contact with your skin.

Talk to your doctor: Tell any health care providers who treat you that you have or had a staph or MRSA skin infection. There are things that can be done to protect people that carry staph/MRSA from getting an infection or spreading it to others when they are in the hospital or have surgery.

Treatment of MRSA Infections

Treatment of MRSA will vary by the type and location of infection.

MRSA Skin Infections

Treatment for MRSA skin infections may include having a health care professional drain the infection and, in some cases, prescribe an antibiotic. Do not attempt to treat an MRSA skin infection by yourself; doing so could worsen or spread it to others. This includes popping, draining, or using disinfectants on the area. If you think you might have an infection, cover the affected skin, wash your hands, and contact your health care provider.

If you are given an antibiotic, be sure to take all of the doses (even if the infection is getting better), unless your health care professional tells you to stop taking it.

If within a few days of visiting your health care provider the infection is not getting better, contact them again. If other people you know or live with get the same infection, tell them to go to their health care provider.

It is possible to get repeat infections with MRSA. If you are cured of an infection, you do not become immune to future infections. Therefore, personal prevention steps are key.

Treating Severe MRSA Infections

For severe infections, consider consulting with an infectious disease specialist. Treatment may include surgical or antimicrobial interventions.

Causes of MRSA Infections

How MRSA Is Spread in the Community

MRSA infections, as with all staph, are usually spread by having contact with someone's skin infection or personal items they have used, like towels, bandages, or razors that touched their infected skin. These infections are most likely to be spread in places where people are in close contact with others—for instance, schools and locker rooms where athletes might share razors or towels.

Factors that have been associated with the spread of MRSA skin infections include: close skin-to-skin contact, openings in the skin such as cuts or abrasions, contaminated items and surfaces, crowded living conditions, and poor hygiene. People may be more at risk in locations where these factors are common, including: athletic facilities, dormitories, military barracks, households, correctional facilities, and day care centers.

Risks from Contaminated Surfaces

MRSA is found on people and not naturally found in the environment (e.g., soil, the ocean, lakes). MRSA could get on objects and surfaces outside the body if someone touches infected skin or certain areas of the body where these bacteria can live (like the nose) and then touches the object or surface. Another way that items can be contaminated with staph and MRSA is if they have direct contact with a person's skin infection. Keeping skin infections covered with bandages is the best way to reduce the chance that surfaces will be contaminated with MRSA.

Even if surfaces have MRSA on them, this does not mean that you will definitely get an infection if you touch these surfaces. MRSA is most likely to cause problems when you have a cut or scrape that is not covered. That's why it's important to cover your cuts and open wounds with bandages. MRSA can also get into small openings in the skin, like the openings at hair follicles. The best defense is good hygiene. Keep your hands clean, use a barrier like clothing or towels between you and any surfaces you share with others (like gym equipment), and shower immediately after activities that involve direct skin contact with others. These are easy ways to decrease your risk of getting MRSA.

Hospitals and Health Care Settings

Health care procedures can leave patients vulnerable to MRSA, which is typically spread in health care settings from patient to patient on unclean hands of health care personnel or through the improper use or reuse of equipment.

Hands may become contaminated with MRSA by contact with the following:

- Colonized or infected patients

- Colonized or infected body sites of the personnel themselves

- Devices, items, or environmental surfaces contaminated with body fluids containing MRSA

Appropriate hand hygiene such as washing with soap and water or using an alcohol-based hand rub can prevent the spread of MRSA.

Section 11.7

Mycoplasma Infection (Walking Pneumonia)

During the school year, it can seem like kids pick up one bug after another. One week it's a runny nose, the next a sore throat, or both. Most of the time, these bugs only last for about a week. But those that linger on for longer can sometimes turn into walking pneumonia.

Walking pneumonia, or atypical pneumonia, is a less serious form of the lung infection pneumonia. It's caused by *Mycoplasma* bacteria, which cause cold-like symptoms in addition to a low-grade fever and a hacking cough.

Most kids with this form of pneumonia will not feel sick enough to stay at home hence, the name "walking" pneumonia—and usually will feel well enough to go to school. But even a child who feels fine needs to stay at home for a few days until antibiotic treatment kicks in and symptoms improve.

Signs and Symptoms

Colds that last longer than 7 to 10 days or respiratory illnesses like respiratory syncytial virus (RSV) can develop into walking pneumonia. Symptoms can come on suddenly or take longer to appear. Those that have a slow onset tend to be more severe.

Here's what to look for:

- Low-grade fever of 101° F (38.5° C) or below
- Headache, chills, sore throat, and other cold or flu-like symptoms
- Rapid breathing or breathing with grunting or wheezing sounds
- Labored breathing that makes the rib muscles retract (when muscles under the ribcage or between ribs draw inward with each breath)
- Hacking cough
- Chest pain or stomach pain
- Malaise
- Vomiting
- Loss of appetite (in older kids) or poor feeding (in infants)

Symptoms usually depend on where in the body the infection is concentrated. A child whose infection is in the top or middle part of the lungs will probably have labored breathing. Another whose infection is concentrated in the lower part of the lungs (near the abdomen) may not have breathing problems at all, but may have an upset stomach, nausea, or vomiting.

Diagnosis

Walking pneumonia is usually diagnosed through a physical examination. The doctor will monitor your child's breathing and listen for a hallmark crackling sound that often indicates walking pneumonia.

If pneumonia is suspected, a chest X-ray, blood test, or bacterial culture of mucus from the throat or nose also might be done to confirm the diagnosis.

Treatment

Antibiotics are an effective treatment for walking pneumonia. A 7- to 10-day course of oral antibiotics is usually recommended. If your doctor prescribes antibiotics, make sure your child takes them on schedule for as long as directed to recover more quickly.

Once on antibiotics, your child has a minimal risk of passing the illness on to other family members, but encourage everyone in your household to wash their hands frequently and correctly (for at least 20 seconds, rubbing hands together with soap and warm water).

Don't let your child share drinking glasses, eating utensils, towels, or toothbrushes, and remind him or her—and everyone else—to wash their hands after touching any used tissues. Also make sure that your kids are up to date on their immunizations to help protect them from future infections.

Home Health

While recovering from walking pneumonia, your child should drink fluids throughout the day to flush the system and rid the body of toxins (especially if he or she has a fever). Ask the doctor before you use a medicine to treat a cough because cough suppressants stop the lungs from clearing mucus, which may not always be helpful for lung infections like walking pneumonia.

If your child has chest pain, try a heating pad or warm compress on the chest area. Take your child's temperature at least once each morning and each evening, and call the doctor if it goes above 102° F (38.9° C) in an older infant or child, or above 100.4° F (38° C) in an infant under six months of age.

With treatment, most types of bacterial pneumonia go away within one to two weeks. However, walking pneumonia can take up to four to six weeks to resolve completely.

Section 11.8

Tetanus

This section excerpted from "Tetanus," Centers for Disease Control and Prevention (www.cdc.gov), March 2011.

Tetanus Symptoms

Tetanus is a bacterial disease. When the tetanus bacteria invade the body through a wound, they produce a toxin, or poison, that causes muscles to become tight, which is very painful. Tetanus mainly affects the neck and abdomen. Tetanus is also known as "lockjaw" because it often causes a person's neck and jaw muscles to lock, making it hard to open the mouth or swallow. It also can cause breathing problems, severe muscle spasms, and seizure-like movements. Complete recovery can take months. If left untreated, tetanus can be fatal.

Causes of Tetanus

Unvaccinated children can get tetanus just by playing outdoors and getting cuts that become infected with the bacteria. That's because tetanus bacteria are common in soil. Tetanus is not like any other vaccine-preventable disease. The main difference is that tetanus enters the body through wounds. It cannot be passed from person to person.

"Parents may have heard this, and it is true: children can get tetanus from stepping on a rusty nail," says Doug Campos-Outcalt of the American Academy of Family Physicians. "Of course, they also can get it from other wounds as well. Deeper and more severe wounds are more likely to become infected with tetanus."

Tetanus: The United States Story

In the United States, widespread vaccination against tetanus has made the disease almost nonexistent. Vaccination to prevent tetanus began in the late 1940s. In 1947 through 1949, before widespread use of the vaccine, an average of 580 cases of tetanus and an average of 472 deaths from tetanus were reported.

Today, tetanus is uncommon in the United States, with an average of 29 reported cases annually from 1996 through 2008. Nearly all cases of tetanus are among people who have never received a tetanus vaccine, or adults who don't stay up to date on their 10-year booster shots. More than half of the reported cases from 2001 through 2008 were among persons younger than 50 years of age, but almost all of the fatal cases were in persons age 65 and older.

"People of all ages can get tetanus," says Dr. Tejpratap Tiwari of the CDC. "Beginning tetanus vaccination on schedule and getting timely boosters is the best way to make sure you keep yourself and your children safe."

Tetanus Vaccine for Baby

Babies get DTaP vaccine to protect them from tetanus and two other diseases caused by bacteria, diphtheria and pertussis. DTaP vaccines are recommended at ages 2 months, 4 months, and 6 months, and at 15 through 18 months old. A DTaP booster is recommended at age 4 through 6 years. To reduce the number of shots needed at a vaccine visit, other vaccines have been combined with DTaP. Your doctor can tell you more about combination vaccines.

Because immunity to tetanus decreases over time, a booster shot (Td) is recommended every 10 years to stay protected. Tetanus is also part of the tetanus-diphtheria-pertussis vaccine (Tdap) that everyone needs to receive one time. Tdap is recommended for all 11- or 12-year-olds. Anyone who does not get the Tdap vaccine at that age should get one dose as a replacement for their 10-year tetanus-diphtheria (Td) booster shot.

Benefits of DTaP Vaccine

In addition to protecting from diphtheria and pertussis (also known as whooping cough), getting the vaccine to protect against tetanus as recommended accomplishes the following:

- Saves lives

- Prevents hospitalizations

- Protects young children, for whom the diseases prevented by this vaccine can be especially serious

- Protects the community by reducing the number of people who may spread diphtheria or pertussis

Risks of DTaP Vaccine

- Mild side effects are fever, redness, swelling or soreness at the site of the injection, fussiness, tiredness or poor appetite, or vomiting.

- Moderate side effects are uncommon. One out of 1,000 children may cry for three or more hours; 1 out of 14,000 children may have a seizure; 1 out of 16,000 children may have high fever.

- Severe side effects are rare. For example, fewer than one in a million children have a severe allergic reaction.

Section 11.9

Tuberculosis

"Tuberculosis: General Information," Centers for Disease Control and Prevention (www.cdc.gov), October 28, 2011.

What is TB?

Tuberculosis (TB) is a disease caused by germs that are spread from person to person through the air. TB usually affects the lungs, but it can also affect other parts of the body, such as the brain, the kidneys, or the spine. A person with TB can die if they do not get treatment.

What are the symptoms of TB?

The general symptoms of TB disease include feelings of sickness or weakness, weight loss, fever, and night sweats. The symptoms of TB disease of the lungs also include coughing, chest pain, and the coughing up of blood. Symptoms of TB disease in other parts of the body depend on the area affected.

How is TB spread?

TB germs are put into the air when a person with TB disease of the lungs or throat coughs, sneezes, speaks, or sings. These germs can stay in the air for several hours, depending on the environment. Persons who breathe in the air containing these TB germs can become infected; this is called latent TB infection.

What is the difference between latent TB infection and TB disease?

People with latent TB infection have TB germs in their bodies, but they are not sick because the germs are not active. These people do not have symptoms of TB disease, and they cannot spread the germs to others. However, they may develop TB disease in the future. They are often prescribed treatment to prevent them from developing TB disease.

People with TB disease are sick from TB germs that are active, meaning that they are multiplying and destroying tissue in their body. They usually have symptoms of TB disease. People with TB disease of the lungs or throat are capable of spreading germs to others. They are prescribed drugs that can treat TB disease.

What should I do if I have spent time with someone with latent TB infection or TB disease?

A person with latent TB infection cannot spread germs to other people. You do not need to be tested if you have spent time with someone with latent TB infection. However, if you have spent time with someone with TB disease or someone with symptoms of TB, you should be tested.

People with TB disease are most likely to spread the germs to people they spend time with every day, such as family members or co-workers. If you have been around someone who has TB disease, you should go to your doctor or your local health department for tests.

How do you get tested for TB?

There are two tests that can be used to help detect TB infection: a skin test or TB blood test. The Mantoux tuberculin skin test is performed by injecting a small amount of fluid (called tuberculin) into the skin in the lower part of the arm. A person given the tuberculin skin test must return within 48 to 72 hours to have a trained health care worker look for a reaction on the arm. The TB blood tests measure how the patient's immune system reacts to the germs that cause TB.

What does a positive test for TB infection mean?

A positive test for TB infection only tells that a person has been infected with TB germs. It does not tell whether or not the person has progressed to TB disease. Other tests, such as a chest X-ray and a sample of sputum, are needed to see whether the person has TB disease.

What is Bacille Calmette-Guérin (BCG)?

BCG is a vaccine for TB disease. BCG is used in many countries, but it is not generally recommended in the United States. BCG vaccination does not completely prevent people from getting TB. It may also cause a false positive tuberculin skin test. However, persons who have been vaccinated with BCG can be given a tuberculin skin test or TB blood test.

Why is latent TB infection treated?

If you have latent TB infection but not TB disease, your doctor may want you to take a drug to kill the TB germs and prevent you from developing TB disease. The decision about taking treatment for latent infection will be based on your chances of developing TB disease. Some people are more likely than others to develop TB disease once they have TB infection. This includes people with HIV infection, people who were recently exposed to someone with TB disease, and people with certain medical conditions.

How is TB disease treated?

TB disease can be treated by taking several drugs for 6 to 12 months. It is very important that people who have TB disease finish the medicine and take the drugs exactly as prescribed. If they stop taking the drugs too soon, they can become sick again; if they do not take the drugs correctly, the germs that are still alive may become resistant to those drugs. TB that is resistant to drugs is harder and more expensive to treat. In some situations, staff of the local health department meet regularly with patients who have TB to watch them take their medications. This is called directly observed therapy (DOT). DOT helps the patient complete treatment in the least amount of time.

Section 11.10

Whooping Cough (Pertussis)

This section excerpted from "Pertussis," Centers for Disease
Control and Prevention (www.cdc.gov), August 26, 2010.

Causes

Pertussis, a respiratory illness commonly known as whooping cough,
is a very contagious disease caused by a type of bacteria called *Bordetella
pertussis*. These bacteria attach to the cilia (tiny, hair-like extensions)
that line part of the upper respiratory system. The bacteria release
toxins, which damage the cilia and cause inflammation (swelling).

Transmission

Pertussis is a very contagious disease only found in humans and
is spread from person to person. People with pertussis usually spread
the disease by coughing or sneezing while in close contact with others,
who then breathe in the pertussis bacteria. Many infants who get pertussis are infected by older siblings, parents, or caregivers who might
not even know they have the disease. Symptoms of pertussis usually
develop within 7–10 days after being exposed, but sometimes not for
as long as six weeks.

Pertussis vaccines are very effective in protecting you from disease,
but no vaccine is 100% effective. If pertussis is circulating in the community, there is a chance that a fully vaccinated person, of any age,
can catch this very contagious disease. If you have been vaccinated,
the infection is usually less severe. If you or your child develops a cold
that includes a severe cough or a cough that lasts for a long time, it
may be pertussis. The best way to know is to contact your doctor.

Signs and Symptoms

Pertussis (whooping cough) can cause serious illness in infants,
children, and adults. The disease usually starts with cold-like symptoms and maybe a mild cough or fever. After one to two weeks, severe

coughing can begin. Unlike the common cold, pertussis can become a series of coughing fits that continues for weeks.

In infants, the cough can be minimal or not even there. Infants may have a symptom known as "apnea." Apnea is a pause in the child's breathing pattern. Pertussis is most dangerous for babies. More than half of infants younger than one year of age who get the disease must be hospitalized.

Pertussis can cause violent and rapid coughing, over and over, until the air is gone from the lungs and you are forced to inhale with a loud "whooping" sound. This extreme coughing can cause you to throw up and be very tired. The "whoop" is often not there and the infection is generally milder (less severe) in teens and adults, especially those who have been vaccinated.

Early symptoms can last for one to two weeks and usually include these symptoms:

- Runny nose
- Low-grade fever (generally minimal throughout the course of the disease)
- Mild, occasional cough
- Apnea—a pause in breathing (in infants)

Because pertussis in its early stages appears to be nothing more than the common cold, it is often not suspected or diagnosed until the more severe symptoms appear. Infected people are most contagious during this time, up to about two weeks after the cough begins. Antibiotics may shorten the amount of time someone is contagious.

As the disease progresses, the traditional symptoms of pertussis appear and include the following:

- Paroxysms (fits) of many, rapid coughs followed by a high-pitched "whoop"
- Vomiting
- Exhaustion (very tired) after coughing fits

The coughing fits can go on for up to 10 weeks or more. Although you are often exhausted after a coughing fit, you usually appear fairly well in-between. Coughing fits generally become more common and severe as the illness continues and can occur more often at night. Recovery from pertussis can happen slowly. The cough becomes less severe and less common. However, coughing fits can return with other respiratory infections for many months after pertussis started.

Diagnosis

Pertussis (whooping cough) can be diagnosed by taking into consideration if you have been exposed to pertussis and by the following procedures:

- History of typical signs and symptoms
- Physical examination
- Laboratory test that involves taking a sample of secretions (with a swab or syringe filled with saline) from the back of the throat through the nose
- Blood test

Treatment

Pertussis is generally treated with antibiotics, and early treatment is very important. Treatment may make your infection less severe if it is started early, before coughing fits begin. Treatment can also help prevent spreading the disease to close contacts (people who have spent a lot of time around the infected person) and is necessary for stopping the spread of pertussis. Treatment after three weeks of illness is unlikely to help because the bacteria are gone from your body, even though you usually will still have symptoms. This is because the bacteria have already done damage to your body.

There are several antibiotics available to treat pertussis. If you or your child is diagnosed with pertussis, your doctor will explain how to treat the infection.

If Your Child Is Treated for Pertussis at Home

Do not give cough medications unless instructed by your doctor. Giving cough medicine probably will not help and is often not recommended for kids younger than four years old.

Manage pertussis and reduce the risk of spreading it to others by taking these actions:

- Follow the schedule for giving antibiotics exactly as your doctor prescribed.
- Keep your home free from irritants—as much as possible—that can trigger coughing, such as smoke, dust, and chemical fumes.

- Use a clean, cool mist vaporizer to help loosen secretions and soothe the cough.

- Practice good hand washing.

- Drink plenty of fluids, including water, juices, and soups, and eat fruits to prevent dehydration (lack of fluids). Report any signs of dehydration to your doctor immediately. These include dry, sticky mouth, sleepiness or tiredness, thirst, decreased urination or fewer wet diapers, few or no tears when crying, muscle weakness, headache, dizziness, or lightheadedness.

- Eat small, frequent meals to help prevent vomiting if occurring.

If Your Child Is Treated for Pertussis in the Hospital

Your child may need help keeping breathing passages clear, which may require suctioning (drawing out) of thick respiratory secretions. Breathing is monitored and oxygen will be given, if needed. Intravenous (IV, through the vein) fluids might be required if your child shows signs of dehydration or has difficulty eating. Precautions, like practicing good hand hygiene and keeping surfaces clean, should be taken.

Prevention

Vaccines

The best way to prevent pertussis (whooping cough) among infants, children, teens, and adults is to get vaccinated. Also, keep infants and other people at high risk for pertussis complications away from infected people.

In the United States, the recommended pertussis vaccine for infants and children is called DTaP. This is a combination vaccine that protects against three diseases: diphtheria, tetanus, and pertussis. For maximum protection against pertussis, children need five DTaP shots. The first three shots are given at 2, 4, and 6 months of age. The fourth shot is given between 15 and 18 months of age, and a fifth shot is given before a child enters school, at four to six years of age. Parents can also help protect infants by keeping them away as much as possible from anyone who has cold symptoms or is coughing.

Vaccine protection for pertussis, tetanus, and diphtheria fades with time. Before 2005, the only booster available contained protection against tetanus and diphtheria (called Td) and was recommended for teens and adults every 10 years. Today there are boosters for preteens,

teens, and adults that contain protection against tetanus, diphtheria, and pertussis (Tdap). Preteens going to the doctor for their regular check-up at age 11 or 12 years should get a dose of Tdap. Teens who did not get this vaccine at the 11- or 12-year-old check-up should get vaccinated at their next visit. Adults who did not get Tdap as a preteen or teen should get one dose of Tdap. Pregnant women who have not been previously vaccinated with Tdap should get one dose of Tdap postpartum before leaving the hospital or birthing center. Adults 65 years and older (grandparents, child care providers, and health care providers) who have close contact with infants should get a dose of Tdap, following the newest vaccine recommendations. Getting vaccinated with Tdap is especially important for families with and caregivers of new infants.

The easiest thing for adults to do is to get Tdap instead of their next regular tetanus booster—that Td shot that they were supposed to get every 10 years. The dose of Tdap can be given earlier than the 10-year mark, so it is a good idea for adults to talk to a health care provider about what is best for their specific situation.

Infection

If your doctor confirms that you have pertussis, your body will have a natural defense (immunity) to future infections. Since this immunity fades and does not offer lifelong protection, routine vaccines are recommended.

Antibiotics

Your local health department may recommend preventive antibiotics (medications that help prevent diseases caused by bacteria) to close contacts, including all household members of a pertussis patient, regardless of age and vaccination status. This might prevent or reduce the chance of getting pertussis. A close contact is anyone who had face-to-face contact or shared a small space for a long period of time with an infected person or had direct contact with respiratory secretions (like from coughing or sneezing) from a person with pertussis.

Chapter 12

Viral Infections

Chapter Contents

Section 12.1

Adenovirus Infections

This section excerpted from "Adenovirus," Centers for Disease Control and Prevention (www.cdc.gov), December 27, 2011.

Adenoviruses are common viruses that can cause illness in humans. But most illnesses are not serious. Adenoviruses most often cause respiratory illness. The viruses may also cause fever, diarrhea, pink eye (conjunctivitis), bladder infection (cystitis), or rash illness.

Anyone can get infected with adenoviruses. Infants and people with weakened immune systems or existing respiratory or cardiac disease are at higher risk of getting sick from an adenovirus infection. You can get infected with adenoviruses by having close contact with people who are infected with these viruses or those who are sick. You can also get infected by touching surfaces or objects that have adenoviruses on them then touching your mouth, nose, or eyes.

Symptoms

Adenoviruses rarely cause serious illness or death. The viruses cause a wide range of illnesses and symptoms:

- Colds

- Sore throat (pharyngitis)

- Bronchitis

- Pneumonia

- Diarrhea

- Pink eye (conjunctivitis)

- Fever

- Bladder inflammation or infection (cystitis)

- Inflammation of stomach and intestines (gastroenteritis)

- Neurologic disease

Some adenoviruses cause different illnesses depending on the way a person is infected. For example, breathing in adenovirus type 7 can cause severe lower respiratory tract illness. But, swallowing the virus usually doesn't cause disease or only mild illness.

You can have persistent adenovirus infections of your tonsils, adenoids, and intestines that do not cause symptoms. The virus can be shed for months or years.

Transmission

Adenoviruses are usually spread from an infected person to others through these methods:

- Close personal contact, such as touching or shaking hands

- The air by coughing and sneezing

- Touching an object or surface with adenoviruses on it then touching your mouth, nose, or eyes before washing your hands

Some adenoviruses can spread through an infected person's stool—for example, during diaper changing. Adenovirus can also spread through the water, such as swimming pools, but this is less common.

Prevention

A vaccine against adenovirus types 4 and 7 was approved by the U.S. Food and Drug Administration in March 2011 for U.S. military personnel only. The vaccine is not available to the general public.

You can protect yourself and others from adenovirus infection by taking these precautions:

- Washing your hands often with soap and water

- Covering your mouth and nose when coughing or sneezing

- Not touching your eyes, nose, or mouth

- Avoiding close contact with people who are sick

- Staying home when you are sick

Frequent hand washing is especially important in child care settings.

To prevent outbreaks of conjunctivitis caused by adenovirus, it is important to keep adequate levels of chlorine in swimming pools.

Treatment

Most adenovirus infections are mild and typically require only treatment of symptoms. There is no specific therapy for adenoviruses. Serious adenovirus infections can only be managed by treating symptoms and health complications of the infection.

Section 12.2

Chickenpox (Varicella)

This section excerpted from "Varicella Disease Questions & Answers," Centers for Disease Control and Prevention (www.cdc.gov), June 1, 2009.

What is varicella (chickenpox)?

Chickenpox is an infectious disease caused by the varicella-zoster virus, which results in a blister-like rash, itching, tiredness, and fever.

The rash appears first on the trunk and face but can spread over the entire body, causing between 250 to 500 itchy blisters in unvaccinated persons. Prior to use of the varicella vaccine, most cases of chickenpox occurred in persons younger than 15 years of age and the disease had annual cycles, peaking in the spring of each year.

How do you get chickenpox?

Chickenpox is highly infectious and spreads from person to person by direct contact or through the air from an infected person's coughing or sneezing or from aerosolization of virus from skin lesions. A person with chickenpox is contagious 1–2 days before the rash appears and until all blisters have formed scabs. It takes from 10–21 days after exposure for someone to develop chickenpox.

Can you get chickenpox if you've been vaccinated?

Yes. About 15%–20% of people who have received one dose of chickenpox vaccine do still get chickenpox if they are exposed, but their disease is usually mild. Vaccinated persons who get chickenpox generally have fewer than 50 spots or bumps, which may resemble bug bites more than typical, fluid-filled chickenpox blisters. In 2006, the Advisory Committee on Immunization Practices (ACIP) voted to recommend routine two-dose varicella vaccination for children. In one study, children who received two doses of the chickenpox vaccine were three times less likely to get chickenpox than individuals who have had only one dose.

What is the chickenpox illness like?

In unvaccinated children, chickenpox most commonly causes an illness that lasts about 5–10 days. Children usually miss 5 or 6 days of school or child care due to their chickenpox and have symptoms such as high fever, severe itching, an uncomfortable rash, and dehydration or headache. In addition, about 1 in 10 unvaccinated children who get the disease will have a complication from chickenpox serious enough to visit a health care provider. These complications include infected skin lesions, other infections, dehydration from vomiting or diarrhea, or more serious complications such as pneumonia and encephalitis. In vaccinated children, chickenpox illness is typically mild, producing no symptoms at all other than a few red bumps. However, about 25% to 30% of vaccinated children who get the disease will develop illness as serious as unvaccinated children.

Certain groups of people are more likely to have more severe illness with serious complications. These include adults, infants, adolescents, and people whose immune systems have been weakened because of illness or medications such as long-term use of steroids.

Serious complications from chickenpox include bacterial infections that can involve many sites of the body including the skin, tissues under the skin, bone, lungs (pneumonia), joints, and blood. Other serious complications are due directly to infection with the varicella-zoster virus and include viral pneumonia, bleeding problems, and infection of the brain (encephalitis). Many people are not aware that before a vaccine was available approximately 10,600 persons were hospitalized and 100 to 150 died as a result of chickenpox in the United States every year.

Can a healthy person who gets varicella die from the disease?

Yes. Many of the deaths and complications from chickenpox occur in previously healthy children and adults. From 1990 to 1994, before a vaccine was available, about 50 children and 50 adults died from chickenpox every year; most of these persons were healthy or did not have a medical illness (such as cancer) that placed them at higher risk of getting severe chickenpox. Since 1999, states have been encouraged to report chickenpox deaths to Centers for Disease Control and Prevention (CDC). These reports have shown that some deaths from chickenpox continue to occur in healthy, unvaccinated children and adults. Most of the healthy adults who died from chickenpox contracted the disease from their unvaccinated children.

Can you get chickenpox more than once?

Yes, but such occurrences are uncommon. For most people, one infection appears to confer lifelong immunity.

Chickenpox in children is usually not serious. Why not let children get the disease?

It is not possible to predict who will have a mild case of chickenpox and who will have a serious or even deadly case of disease. Now that there is a safe and effective vaccine, it is not worth taking this chance.

Section 12.3

Common Cold

"Common Cold and Runny Nose," Centers for
Disease Control and Prevention (www.cdc.gov), June 30, 2009.

A cold usually includes a runny nose, sore throat, sneezing, and coughing. These symptoms can last for up to two weeks.

- Over 200 viruses can cause the common cold.

- The rhinovirus is the most common type of virus that causes colds.

Runny Nose during a Cold

When germs that cause colds first infect the nose and sinuses, the nose makes clear mucus. This helps wash the germs from the nose and sinuses. After two or three days, the body's immune cells fight back, changing the mucus to a white or yellow color. As the bacteria that live in the nose grow back, they may also be found in the mucus, which changes the mucus to a greenish color. This is normal and does not mean you or your child needs antibiotics.

Signs and Symptoms of the Common Cold

- Sneezing
- Stuffy or runny nose
- Sore throat
- Coughing
- Watery eyes
- Mild headache
- Mild body aches

See a health care provider if you or your child has any of the following:

- Temperature higher than 100.4° F
- Symptoms that last more than 10 days
- Symptoms that are not relieved by over-the-counter medicines

Your health care provider can determine if you or your child has a cold and can recommend symptomatic therapy. If your child is younger than three months of age and has a fever, it's important to always call your health care provider right away.

Treatment

When Antibiotics Are Needed

Antibiotics are needed only if your health care provider tells you that you or your child has a bacterial infection. Your health care provider may prescribe other medicine or give tips to help with a cold's symptoms, but antibiotics are not needed to treat a cold or runny nose.

When Antibiotics Will Not Help

Since the common cold is caused by a virus, antibiotics will not help it get better. A runny nose or cold almost always gets better on its own, so it is better to wait and take antibiotics only when they are needed. Taking antibiotics when they are not needed can be harmful.

Each time you or your child takes an antibiotic, the bacteria that normally live in your body (on the skin, in the intestine, in the mouth and nose, etc.) are more likely to become resistant to antibiotics. Common antibiotics cannot kill infections caused by these resistant germs.

How to Feel Better

Rest, over-the-counter medicines, and other self-care methods may help you or your child feel better. For more information about symptomatic relief, talk to your health care provider or pharmacist. Remember, always use over-the-counter products as directed. Many over-the-counter products are not recommended for children younger than certain ages.

Preventing the Common Cold

- Practice good hand hygiene.
- Avoid close contact with people who have colds or other upper respiratory infections.

Section 12.4

Croup

About Croup

Croup is a condition that causes an inflammation of the upper airways—the voice box (larynx) and windpipe (trachea). It often leads to a barking cough or hoarseness, especially when a child cries.

Most cases of croup are caused by viruses. Those involved are usually parainfluenza virus (which accounts for most cases), adenovirus, and respiratory syncytial virus (RSV). Croup is most common—and symptoms are most severe—in children six months to three years old, but can affect older kids, too.

Most cases of viral croup are mild and can be treated at home, though rarely it can be severe and even life-threatening. Some children are more prone to developing croup when they get a viral upper respiratory infection.

The term spasmodic croup refers to a type of croup that develops quickly and may happen in a child with a mild cold. The barking cough usually begins at night and is not accompanied by fever. Spasmodic croup has a tendency to come back again (recur).

Symptoms are treated the same for either form of croup.

Signs and Symptoms

At first, a child may have cold symptoms, like a stuffy or runny nose and a fever. As the upper airway (the lining of the windpipe and the voice box) becomes progressively inflamed and swollen, the child may become hoarse, with a harsh, barking cough. This loud cough, which is characteristic of croup, often sounds like the barking of a seal.

If the upper airway becomes increasingly swollen, it becomes even more difficult for a child to breathe, and you may hear a high-pitched or squeaking noise when a child inhales (this is called stridor). A child also may tend to breathe very fast and might have retractions (when the skin between the ribs pulls in during breathing). In the most serious cases, a child may appear pale or have a bluish tinge around the mouth due to a lack of oxygen.

Symptoms of croup are often worse at night and when children are upset or crying. Besides the effects on the upper airway, the viruses that cause croup can cause inflammation farther down the airway and affect the bronchi (large breathing tubes that connect to the windpipe).

Contagiousness

Outbreaks of croup tend to occur in the fall and early winter when the viruses that cause it peak. Many children who come in contact with the viruses that cause croup will not get croup, but will instead have symptoms of a common cold.

Diagnosis

Doctors can usually diagnose croup by listening for the telltale barking cough and stridor. They will also ask if your child has had any recent illnesses with a fever, runny nose, and congestion, and if your child has a history of croup or upper airway problems.

If a child's croup is severe and slow to respond to treatment, a neck X-ray may be taken to rule out any other reasons for the breathing difficulty, such as a foreign object lodged in the throat, an abscess behind the throat, or epiglottitis (a inflammation of the epiglottis, the flap of tissue that covers the windpipe). Typical findings on an X-ray if a child has croup includes the top of the airway narrowing to a point, which doctors call a "steeple sign."

Treatment

Most, though not all, cases of viral croup are mild. Breathing in moist air seems to make kids feel better. And ibuprofen or acetaminophen can make a child feel more comfortable. Doctors will also sometimes treat with steroids, which help with the airway swelling.

The best way to expose your child to moist air is to use a cool mist humidifier, or run a hot shower to create a steam-filled bathroom where you can sit with your child for 10 minutes. Breathing in the mist will sometimes stop a child from severe coughing. In the cooler months, try taking your child outside for a few minutes to breath in the cool air—this may also alleviate symptoms. You can also try driving your child around in the car with the windows down.

When your child is sick, you might also want to consider sleeping overnight in the same room to provide close observation. If you are not able to break your child's fast breathing and croupy cough, call your child's doctor or seek medical attention as soon as possible.

Medical professionals will need to evaluate your child if the croup appears serious or if there's any suspicion of airway blockage. If the croup becomes severe, doctors will give a breathing treatment that contains epinephrine (adrenalin). This reduces swelling in the airway quickly. Oxygen may also be given, and sometimes a child with croup will remain in the hospital overnight for observation. As with most illnesses, rest and plenty of fluids are recommended.

Duration

The symptoms of croup generally peak two to three days after the symptoms of infection with a virus start. Viral croup usually lasts three to seven days.

Complications

The vast majority of children recover from croup with no complications. Rarely, children will develop a bacterial infection of the upper airway, or pneumonia. Dehydration may occur due to inadequate fluid intake.

Children who were born prematurely or who have a history of lung disease (such as asthma), or neuromuscular disease like cerebral palsy, are more likely to develop severe symptoms of croup and often require hospitalization. Croup rarely causes any long-term complications.

Prevention

Frequent hand washing and avoiding contact with people who have respiratory infections are the best ways to reduce the chance of spreading the viruses that cause croup.

When to Call the Doctor

Immediately call your doctor or seek medical attention if your child has:

- difficulty breathing, including rapid or labored breathing;

- retractions (when the skin between the ribs pulls in with each breath);

- stridor (high-pitched or squeaking noise when inhaling);

- a pale or bluish color around the mouth;

- drooling or difficulty swallowing;

- a fatigued appearance;

- signs of dehydration;

- a very sick appearance.

Section 12.5

Fifth Disease

"Parvovirus B19 (Fifth Disease)," Centers for Disease Control and Prevention (www.cdc.gov), February 25, 2011.

What is "fifth disease?"

Fifth disease is a mild rash illness that occurs most commonly in children. The ill child typically has a "slapped-cheek" rash on the face and a lacy red rash on the trunk and limbs. Occasionally, the rash may itch. An ill child may have a low-grade fever, malaise, or a "cold" a few days before the rash breaks out. The child is usually not very ill, and the rash resolves in 7 to 10 days.

What causes fifth disease?

Fifth disease is caused by infection with human parvovirus B19. This virus infects only humans. Pet dogs or cats may be immunized against "parvovirus," but these are animal parvoviruses that do not infect humans. Therefore, a child cannot "catch" parvovirus from a pet dog or cat, and a pet cat or dog cannot catch human parvovirus B19 from an ill child.

Can adults get fifth disease?

Yes, they can. An adult who is not immune can be infected with parvovirus B19 and either have no symptoms or develop the typical rash of fifth disease, joint pain or swelling, or both. Usually, joints on both sides of the body are affected. The joints most frequently affected are the hands, wrists, and knees. The joint pain and swelling usually resolve in a week or two, but they may last several months. About 50% of adults, however, have been previously infected with parvovirus B19, have developed immunity to the virus, and cannot get fifth disease.

Is fifth disease contagious?

Yes. A person infected with parvovirus B19 is contagious during the early part of the illness, before the rash appears. By the time a child has the characteristic "slapped cheek" rash of fifth disease, for example, he or she is probably no longer contagious and may return to school or child care center. This contagious period is different than that for many other rash illnesses, such as measles, for which the child is contagious while he or she has the rash.

How does someone get infected with parvovirus B19?

Parvovirus B19 has been found in the respiratory secretions (e.g., saliva, sputum, or nasal mucus) of infected persons before the onset of rash, when they appear to "just have a cold." The virus is probably spread from person to person by direct contact with those secretions, such as sharing drinking cups or utensils. In a household, as many as 50% of susceptible persons exposed to a family member who has fifth disease may become infected. During school outbreaks, 10% to 60% of students may get fifth disease.

A susceptible person usually becomes ill 4 to 14 days after being infected with the virus, but may become ill for as long as 20 days after infection.

Does everyone who is infected with parvovirus B19 become ill?

No. During outbreaks of fifth disease, about 20% of adults and children who are infected with parvovirus B19 do not develop any symptoms. Furthermore, other persons infected with the virus will have a nonspecific illness that is not characteristic of fifth disease. Persons infected with the virus, however, do develop lasting immunity that protects them against infection in the future.

143

How is fifth disease diagnosed?

A physician can often diagnose fifth disease by seeing the typical rash during a physical examination. In cases in which it is important to confirm the diagnosis, a blood test may be done to look for antibodies to parvovirus. Antibodies are proteins produced by the immune system in response to parvovirus B19 and other germs. If immunoglobulin M (IgM) antibody to parvovirus B19 is detected, the test result suggests that the person has had a recent infection.

Is fifth disease serious?

Fifth disease is usually a mild illness that resolves on its own among children and adults who are otherwise healthy. Joint pain and swelling in adults usually resolve without long-term disability.

Parvovirus B19 infection may cause a serious illness in persons with sickle-cell disease or similar types of chronic anemia. In such persons, parvovirus B19 can cause an acute, severe anemia. The ill person may be pale, weak, and tired and should see his or her physician for treatment. (The typical rash of fifth disease is rarely seen in these persons.) Once the infection is controlled, the anemia resolves. Furthermore, persons who have problems with their immune systems may also develop a chronic anemia with parvovirus B19 infection that requires medical treatment. People who have leukemia or cancer, who are born with immune deficiencies, who have received an organ transplant, or who have human immunodeficiency virus (HIV) infection are at risk for serious illness due to parvovirus B19 infection.

How are parvovirus B19 infections treated?

Treatment of symptoms such as fever, pain, or itching is usually all that is needed for fifth disease. Adults with joint pain and swelling may need to rest, restrict their activities, and take medicines such as aspirin or ibuprofen to relieve symptoms. The few people who have severe anemia caused by parvovirus B19 infection may need to be hospitalized and receive blood transfusions. Persons with immune problems may need special medical care, including treatment with immune globulin (antibodies), to help their bodies get rid of the infection.

Can parvovirus B19 infection be prevented?

There is no vaccine or medicine that prevents parvovirus B19 infection. Frequent handwashing is recommended as a practical and probably effective method to decrease the chance of becoming infected. Excluding persons with fifth disease from work, child care centers, or schools is not likely to prevent the spread of the virus, since people are contagious before they develop the rash.

Section 12.6

Hand, Foot, and Mouth Disease

"Hand, Foot, and Mouth Disease," Centers for Disease Control and Prevention (www.cdc.gov), July 5, 2011.

Hand, foot, and mouth disease (HFMD) is a contagious viral illness that commonly affects infants and children in the U.S. and abroad. In the U.S. and other countries with temperate climates, HFMD occurs most often in summer and early autumn. While there is no vaccine to prevent the disease, there are simple steps you and your family can take to reduce the risk of getting sick.

The following are characteristics of HFMD:

- Usually causes fever, sores in the mouth, and a rash with blisters

- Is moderately contagious

- Mostly affects children younger than 10 years of age, but people of any age can be infected

- Has no specific treatment

- Infection risk can be reduced by practicing good hygiene, such as washing hands frequently

- Is not the same as foot-and-mouth disease

What are the symptoms of HFMD?

Symptoms usually begin with a fever, poor appetite, malaise (feeling vaguely unwell), and often a sore throat. A couple of days after the fever starts, painful sores can develop in the mouth. A skin rash with flat or raised red spots can also develop, usually on the palms of the hands and soles of the feet and sometimes on the buttocks. This rash may blister, but it will not itch.

Some people with HFMD may only have a rash; others may only have mouth sores. Other people with HFMD may show no symptoms at all.

Is HFMD serious?

HFMD is usually not serious. The illness is typically mild, and nearly all patients recover in 7–10 days without medical treatment. Complications are uncommon. Rarely, an infected person can develop viral meningitis (characterized by fever, headache, stiff neck, or back pain) and may need to be hospitalized for a few days. Other rare complications can include polio-like paralysis or encephalitis (brain inflammation), which can be fatal.

Is HFMD contagious?

Yes, HFMD is moderately contagious. The disease is spread by direct contact with nose and throat discharges, saliva, fluid from blisters, or the stool of infected persons.

People with HFMD are most contagious during the first week of their illness, but they can spread the virus that causes HFMD weeks after symptoms have gone away. It is also important to remember that people who get HFMD and show no symptoms of the disease can still spread the viruses that cause it.

Who is at risk for HFMD?

HFMD mostly infects children younger than 10 years of age, but older children and adults can also get the disease. Individuals who get HFMD develop immunity to the specific virus that caused their infection. However, because HFMD can be caused by several different viruses, people can get the disease again if they are infected by one of the other HFMD-causing viruses.

Can HFMD be treated?

There is no specific treatment for HFMD. Fever and pain can be managed with over-the-counter fever reducers/pain relievers, such as acetaminophen or ibuprofen. In addition, individuals with HFMD should drink enough fluids to prevent dehydration (loss of body fluids).

Can HFMD be prevented?

There is no vaccine to protect against HFMD. However, the risk of getting the disease can be reduced by these precautions:

- Frequently washing hands, especially after diaper changes

- Thoroughly cleaning objects and surfaces (toys, doorknobs, etc.) that may be contaminated with a virus that causes HFMD

- Avoiding close contact (like kissing and hugging) with people who are infected

Is HFMD the same as foot-and-mouth disease?

No. HFMD is often confused with foot-and-mouth (also called hoof-and-mouth) disease, which affects cattle, sheep, and swine. For information on foot-and-mouth disease, visit the website of the U.S. Department of Agriculture.

Section 12.7

Infectious Mononucleosis

Mononucleosis is a viral infection causing fever, sore throat, and swollen lymph glands, especially in the neck.

Causes

Mononucleosis, or mono, is often spread by saliva and close contact. It is known as "the kissing disease," and occurs most often in those age 15 to 17. However, the infection may develop at any age.

Mono is usually linked to the Epstein-Barr virus (EBV), but can also be caused by other organisms such as cytomegalovirus (CMV).

Symptoms

Mono may begin slowly with fatigue, a general ill feeling, headache, and sore throat. The sore throat slowly gets worse. Your tonsils become swollen and develop a whitish-yellow covering. The lymph nodes in the neck are frequently swollen and painful.

A pink, measles-like rash can occur and is more likely if you take the medicines ampicillin or amoxicillin for a throat infection. (Antibiotics should *not* be given without a positive Strep test.)

Symptoms of mononucleosis include:

- drowsiness;

- fever;

- general discomfort, uneasiness, or ill feeling;

- loss of appetite;

- muscle aches or stiffness;

- rash;

- sore throat;

- swollen lymph nodes, especially in the neck and armpit;

- swollen spleen.

Less frequently occurring symptoms include:

- chest pain;

- cough;

- fatigue;

- headache;

- hives;

- jaundice (yellow color to the skin);

- neck stiffness;

- nosebleed;

- rapid heart rate;

- sensitivity to light;

- shortness of breath.

Exams and Tests

During a physical examination, the doctor may find swollen lymph nodes in the front and back of your neck, as well as swollen tonsils with a whitish-yellow covering.

The doctor might also feel a swollen liver or swollen spleen when pushing on your belly. There may be a skin rash.

Blood work often reveals a higher-than-normal white blood cell (WBC) count and unusual-looking white blood cells called atypical lymphocytes, which are seen when blood is examined under a microscope. Atypical lymphocytes and abnormal liver function tests are a hallmark sign of the disease.

- A monospot test will be positive for infectious mononucleosis.

- A special test called an antibody titer can help your doctor distinguish a current (acute) EBV infection from one that occurred in the past.

Treatment

The goal of treatment is to relieve symptoms. Medicines such as steroids (prednisone) and antivirals (such as acyclovir) have little or no benefit.

To relieve typical symptoms:

- Drink plenty of fluids.

- Gargle with warm salt water to ease a sore throat.

- Get plenty of rest.

- Take acetaminophen or ibuprofen for pain and fever.

You should also avoid contact sports while the spleen is swollen (to prevent it from rupturing).

Outlook (Prognosis)

The fever usually drops in 10 days, and swollen lymph glands and spleen heal in four weeks. Fatigue usually goes away within a few weeks, but may linger for two to three months.

When to Contact a Medical Professional

The initial symptoms of mono feel very much like a typical viral illness. It is not necessary to contact a health care provider unless symptoms last longer than 10 days or you develop the following:

- Abdominal pain

- Breathing difficulty

- Persistent high fevers (more than 101.5° F)
- Severe headache
- Severe sore throat or swollen tonsils
- Weakness in the arm or legs
- Yellow discoloration of your eyes or skin

Call 911 or go to an emergency room if you develop:

- sharp, sudden, severe abdominal pain;
- significant difficulty swallowing or breathing; or
- stiff neck or severe weakness.

Prevention

Persons with mononucleosis may be contagious while they have symptoms and for up to a few months afterwards. How long someone with the disease is contagious varies. The virus can live for several hours outside the body. Avoid kissing or sharing utensils if you or someone close to you has mono.

Section 12.8

Influenza

This section excerpted from "Key Facts about Influenza (Flu) & Flu Vaccine," Centers for Disease Control and Prevention (www.cdc.gov), October 4, 2011.

What is influenza (also called flu)?

The flu is a contagious respiratory illness caused by influenza viruses that infect the nose, throat, and lungs. It can cause mild to severe illness, and at times can lead to death. The best way to prevent the flu is by getting a flu vaccine each year.

What are the signs and symptoms of flu?

People who have the flu often feel some or all of these signs and symptoms:

- Fever or feeling feverish/chills (it's important to note that not everyone with flu will have a fever)
- Cough
- Sore throat
- Runny or stuffy nose
- Muscle or body aches
- Headaches
- Fatigue (very tired)
- Vomiting and diarrhea, though this is more common in children than adults

How does flu spread?

Most experts believe that flu viruses spread mainly by droplets made when people with flu cough, sneeze, or talk. These droplets can land in the mouths or noses of people who are nearby. Less often, a person might also get flu by touching a surface or object that has flu virus on it and then touching their own mouth, eyes, or possibly their nose.

How long are you contagious?

You may be able to pass on the flu to someone else before you know you are sick, as well as while you are sick. Most healthy adults may be able to infect others beginning one day before symptoms develop and up to five to seven days after becoming sick. Some people, especially young children and people with weakened immune systems, might be able to infect others for an even longer time.

How serious is the flu?

Flu is unpredictable, and how severe it is can vary widely from one season to the next depending on many things, including the following:

- What flu viruses are spreading
- How much flu vaccine is available
- When vaccine is available
- How many people get vaccinated
- How well the flu vaccine is matched to flu viruses that are causing illness

Certain people are at greater risk for serious complications if they get the flu. This includes older people, young children, pregnant women and people with certain health conditions (such as asthma, diabetes, or heart disease), and persons who live in facilities like nursing homes.

Flu seasons are unpredictable and can be severe. Over a period of 30 years, between 1976 and 2006, estimates of flu-associated deaths in the United States range from a low of about 3,000 to a high of about 49,000 people.

What are the complications of flu?

Complications of flu can include bacterial pneumonia, ear infections, sinus infections, dehydration, and worsening of chronic medical conditions, such as congestive heart failure, asthma, or diabetes.

How do you prevent seasonal flu?

The single best way to prevent the flu is to get a flu vaccine each season. There are two types of flu vaccines:

- "Flu shots" are inactivated vaccines (containing killed virus) that are given with a needle. There are three flu shots being produced for the United States market now.

- The nasal-spray flu vaccine, a vaccine made with live, weakened flu viruses, is given as a nasal spray (sometimes called LAIV for "Live Attenuated Influenza Vaccine"). The viruses in the nasal spray vaccine do not cause the flu. LAIV is approved for use in healthy people 2 to 49 years of age who are not pregnant.

About two weeks after vaccination, antibodies develop that protect against influenza virus infection. Flu vaccines will not protect against flu-like illnesses caused by non-influenza viruses.

The seasonal flu vaccine protects against the three influenza viruses that research suggests will be most common.

Yearly flu vaccination should begin in September, or as soon as vaccine is available, and continue throughout the flu season, which can last as late as May. This is because the timing and duration of flu seasons vary. While flu season can begin early as October, most of the time seasonal flu activity peaks in January, February, or later.

Who should get vaccinated?

Everyone six months and older should get a flu vaccine each year. This recommendation has been in place since February 24, 2010, when CDC's Advisory Committee on Immunization Practices (ACIP) voted for "universal" flu vaccination in the U.S. to expand protection against the flu to more people. While everyone should get a flu vaccine each flu season, it's especially important that certain people get vaccinated either because they are at high risk of having serious flu-related complications or because they live with or care for people at high risk for developing flu-related complications.

Who is at high risk for developing flu-related complications?

- Children younger than 5, but especially children younger than 2 years old

- Adults 65 years of age and older

- Pregnant women
- American Indians and Alaskan Natives seem to be at higher risk of flu complications
- People who have certain medical conditions

Who else should get vaccinated?

Other people for whom vaccination is especially important are the following:

- People who live in nursing homes and other long-term care facilities
- People who live with or care for those at high risk for complications from flu, including health care workers, household contacts of persons at high risk for complications, and household contacts and caregivers of children younger than five years of age with particular emphasis on vaccinating contacts of children younger than six months of age (who are at highest risk of flu-related complications but are too young to get vaccinated)

Who should not be vaccinated against seasonal flu?

Some people should not be vaccinated without first consulting a physician. They include the following:

- People who have a severe allergy to chicken eggs
- People who have had a severe reaction to an influenza vaccination in the past
- Children younger than six months of age (influenza vaccine is not approved for use in this age group)
- People who currently have a moderate or severe illness with a fever
- People with a history of Guillain-Barré syndrome (a severe paralytic illness) that occurred after receiving influenza vaccine and who are not at risk for severe illness from influenza

If you have questions about whether you should get a flu vaccine, consult your health care provider.

Section 12.9

Measles

This section excerpted from "Overview of Measles Disease," Centers for Disease Control and Prevention (www.cdc.gov), May 6, 2011.

Cause

Measles is a respiratory disease caused by a virus. The disease of measles and the virus that causes it share the same name. The disease is also called rubeola. Measles virus normally grows in the cells that line the back of the throat and lungs.

Measles Incidence

Measles is very rare in countries and regions of the world that are able to keep vaccination coverage high. In North and South America, Finland, and some other areas, endemic measles transmission is considered to have been interrupted through vaccination. There are still sporadic cases of measles in the United States because visitors from other countries or U.S. citizens traveling abroad can become infected before or during travel and spread the infection to unvaccinated or unprotected persons.

Worldwide, there are estimated to be 20 million cases and 197,000 deaths each year. More than half of the deaths occur in India.

Signs and Symptoms

The symptoms of measles generally begin about 7–14 days after a person is infected and include the following:

- Blotchy rash
- Fever
- Cough
- Runny nose
- Red, watery eyes (conjunctivitis)

- Feeling run down, achy (malaise)

- Tiny white spots with bluish-white centers found inside the mouth (Koplik spots)

A typical case of measles begins with mild to moderate fever, cough, runny nose, red eyes, and sore throat. Two or three days after symptoms begin, tiny white spots (Koplik spots) may appear inside the mouth.

Three to five days after the start of symptoms, a red or reddish-brown rash appears. The rash usually begins on a person's face at the hairline and spreads downward to the neck, trunk, arms, legs, and feet. When the rash appears, a person's fever may spike to more than 104° F.

After a few days, the fever subsides and the rash fades.

Transmission of Measles

Measles is highly contagious and can be spread to others from four days before to four days after the rash appears. Measles is so contagious that if one person has it, 90% of the people close to that person who are not immune will also become infected with the measles virus.

The virus lives in the mucus in the nose and throat of the infected person. When that person sneezes or coughs, droplets spray into the air. The droplets can get into other people's noses or throats when they breathe or put their fingers in their mouth or nose after touching an infected surface. The virus can live on infected surfaces for up to two hours and spreads so easily that people who are not immune will probably get it when they come close to someone who is infected.

Measles is a disease of humans; measles virus is not spread by any other animal species.

Complications of Measles

About 30% of measles cases develop one or more complications, including the following:

- Pneumonia, which is the complication that is most often the cause of death in young children.

- Ear infections occur in about 1 in 10 measles cases, and permanent loss of hearing can result.

- Diarrhea is reported in about 8% of cases.

These complications are more common among children under 5 years of age and adults over 20 years old.

Even in previously healthy children, measles can be a serious illness requiring hospitalization. As many as 1 out of every 20 children with measles gets pneumonia, and about 1 child in every 1,000 who get measles will develop encephalitis (an inflammation of the brain that can lead to convulsions and can leave the child deaf or mentally retarded). For every 1,000 children who get measles, 1 or 2 will die from it. Measles also can make a pregnant woman have a miscarriage, give birth prematurely, or have a low-birth-weight baby.

Measles Vaccination

Measles can be prevented by the combination MMR (measles, mumps, and rubella) vaccine. In the decade before the measles vaccination program began, an estimated 3–4 million people in the United States were infected each year, of whom 400–500 died, 48,000 were hospitalized, and another 1,000 developed chronic disability from measles encephalitis. Widespread use of measles vaccine has led to a greater than 99% reduction in measles cases in the United States compared with the prevaccine era, and in 2009, only 71 cases of measles were reported in the United States.

Section 12.10

Mumps

This section excerpted from "Overview of Mumps," Centers for Disease Control and Prevention (www.cdc.gov), March 14, 2010.

Mumps is a contagious disease that is caused by the mumps virus. Mumps typically starts with a few days of fever, headache, muscle aches, tiredness, and loss of appetite and is followed by swelling of salivary glands. Anyone who is not immune from either previous mumps infection or from vaccination can get mumps.

Before the routine vaccination program was introduced in the United States, mumps was a common illness in infants, children, and young adults. Because most people have now been vaccinated, mumps has become a rare disease in the United States.

Currently, there is no specific treatment for mumps. Supportive care should be given as needed. If someone becomes very ill, they should seek medical attention. If someone seeks medical attention, they should call their doctor in advance so that they don't have to sit in the waiting room for a long time and possibly infect other patients.

Signs and Symptoms of Mumps

Up to half of people who get mumps have very mild or no symptoms, and therefore do not know they were infected with mumps. The most common symptoms include the following:

- Fever
- Headache
- Muscle aches
- Tiredness
- Loss of appetite
- Swollen and tender salivary glands under the ears on one or both sides (parotitis)

Symptoms typically appear 16–18 days after infection, but this period can range from 12–25 days after infection.

Complications of Mumps

Mumps is best known for the swelling of the cheeks and jaw that it causes, which is a result of swelling of the salivary glands. It is usually a mild disease but can occasionally cause serious complications.

The most common complication is inflammation of the testicles (orchitis) in males who have reached puberty; rarely does this lead to fertility problems.

Other rare complications include the following:

- Inflammation of the brain and/or tissue covering the brain and spinal cord (encephalitis/meningitis)

- Inflammation of the ovaries (oophoritis) and/or breasts (mastitis) in females who have reached puberty

- Deafness

Transmission of Mumps

Mumps has not disappeared in the United States, and the MMR vaccine is the best way to prevent the disease.

- Check your child's immunization record or contact the doctor to see whether your child has already received the MMR vaccine.

- Get your child vaccinated on time.

- Remember that some older children and adults also need MMR vaccine.

- Recognize the signs and symptoms of mumps.

- Report suspect mumps cases to your doctor right away.

Mumps is spread by droplets of saliva or mucus from the mouth, nose, or throat of an infected person, usually when the person coughs, sneezes, or talks. Items used by an infected person, such as soft drink cans or eating utensils, can also be contaminated with the virus, which may spread to others if those items are shared. In addition, the virus may spread when someone with mumps touches items or surfaces without washing their hands and someone else then touches the same surface and rubs their mouth or nose.

Most mumps transmission likely occurs before the salivary glands begin to swell and up to 5 days after the swelling begins. Therefore, the CDC recommends isolation of mumps patients for 5 days after their glands begin to swell. The incubation time (how long it takes for symptoms to appear after a person is exposed to the virus) can range from 12–25 days.

Some things people can do to help prevent the spread of mumps and other infections include these steps:

- Wash hands well and often with soap, and teach children to wash their hands too.

- Do not share eating or drinking utensils.

- Clean surfaces that are frequently touched (such as toys, door-knobs, tables, and counters) regularly with soap and water or with cleaning wipes.

- Minimize close contact with other people if you are sick.

- Cover your mouth and nose with a tissue when you cough or sneeze, and put your used tissue in the trash can; if you don't have a tissue, cough or sneeze into your upper sleeve or elbow, not your hands.

Mumps Vaccination

Mumps vaccine, which is included in the combination MMR and measles-mumps-rubella-varicella (MMRV) vaccines, is the best way to prevent mumps. Mumps vaccine effectiveness has been estimated at 62%–91% for one dose and 76%–95% for two doses. The first vaccine against mumps was licensed in the United States in 1967, and by 2005, high two-dose childhood vaccination coverage reduced disease rates by 99%.

Children should receive the first dose of mumps-containing vaccine at 12–15 months and the second dose at 4–6 years. All adults born during or after 1957 should have documentation of one dose. Adults at higher risk, such as university students, health care personnel, international travelers, and persons with potential mumps outbreak exposure, should have documentation of two doses of mumps vaccine or other proof of immunity to mumps.

Section 12.11

Rabies

This section excerpted from "Rabies," Centers for Disease
Control and Prevention (www.cdc.gov), 2011.

Rabies is a preventable viral disease of mammals most often transmitted through the bite of a rabid animal. The vast majority of rabies cases reported to the CDC each year occur in wild animals like raccoons, skunks, bats, and foxes.

The rabies virus infects the central nervous system, ultimately causing disease in the brain and death. The early symptoms of rabies in people are similar to that of many other illnesses, including fever, headache, and general weakness or discomfort. As the disease progresses, more specific symptoms appear and may include insomnia, anxiety, confusion, slight or partial paralysis, excitation, hallucinations, agitation, hypersalivation (increase in saliva), difficulty swallowing, and hydrophobia (fear of water). Death usually occurs within days of the onset of these symptoms.

When should I seek medical attention?

The rabies virus is transmitted through saliva or brain/nervous system tissue. You can only get rabies by coming in contact with these specific bodily excretions and tissues.

It's important to remember that rabies is a medical urgency but not an emergency. Decisions should not be delayed.

Wash any wounds immediately. One of the most effective ways to decrease the chance for infection is to wash the wound thoroughly with soap and water.

See your doctor for attention for any trauma due to an animal attack before considering the need for rabies vaccination.

Your doctor, possibly in consultation with your state or local health department, will decide if you need a rabies vaccination. Decisions to start vaccination, known as postexposure prophylaxis (PEP), will be based on your type of exposure and the animal you were exposed to, as well as laboratory and surveillance information for the geographic area where the exposure occurred.

In the United States, postexposure prophylaxis consists of a regimen of one dose of immune globulin and four doses of rabies vaccine over a 14-day period. Rabies immune globulin and the first dose of rabies vaccine should be given by your health care provider as soon as possible after exposure. Additional doses of rabies vaccine should be given on days 3, 7, and 14 after the first vaccination. Current vaccines are relatively painless and are given in your arm, like a flu or tetanus vaccine.

What are the signs and symptoms of rabies?

The first symptoms of rabies may be very similar to those of the flu, including general weakness or discomfort, fever, or headache. These symptoms may last for days.

There may be also discomfort or a prickling or itching sensation at the site of the bite, progressing within days to symptoms of cerebral dysfunction, anxiety, confusion, and agitation. As the disease progresses, the person may experience delirium, abnormal behavior, hallucinations, and insomnia.

The acute period of disease typically ends after 2 to 10 days. Once a person begins to exhibit signs of the disease, survival is rare. To date less than 10 documented cases of human survival from clinical rabies have been reported and only 2 have not had a history of pre- or postexposure prophylaxis.

How is rabies transmitted?

All species of mammals are susceptible to rabies virus infection, but only a few species are important as reservoirs for the disease. In the United States, distinct strains of rabies virus have been identified in raccoons, skunks, foxes, and coyotes. Several species of insectivorous bats are also reservoirs for strains of the rabies virus.

Transmission of rabies virus usually begins when infected saliva of a host is passed to an uninfected animal. The most common mode of rabies virus transmission is through the bite and virus-containing saliva of an infected host. Transmission has been rarely documented via other routes such as contamination of mucous membranes (i.e., eyes, nose, mouth), aerosol transmission, and corneal and organ transplantations.

How is rabies diagnosed in humans?

Several tests are necessary to diagnose rabies antemortem (before death) in humans; no single test is sufficient. Tests are performed on samples of saliva, serum, spinal fluid, and skin biopsies of hair follicles at the nape of the neck.

How is rabies prevented?

Rabies in humans is 100% preventable through prompt appropriate medical care. Yet, more than 55,000 people, mostly in Africa and Asia, die from rabies every year.

The most important global source of rabies in humans is from uncontrolled rabies in dogs. Children are often at greatest risk from rabies. They are more likely to be bitten by dogs, and are also more likely to be severely exposed through multiple bites in high-risk sites on the body. Severe exposures make it more difficult to prevent rabies unless access to good medical care is immediately available.

Section 12.12

Rubella
(German Measles)

This section excerpted from "Rubella: Make Sure Your Child Is Fully Immunized," Centers for Disease Control and Prevention (www.cdc.gov), January 3, 2011.

Rubella—also known as German measles or three-day measles—is a contagious viral infection. But don't confuse rubella with measles, which is sometimes called rubeola. The two illnesses share similar features, including a characteristic red rash, but they are caused by different viruses.

Rubella virus "lives" in the respiratory secretions of infected persons and is usually spread to others through sneezing or coughing.

In young children, rubella is usually mild, with few noticeable symptoms. They may feel feverish and have a sore throat. Adults are more likely to experience headache, pink eye, and general discomfort one to five days before the rash appears. Adults also tend to have more complications, including sore, swollen joints and, less commonly, arthritis, especially in women. A brain infection called encephalitis is a rare, but serious, complication affecting adults with rubella. However, the most serious consequence from rubella infection is the harm it can cause to a pregnant woman's unborn baby.

Rubella Is Dangerous for Unborn Babies

Rubella infection during pregnancy, especially in the first 12 weeks, can lead to miscarriage, premature delivery, and serious birth defects, including heart problems, hearing and sight problems, cognitive impairment, and liver or spleen damage. Preventing rubella infection in a pregnant woman is the best way to protect her unborn baby. And vaccination is the best way to prevent rubella infection.

Any woman who might become pregnant should be vaccinated, unless a blood test shows she is already immune to the disease. And, even though children may only have mild rubella disease, they should be vaccinated on schedule to help stop the spread of rubella to pregnant women.

MMR Vaccine: Preventing Rubella Disease and Birth Defects since the 1960s

Rubella vaccine is included in MMR, a combination vaccine that provides protection against three viral diseases: measles, mumps, and rubella. MMR vaccine is safe and effective and has been widely used in the United States for over 20 years.

In the United States, two doses are recommended for children:

- The first dose at 12–15 months of age

- The second dose before entering school, at four to six years of age

In 2004 a second combination vaccine, MMRV, was licensed. Your child's doctor can help you choose between getting the MMR vaccine plus the varicella (chickenpox) vaccine or the single MMRV vaccine.

Immunizing your child on schedule is the best way to protect your child and others, including pregnant women and their unborn babies, from rubella infection.

MMR Vaccine for Adults: The Responsible Choice

In 2004, the United States declared that rubella had been eliminated. But the virus can be brought into the country at any time by visitors from other countries where the disease is still present. In addition, unvaccinated U.S. residents traveling to these countries can become infected and unknowingly bring the disease back home with them.

Anyone born during or after 1957 who has not had rubella or has not been vaccinated against the disease should receive at least one dose of MMR vaccine. If you're unsure, ask your health care provider to test your blood to see if you are immune to rubella.

Chapter 13

Parasitic and Fungal Infections

Chapter Contents

Section 13.1

Ascariasis and Hookworm Infection

This section excerpted from "Ascariasis FAQs" and "Hookworm FAQs,"
Centers for Disease Control and Prevention (www.cdc.gov), November 2, 2010.

Ascariasis

What is ascariasis?

Ascaris is an intestinal parasite of humans. It is the most common human worm infection. The larvae and adult worms live in the small intestine and can cause intestinal disease.

How is ascariasis spread?

Ascaris lives in the intestine and *Ascaris* eggs are passed in the feces of infected persons. If the infected person defecates outside (near bushes, in a garden or field), or if the feces of an infected person are used as fertilizer, then eggs are deposited on the soil. They can then mature into a form that is infective. Ascariasis is caused by ingesting infective eggs. This can happen when hands or fingers that have contaminated dirt on them are put in the mouth or by consuming vegetables or fruits that have not been carefully cooked, washed, or peeled.

Who is at risk for infection?

Infection occurs worldwide in warm and humid climates where sanitation and hygiene are poor, including in temperate zones during warmer months. Persons in these areas are at risk if soil contaminated with human feces enters their mouths or if they eat vegetables or fruit that have not been carefully washed, peeled, or cooked. Ascariasis is now uncommon in the United States.

What are the symptoms of ascariasis?

People infected with *Ascaris* often show no symptoms. If symptoms do occur they can be light and include abdominal discomfort. Heavy infections can cause intestinal blockage and impair growth in children. Other symptoms such as cough are due to migration of the worms through the body.

How is ascariasis diagnosed?

Health care providers can diagnose ascariasis by taking a stool sample and using a microscope to look for the presence of eggs. Some people notice infection when a worm is passed in their stool or is coughed up. If this happens, bring in the worm specimen to your health care provider for diagnosis.

How can I prevent infection?

- Avoid contact with soil that may be contaminated with human feces, including with human fecal matter ("night soil") used to fertilize crops.

- Wash your hands with soap and warm water before handling food.

- Teach children the importance of washing hands to prevent infection.

- Wash, peel, or cook all raw vegetables and fruits before eating, particularly those that have been grown in soil that has been fertilized with manure.

Transmission of infection to others can be prevented by not defecating outdoors and by effective sewage disposal systems.

What is the treatment for ascariasis?

Anthelminthic medications (drugs that rid the body of parasitic worms), such as albendazole and mebendazole, are the drugs of choice for treatment. Infections are generally treated for one to three days. The recommended medications are effective.

Hookworm

What is hookworm?

Hookworm is an intestinal parasite of humans. The larvae and adult worms live in the small intestine and can cause intestinal disease. The two main species of hookworm infecting humans are *Anclostoma duodenale* and *Necator americanus*.

How is hookworm spread?

Hookworm eggs are passed in the feces of an infected person. If an infected person defecates outside (near bushes, in a garden or field) or if the feces from an infected person are used as fertilizer, eggs are deposited on soil. They can then mature and hatch, releasing larvae (immature worms). The larvae mature into a form that can penetrate the skin of humans. Hookworm infection is transmitted primarily by walking barefoot on contaminated soil. One kind of hookworm (*Anclostoma duodenale*) can also be transmitted through the ingestion of larvae.

Who is at risk for infection?

People living in areas with warm and moist climates and where sanitation and hygiene are poor are at risk for hookworm infection if they walk barefoot or in other ways allow their skin to have direct contact with contaminated soil. Children who play in contaminated soil may also be at risk.

What are the signs and symptoms of hookworm?

Itching and a localized rash are often the first signs of infection. These symptoms occur when the larvae penetrate the skin. A person with a light infection may have no symptoms. A person with a heavy infection may experience abdominal pain, diarrhea, loss of appetite, weight loss, fatigue, and anemia. The physical and cognitive growth of children can be affected.

How is hookworm diagnosed?

Health care providers can diagnose hookworm by taking a stool sample and using a microscope to look for the presence of hookworm eggs.

How can I prevent infection?

Do not walk barefoot in areas where hookworm is common and where there may be fecal contamination of the soil. Avoid other skin-to-soil contact and avoid ingesting such soil.

The infection of others can be prevented by not defecating outdoors or using human feces as fertilizer and by effective sewage disposal systems.

What is the treatment for hookworm?

Hookworm infections are generally treated for one to three days with medication prescribed by your health care provider. The drugs are effective and appear to have few side effects. Iron supplements may be prescribed if you have anemia.

Preventive Treatment for Ascariasis and Hookworm

In developing countries, groups at higher risk for soil-transmitted helminth infections (hookworm, *Ascaris*, and whipworm) are often treated without a prior stool examination. Treating in this way is called preventive treatment (or "preventive chemotherapy"). The high-risk groups identified by the World Health Organization are preschool and school-age children, women of childbearing age (including pregnant women in the second and third trimesters and lactating women), and adults in occupations where there is a high risk of heavy infections. School-age children are often treated through school-health programs and preschool children and pregnant women at visits to health clinics.

What is mass drug administration (MDA)?

The soil-transmitted helminths and four other "neglected tropical diseases" (river blindness, lymphatic filariasis, schistosomiasis, and trachoma) are sometimes treated through mass drug administrations. Since the drugs used are safe and inexpensive or donated, entire risk groups are offered preventive treatment. Mass drug administrations are conducted periodically (often annually), commonly with drug distributors who go door to door. Multiple neglected tropical diseases are often treated simultaneously using MDAs.

Section 13.2

Baylisascaris *Infection*

"Baylisascaris FAQs," Centers for Disease Control
and Prevention (www.cdc.gov), March 3, 2011.

What is Baylisascaris?

Baylisascaris worms are intestinal parasites found in a wide variety
of animals. Different species of *Baylisascaris* are associated with different animal hosts. For example, *Baylisascaris procyonis* is found in
raccoons and *Baylisascaris columnaris* is an intestinal parasite found
in skunks. Cases of *Baylisascaris* infection in people are not frequently
reported, but can be severe. *Baylisascaris procyonis* is thought to pose
the greatest risk to humans because of the often close association of
raccoons to human dwellings.

In what parts of the world is Baylisascaris *found?*

Baylisascaris procyonis has been identified in the United States,
Europe, and Japan. Some evidence of infection in animals has been
reported in South America.

In the United States, infected raccoons have been found in a number
of states, especially in the mid-Atlantic, northeastern, and Midwestern
states and parts of California.

How do people get infected?

People become infected by ingesting infectious eggs. Most infections
are in children and others who are more likely to put dirt or animal
waste in their mouth by mistake.

How can I prevent Baylisascaris *infection?*

Eggs passed in raccoon feces are not immediately infectious. In
the environment, eggs take two to four weeks to become infectious.
If raccoons have set up a den or a latrine in your yard, raccoon feces
and material contaminated with raccoon feces should be removed

carefully and burned, buried, or sent to a landfill. Care should be taken to avoid contaminating hands and clothes. Treat decks, patios, and other surfaces with boiling water or a propane flame-gun (exercise proper precautions). Prompt removal and destruction of raccoon feces before the eggs become infectious will reduce risk for exposure and possible infection.

Do not keep, feed, or adopt wild animals, including raccoons, as pets.

Washing your hands after working or playing outdoors is good practice for preventing a number of diseases.

What are the symptoms and signs of Baylisascaris *infection?*

The incubation period (time from exposure to symptoms) is usually one to four weeks. If present, signs and symptoms can include the following:

- Nausea

- Tiredness

- Liver enlargement

- Loss of coordination

- Lack of attention to people and surroundings

- Loss of muscle control

- Blindness

- Coma

What should I do if I think I am infected with Baylisascaris?

You should discuss your concerns with your health care provider, who will examine you and ask you questions (for example, about your interactions with raccoons or other wild animals). *Baylisascaris* infection is difficult to diagnosis in humans. There are no widely available tests, so the diagnosis is often made by ruling out other diseases.

How is Baylisascaris *infection treated?*

A health care provider can discuss treatment options with you. No drug has been found to be completely effective against *Baylisascaris* infection in people. Albendazole has been recommended for some cases.

If I have Baylisascaris *infection, should my family members be tested for the infection?*

Baylisascaris infection is not contagious, so one person cannot give the infection to another. However, if your family may have been exposed the same way you were (such as contact with or exposure to an environment contaminated with raccoon or exotic pet feces), they should consult with a health care provider.

Section 13.3

Cryptosporidiosis

This section excerpted from "Cryptosporidiosis: General Information: Infection—General Public," Centers for Disease Control and Prevention (www.cdc.gov), November 2, 2010.

What is cryptosporidiosis?

Cryptosporidiosis is a diarrheal disease caused by microscopic parasites, *Cryptosporidium*, that can live in the intestine of humans and animals and are passed in the stool of an infected person or animal. Both the disease and the parasite are commonly known as "Crypto." The parasite is protected by an outer shell that allows it to survive outside the body for long periods of time and makes it very resistant to chlorine-based disinfectants. During the past two decades, Crypto has become recognized as one of the most common causes of waterborne disease (recreational water and drinking water) in humans in the United States. The parasite is found in every region of the United States and throughout the world.

How is cryptosporidiosis spread?

Cryptosporidium lives in the intestine of infected humans or animals. An infected person or animal sheds Crypto parasites in the stool. Millions of Crypto germs can be released in a bowel movement from an infected human or animal. Shedding of Crypto in the stool begins when the symptoms begin and can last for weeks after the symptoms (e.g., diarrhea) stop. You can become infected after accidentally swallowing the parasite. *Cryptosporidium* may be found in soil, food, water, or surfaces that have been contaminated with the feces from infected humans or animals. Crypto is not spread by contact with blood.

Crypto can be spread in a number of ways:

- By putting something in your mouth or accidentally swallowing something that has come into contact with stool of a person or animal infected with Crypto

- By swallowing recreational water contaminated with Crypto (recreational water is water in swimming pools, hot tubs, Jacuzzis, fountains, lakes, rivers, springs, ponds, or streams)

- By swallowing water or beverages contaminated with stool from infected humans or animals

- By eating uncooked food contaminated with Crypto

- By touching your mouth with contaminated hands (hands can become contaminated through a variety of activities, such as touching surfaces that have been contaminated by stool from an infected person, changing diapers, caring for an infected person, and handling an infected cow or calf)

- By exposure to human feces through sexual contact

What are the symptoms of cryptosporidiosis?

The most common symptom of cryptosporidiosis is watery diarrhea. Other symptoms include these:

- Stomach cramps or pain

- Dehydration

- Nausea

- Vomiting

- Fever

- Weight loss

Some people with Crypto will have no symptoms at all. While the small intestine is the site most commonly affected, Crypto infections could possibly affect other areas of the digestive tract or the respiratory tract.

How long after infection do symptoms appear?

Symptoms of cryptosporidiosis generally begin 2 to 10 days (average 7 days) after becoming infected with the parasite.

How long will symptoms last?

In persons with healthy immune systems, symptoms usually last about one to two weeks. The symptoms may go in cycles in which you may seem to get better for a few days, then feel worse again before the illness ends.

Who is most at risk for cryptosporidiosis?

People who are most likely to become infected with *Cryptosporidium* include the following:

- Children who attend day care centers, including diaper-aged children
- Child care workers
- Parents of infected children
- People who take care of other people with cryptosporidiosis
- International travelers
- Backpackers, hikers, and campers who drink unfiltered, untreated water
- People who drink from untreated shallow, unprotected wells
- People, including swimmers, who swallow water from contaminated sources
- People who handle infected cattle
- People exposed to human feces through sexual contact

Who is most at risk for getting seriously ill with cryptosporidiosis?

Although Crypto can infect all people, some groups are likely to develop more serious illness.

- Young children and pregnant women may be more susceptible to the dehydration resulting from diarrhea and should drink plenty of fluids while ill.

• If you have a severely weakened immune system, you are at risk for more serious disease. Your symptoms may be more severe and could lead to serious or life-threatening illness.

How is a cryptosporidiosis diagnosed?

If you suspect that you have cryptosporidiosis, see your health care provider. Your health care provider will ask you to submit stool samples to see if you are infected. Because testing for Crypto can be difficult, you may be asked to submit several stool specimens over several days. Tests for Crypto are not routinely done in most laboratories. Therefore, your health care provider should specifically request testing for the parasite.

What is the treatment for cryptosporidiosis?

Nitazoxanide has been approved by the FDA (U.S. Food and Drug Administration) for treatment of diarrhea caused by *Cryptosporidium* in people with healthy immune systems and is available by prescription. Consult with your health care provider for more information. Most people who have healthy immune systems will recover without treatment. Diarrhea can be managed by drinking plenty of fluids to prevent dehydration. Young children and pregnant women may be more susceptible to dehydration. Rapid loss of fluids from diarrhea may be especially life threatening to babies. Therefore, parents should talk to their health care provider about fluid replacement therapy options for infants. Antidiarrheal medicine may help slow down diarrhea, but a health care provider should be consulted before such medicine is taken.

People who are in poor health or who have weakened immune systems are at higher risk for more severe and more prolonged illness. The effectiveness of nitazoxanide in immunosuppressed individuals is unclear. HIV-positive individuals who suspect they have Crypto should contact their health care provider. For persons with AIDS, antiretroviral therapy that improves immune status will also decrease or eliminate symptoms of Crypto. However, even if symptoms disappear, cryptosporidiosis is often not curable and the symptoms may return if the immune status worsens.

I have been diagnosed with cryptosporidiosis, should I worry about spreading the infection to others?

Yes, *Cryptosporidium* can be very contagious. Infected individuals should follow these guidelines to avoid spreading the disease to others:

- Wash your hands frequently with soap and water, especially after using the toilet, after changing diapers, and before eating or preparing food.

- Do not swim in recreational water if you have cryptosporidiosis and for at least two weeks after the diarrhea stops. You can pass Crypto in your stool and contaminate water for several weeks after your symptoms have ended. You do not even need to have a fecal accident in the water. Immersion in the water may be enough for contamination to occur.

- Avoid sexual practices that might result in oral exposure to stool (e.g., oral-anal contact).

- Avoid close contact with anyone who has a weakened immune system.

- Children with diarrhea should be excluded from child care settings until the diarrhea has stopped.

Note: You may not be protected in a chlorinated recreational water venue (e.g., swimming pool, water park, splash pad, spray park) because *Cryptosporidium* is chlorine-resistant and can live for days in chlorine-treated water.

Section 13.4

Giardiasis

This section excerpted from "Giardiasis Frequently
Asked Questions (FAQs)," Centers for Disease Control and
Prevention (www.cdc.gov), March 17, 2011.

What is giardiasis?

Giardiasis is a diarrheal disease caused by the microscopic parasite *Giardia*. A parasite is an organism that feeds off of another to survive. Once a person or animal (for example, cats, dogs, cattle, deer, and beavers) has been infected with *Giardia*, the parasite lives in the intestines and is passed in feces. Once outside the body, *Giardia* can sometimes survive for weeks or months. *Giardia* can be found within every region of the U.S. and around the world.

How do you get giardiasis and how is it spread?

Giardiasis can be spread by the following methods:

- Swallowing *Giardia* picked up from surfaces (such as bathroom handles, changing tables, diaper pails, or toys) that contain stool from an infected person or animal

- Drinking water or using ice made from water sources where *Giardia* may live (for example, untreated or improperly treated water from lakes, streams, or wells)

- Swallowing water while swimming or playing in water where *Giardia* may live, especially in lakes, rivers, springs, ponds, and streams

- Eating uncooked food that contains *Giardia* organisms

- Having contact with someone who is ill with giardiasis

- Traveling to countries where giardiasis is common

Anything that comes into contact with feces from infected humans or animals can become contaminated with the *Giardia* parasite. People become infected when they swallow the parasite. It is not possible to become infected through contact with blood.

What are the symptoms of giardiasis?

Giardia infection can cause a variety of intestinal symptoms:

- Diarrhea
- Gas or flatulence
- Greasy stool that can float
- Stomach or abdominal cramps
- Upset stomach or nausea
- Dehydration

These symptoms may also lead to weight loss. Some people with *Giardia* infection have no symptoms at all.

How long after infection do symptoms appear?

Symptoms of giardiasis normally begin one to three weeks after becoming infected.

How long will symptoms last?

In otherwise healthy people, symptoms of giardiasis may last two to six weeks. Occasionally, symptoms last longer. Medications can help decrease the amount of time symptoms last.

Who is most at risk of getting giardiasis?

Though giardiasis is commonly thought of as a camping or backpacking-related disease and is sometimes called "Beaver Fever," anyone can get giardiasis. People more likely to become infected include the following:

- Children in child care settings, especially diaper-aged children
- Close contacts (for example, people living in the same household) or people who care for those sick with giardiasis
- People who drink water or use ice made from places where *Giardia* may live (for example, untreated or improperly treated water from lakes, streams, or wells)

- Backpackers, hikers, and campers who drink unsafe water or who do not practice good hygiene (for example, proper handwashing)
- People who swallow water while swimming and playing in recreational water where *Giardia* may live, especially in lakes, rivers, springs, ponds, and streams
- International travelers
- People exposed to human feces through sexual contact

How is giardiasis diagnosed?

Contact your health care provider if you think you may have giardiasis. Your health care provider will ask you to submit stool samples to see if you are infected. Because testing for giardiasis can be difficult, you may be asked to submit several stool specimens collected over several days.

What is the treatment for giardiasis?

Many prescription drugs are available to treat giardiasis. Although the *Giardia* parasite can infect all people, infants and pregnant women may be more likely to experience dehydration from the diarrhea caused by giardiasis. To prevent dehydration, infants and pregnant women should drink a lot of fluids while ill. Dehydration can be life threatening for infants, so it is especially important that parents talk to their health care providers about treatment options for their infants.

My child does not have diarrhea, but was recently diagnosed as having Giardia infection. My health care provider says treatment is not necessary. Is this correct?

Your child does not usually need treatment if he or she has no symptoms. However, there are a few exceptions. If your child does not have diarrhea, but does have other symptoms such as nausea or upset stomach, tiredness, weight loss, or a lack of hunger, you and your health care provider may need to think about treatment. The same is true if many family members are ill, or if a family member is pregnant and unable to take the most effective medications to treat *Giardia*. Contact your health care provider for specific treatment recommendations.

What can I do to prevent and control giardiasis?

To prevent and control infection with the *Giardia* parasite, it is important to take the following precautions:

- Practice good hygiene.

- Avoid water (drinking or recreational) that may be contaminated.

- Avoid eating food that may be contaminated.

- Prevent contact and contamination with feces during sex.

Section 13.5

Hymenolepis
(Dwarf Tapeworm) Infection

"Hymenolepiasis FAQs," Centers for Disease Control and
Prevention (www.cdc.gov), November 2, 2010.

What is Hymenolepis nana *infection?*

The dwarf tapeworm or *Hymenolepis nana* is found worldwide. Infection is most common in children, in persons living in institutional settings, and in people who live in areas where sanitation and personal hygiene is inadequate.

How did I get infected?

One becomes infected by accidentally ingesting dwarf tapeworm eggs. This can happen by ingesting fecally contaminated foods or water, by touching your mouth with contaminated fingers, or by ingesting contaminated soil. People can also become infected if they accidentally ingest an infected arthropod (intermediate host, such as a small beetle or mealworm) that has gotten into food.

Adult dwarf tapeworms are very small in comparison with other tapeworms and may reach 15–40 mm (up to 2 inches) in length. The adult dwarf tapeworm is made up of many small segments, called proglottids. As the dwarf tapeworm matures inside the intestine, these segments break off and pass into the stool. An adult dwarf tapeworm can live for four to six weeks. However, once you are infected, the dwarf tapeworm may reproduce inside the body (autoinfection) and continue the infection.

What are the symptoms of a dwarf tapeworm infection?

Most people who are infected do not have any symptoms. Those who have symptoms may experience nausea, weakness, loss of appetite, diarrhea, and abdominal pain. Young children, especially those with a heavy infection, may develop a headache, itchy bottom, or have difficulty sleeping. Sometimes infection is misdiagnosed as a pinworm infection.

Contrary to popular belief, a dwarf tapeworm infection does not generally cause weight loss. You cannot feel the dwarf tapeworm inside your body.

How is dwarf tapeworm infection diagnosed?

Diagnosis is made by identifying dwarf tapeworm eggs in stool. Your health care provider will ask you to submit stool specimens collected over several days to see if you are infected.

Is a dwarf tapeworm infection serious?

No. Infection with the dwarf tapeworm is generally not serious. However, prolonged infection can lead to more severe symptoms; therefore, medical attention is needed to eliminate the dwarf tapeworm.

How is a dwarf tapeworm infection treated?

Treatment is available. A prescription drug called praziquantel is given. The medication causes the dwarf tapeworm to dissolve within the intestine. Praziquantel is generally well tolerated. Sometimes more than one treatment is necessary.

Can infection be spread to other family members?

Yes. Eggs are infectious (meaning they can reinfect you or infect others) immediately after being shed in feces.

How can dwarf tapeworm infection be prevented?

To reduce the likelihood of infection you should take the following precautions:

- Wash your hands with soap and warm water after using the toilet, changing diapers, and before preparing foods.

- Teach children the importance of washing hands to prevent infection.

- When traveling in countries where food is likely to be contaminated, wash, peel or cook all raw vegetables and fruits with safe water before eating.

Section 13.6

Pediculosis Capitis *(Head Lice)*

This section excerpted from "Lice: Head Lice: General Information—
Frequently Asked Questions (FAQs)" and "Lice: Head Lice: Treatment," Centers for Disease Control and Prevention (www.cdc.gov), November 2, 2010.

Head Lice: Frequently Asked Questions

What are head lice?

The head louse, or *Pediculus humanus capitis*, is a parasitic insect that can be found on the head, eyebrows, and eyelashes of people. Head lice feed on human blood several time a day and live close to the human scalp. Head lice are not known to spread disease.

Who is at risk for getting head lice?

Head lice are found worldwide. In the United States, infestation with head lice is most common among preschool children attending child care, elementary school children, and the household members of infested children. Although reliable data on how many people in the United States get head lice each year are not available, an estimated 6 million to 12 million infestations occur each year in the United States among children 3 to 11 years of age.

Head lice move by crawling; they cannot hop or fly. Head lice are spread by direct contact with the hair of an infested person. Anyone who comes in head-to-head contact with someone who already has head lice is at greatest risk. Spread by contact with clothing (such as hats, scarves, coats) or other personal items (such as combs, brushes, or towels) used by an infested person is uncommon. Personal hygiene or cleanliness in the home or school has nothing to do with getting head lice.

What do head lice look like?

Head lice have three forms: the egg (also called a nit), the nymph, and the adult.

Egg/Nit: Nits are lice eggs laid by the adult female head louse at the base of the hair shaft nearest the scalp. Nits are firmly attached to the hair shaft and are oval-shaped and very small (about the size of a knot in thread) and hard to see. Nits are often confused with dandruff, scabs, or hair spray droplets. Head lice nits usually take about 8–9 days to hatch.

Nymph: A nymph is an immature louse that hatches from the nit. A nymph looks like an adult head louse but is smaller. To live, a nymph must feed on blood. Nymphs mature into adults about 9–12 days after hatching from the nit.

Adult: The fully grown and developed adult louse is about the size of a sesame seed, has six legs, and is tan to grayish-white in color. To survive, adult head lice must feed on blood. An adult head louse can live about 30 days on a person's head but will die within one or two days if it falls off a person. Adult female head lice are usually larger than males and can lay about six eggs each day.

Where are head lice most commonly found?

Head lice and head lice nits are found almost exclusively on the scalp, particularly around and behind the ears and near the neckline at the back of the head. Head lice or head lice nits sometimes are found on the eyelashes or eyebrows, but this is uncommon. Head lice hold tightly to hair with hook-like claws at the end of each of their six legs. Head lice nits are cemented firmly to the hair shaft and can be difficult to remove even after the nymphs hatch and empty casings remain.

What are the signs and symptoms of head lice infestation?

- Tickling feeling of something moving in the hair

- Itching, caused by an allergic reaction to the bites of the head louse

- Irritability and difficulty sleeping (head lice are most active in the dark)

- Sores on the head caused by scratching; these sores can sometimes become infected with bacteria found on the person's skin

How did my child get head lice?

Head-to-head contact with an already infested person is the most common way to get head lice. Head-to-head contact is common during play at school, at home, and elsewhere (sports activities, playground, slumber parties, camp).

Although uncommon, head lice can be spread by sharing clothing or belongings. Dogs, cats, and other pets do not play a role in the spread of head lice.

How is head lice infestation diagnosed?

The diagnosis of a head lice infestation is best made by finding a live nymph or adult louse on the scalp or hair of a person. Because nymphs and adult lice are very small, move quickly, and avoid light, they can be difficult to find. Use of a magnifying lens and a fine-toothed comb may be helpful to find live lice. If crawling lice are not seen, finding nits firmly attached within a ¼ inch of base of the hair shafts strongly suggests, but does not confirm, that a person is infested and should be treated. If no live nymphs or adult lice are seen, and the only nits found are more than ¼ inch from the scalp, the infestation is probably old and no longer active and does not need to be treated.

If you are not sure if a person has head lice, the diagnosis should be made by their health care provider, local health department, or other person trained to identify live head lice.

Do head lice spread disease?

Head lice should not be considered as a medical or public health hazard. Head lice are not known to spread disease. Head lice can be an annoyance because their presence may cause itching and loss of sleep. Sometimes the itching can lead to excessive scratching that can sometimes increase the chance of a secondary skin infection.

Can head lice be spread by sharing sports helmets or head-phones?

Head lice are spread most commonly by direct contact with the hair of an infested person. Spread by contact with inanimate objects and personal belongings may occur but is very uncommon. Head lice would have difficulty attaching firmly to smooth or slippery surfaces like plastic, metal, polished synthetic leathers, and other similar materials.

Can wigs or hair pieces spread lice?

Head lice and their eggs (nits) soon perish if separated from their human host. For these reasons, the risk of transmission of head lice from a wig or other hairpiece is extremely small, particularly if the wig or hairpiece has not been worn within the preceding 48 hours by someone who is actively infested with live head lice.

Can swimming spread lice?

Data show that head lice can survive under water for several hours but are unlikely to be spread by the water in a swimming pool. Head lice have been seen to hold tightly to human hair and not let go when submerged under water.

Head lice may be spread by sharing towels or other items that have been in contact with an infested person's hair, although such spread is uncommon. Children should be taught not to share towels, hair brushes, and similar items either at poolside or in the changing room.

Head Lice: Treatment

Treatment for head lice is recommended for persons diagnosed with an active infestation. All household members and other close contacts should be checked; those persons with evidence of an active infestation should be treated. Some experts believe prophylactic treatment is prudent for persons who share the same bed with actively-infested individuals. All infested persons (household members and close contacts) and their bedmates should be treated at the same time.

Retreatment of head lice usually is recommended because no approved pediculicide is completely ovicidal. To be most effective, retreatment should occur after all eggs have hatched but before new eggs are produced. The retreatment schedule can vary depending on whether the pediculicide used is ovicidal (whether it can kill lice eggs).

When treating head lice, supplemental measures can be combined with recommended medicine; however, such additional measures generally are not required to eliminate a head lice infestation. For example, hats, scarves, pillow cases, bedding, clothing, and towels worn or used by the infested person in the two-day period just before treatment is started can be machine washed and dried using the hot water and hot air cycles because lice and eggs are killed by exposure for five minutes to temperatures greater than 53.5° C (128.3° F). Items that cannot be laundered may be dry-cleaned or sealed in a plastic bag for two weeks. Items such as hats, grooming aids, and towels that come in contact with the hair of an infested person should not be shared. Vacuuming furniture and floors can remove an infested person's hairs that might have viable nits attached.

Treat the infested person with an over-the-counter (OTC) or prescription medication. Follow these treatment steps:

1. Before applying treatment, it may be helpful to remove clothing that can become wet or stained during treatment.

2. Apply lice medicine, also called pediculicide, according to the instructions contained in the box or printed on the label. If the infested person has very long hair (longer than shoulder length), it may be necessary to use a second bottle.

    Warning: Do not use a combination shampoo/conditioner or conditioner before using lice medicine. Do not rewash the hair for one to two days after the lice medicine is removed.

3. Have the infested person put on clean clothing after treatment.

4. If a few live lice are still found 8–12 hours after treatment, but are moving more slowly than before, do not re-treat. The medicine may take longer to kill all the lice. Comb dead and any remaining live lice out of the hair using a fine-toothed nit comb. Many flea combs made for cats and dogs are also effective.

5. If, after 8–12 hours of treatment, no dead lice are found and lice seem as active as before, the medicine may not be working. Do not re-treat until speaking with your health care provider; a different lice medicine may be necessary.

6. After each treatment, checking the hair and combing with a nit comb to remove nits and lice every two to three days may decrease the chance of self-reinfestation. Continue to check for two to three weeks to be sure all lice and nits are gone.

7. Retreatment generally is recommended for most drugs on day nine in order to kill any surviving hatched lice before they produce new eggs. However, if using the prescription drug malathion, which is ovicidal, retreatment is recommended after seven to nine days *only* if crawling bugs are found.

Section 13.7

Enterobiasis (Pinworm Infection)

This section excerpted from "Pinworm Infection FAQs," Centers for Disease Control and Prevention (www.cdc.gov), November 2, 2010.

What is a pinworm?

A pinworm ("threadworm") is a small, thin, white roundworm (nematode) called *Enterobius vermicularis* that sometimes lives in the colon and rectum of humans. Pinworms are about the length of a staple. While an infected person sleeps, female pinworms leave the intestine through the anus and deposit their eggs on the surrounding skin.

What are the symptoms of a pinworm infection?

Pinworm infection (called enterobiasis or oxyuriasis) causes itching around the anus that can lead to difficulty sleeping and restlessness. Symptoms of pinworm infection usually are mild and some infected people have no symptoms.

Who is at risk for pinworm infection?

Pinworm infection occurs worldwide and affects persons of all ages and socioeconomic levels. It is the most common worm infection in the United States. Pinworm infection occurs most commonly among school-aged and preschool-aged children, institutionalized persons, and household members and caretakers of persons with pinworm infection.

Pinworm infection often occurs in more than one person in household and institutional settings. Child care centers often are the site of cases of pinworm infection.

How is pinworm infection spread?

Pinworm infection is spread by the fecal-oral route—that is, by the transfer of infective pinworm eggs from the anus to someone's mouth, either directly by hand or indirectly through contaminated clothing, bedding, food, or other articles.

Pinworm eggs become infective within a few hours after being deposited on the skin around the anus and can survive for two to three weeks on clothing, bedding, or other objects. People become infected, usually unknowingly, by swallowing (ingesting) infective pinworm eggs that are on fingers, under fingernails, or on clothing, bedding, and other contaminated objects and surfaces. Because of their small size, pinworm eggs sometimes can become airborne and ingested while breathing.

Can my family become infected with pinworms from swimming pools?

Pinworm infections are rarely spread through the use of swimming pools. Although chlorine levels found in pools are not high enough to kill pinworm eggs, the presence of a small number of pinworm eggs in thousands of gallons of water (the amount typically found in pools) makes the chance of infection unlikely.

How is pinworm infection diagnosed?

Itching during the night in a child's perianal area strongly suggests pinworm infection. Diagnosis is made by identifying the worm or its eggs. Worms can sometimes be seen on the skin near the anus or on underclothing, pajamas, or sheets about two to three hours after falling asleep.

Pinworm eggs can be collected and examined using the "tape test" as soon as the person wakes up. This test is done by firmly pressing the adhesive side of clear, transparent cellophane tape to the skin around the anus. The eggs stick to the tape and the tape can be placed on a slide and looked at under a microscope. This test should be done as soon as the person wakes up in the morning before they wash, bathe, go to the toilet, or get dressed. The tape test should be done on three consecutive mornings to increase the chance of finding pinworm eggs.

Because itching and scratching of the anal area is common in pinworm infection, samples taken from under the fingernails may also contain eggs. Pinworm eggs rarely are found in routine stool or urine samples.

How is pinworm infection treated?

Pinworm can be treated with either prescription or over-the-counter medications. A health care provider should be consulted before treating a suspected case of pinworm infection.

Treatment involves two doses of medication with the second dose being given two weeks after the first dose. All household contacts and caretakers of the infected person should be treated at the same time. Reinfection can occur easily so strict observance of good hand hygiene is essential (e.g., proper handwashing, maintaining clean short fingernails, avoiding nail biting, avoiding scratching the perianal area).

Daily morning bathing and daily changing of underwear helps removes a large proportion of eggs. Showering may be preferred to avoid possible contamination of bath water. Careful handling and frequent changing of underclothing, night clothes, towels, and bedding can help reduce infection, reinfection, and environmental contamination with pinworm eggs. These items should be laundered in hot water, especially after each treatment of the infected person and after each usage of washcloths until infection is cleared.

What should be done if the pinworm infection occurs again?

Reinfection occurs easily. Prevention always should be discussed at the time of treatment. Good hand hygiene is the most effective means of prevention. If pinworm infection occurs again, the infected person should be retreated with the same two-dose treatment. The infected person's household contacts and caretakers also should be treated. If pinworm infection continues to occur, the source of the infection should be sought and treated. Playmates, schoolmates, close contacts outside the home, and household members should be considered possible sources of infection.

How can pinworm infection and reinfection be prevented?

Strict observance of good hand hygiene is the most effective means of preventing pinworm infection. This includes washing hands with soap and warm water after using the toilet, changing diapers, and before handling food. Keep fingernails clean and short, avoid fingernail-biting, and avoid scratching the skin in the perianal area. Teach children the importance of washing hands to prevent infection.

Daily morning bathing and changing of underclothes helps remove a large proportion of pinworm eggs and can help prevent infection and reinfection. Showering may be preferred to avoid possible contamination of bath water. Careful handling (avoid shaking) and frequent laundering of underclothes, night clothes, towels, and bed sheets using hot water also helps reduce the chance of infection and reinfection by reducing environmental contamination with eggs.

189

Control can be difficult in child care centers and schools because the rate of reinfection is high. In institutions, mass and simultaneous treatment, repeated in two weeks, can be effective. Hand hygiene is the most effective method of prevention. Trimming and scrubbing the fingernails and bathing after treatment is important to help prevent reinfection and spread of pinworms.

Section 13.8

Scabies

This section excerpted from "Scabies Frequently Asked Questions (FAQs)," Centers for Disease Control and Prevention (www.cdc.gov), November 2, 2010.

What is scabies?

Scabies is an infestation of the skin by the human itch mite (*Sarcoptes scabiei* var. *hominis*). The microscopic scabies mite burrows into the upper layer of the skin where it lives and lays its eggs. The most common symptoms of scabies are intense itching and a pimple-like skin rash. The scabies mite usually is spread by direct, prolonged, skin-to-skin contact with a person who has scabies.

Scabies is found worldwide and affects people of all races and social classes. Scabies can spread rapidly under crowded conditions where close body and skin contact is frequent. Institutions such as nursing homes, extended-care facilities, and prisons are often sites of scabies outbreaks. Child care facilities also are a common site of scabies infestations.

What is crusted (Norwegian) scabies?

Crusted scabies is a severe form of scabies that can occur in some persons who are immunocompromised (have a weak immune system), elderly, disabled, or debilitated. It is also called Norwegian scabies. Persons with crusted scabies have thick crusts of skin that contain large numbers of scabies mites and eggs. Persons with crusted scabies are very contagious to other persons and can spread the infestation easily both by direct skin-to-skin contact and by contamination of items such as their clothing, bedding, and furniture. Persons with crusted scabies may not show the usual signs and symptoms of scabies such as the characteristic rash or itching (pruritus). Persons with crusted scabies should receive quick and aggressive medical treatment for their infestation to prevent outbreaks of scabies.

How soon after infestation do symptoms of scabies begin?

If a person has never had scabies before, symptoms may take as long as four to six weeks to begin. It is important to remember that an infested person can spread scabies during this time, even if he/she does not have symptoms yet.

In a person who has had scabies before, symptoms usually appear much sooner (one to four days) after exposure.

What are the signs and symptoms of scabies infestation?

The most common signs and symptoms of scabies are intense itching (pruritus), especially at night, and a pimple-like (papular) itchy rash. The itching and rash each may affect much of the body or be limited to common sites such as the wrist, elbow, armpit, webbing between the fingers, nipple, penis, waist, belt-line, and buttocks. The rash also can include tiny blisters (vesicles) and scales. Scratching the rash can cause skin sores; sometimes these sores become infected by bacteria.

Tiny burrows sometimes are seen on the skin; these are caused by the female scabies mite tunneling just beneath the surface of the skin. These burrows appear as tiny raised and crooked (serpiginous) grayish-white or skin-colored lines on the skin surface. Because mites are often few in number (only 10–15 mites per person), these burrows may be difficult to find. They are found most often in the webbing between the fingers, in the skin folds on the wrist, elbow, or knee, and on the penis, breast, or shoulder blades.

The head, face, neck, palms, and soles often are involved in infants and very young children, but usually not adults and older children.

How did I get scabies?

Scabies usually is spread by direct, prolonged, skin-to-skin contact with a person who has scabies. Contact generally must be prolonged; a quick handshake or hug usually will not spread scabies. Scabies is spread easily to sexual partners and household members. Scabies in adults frequently is sexually acquired. Scabies sometimes is spread indirectly by sharing articles such as clothing, towels, or bedding used by an infested person; however, such indirect spread can occur much more easily when the infested person has crusted scabies.

How is scabies infestation diagnosed?

Diagnosis of a scabies infestation usually is made based on the customary appearance and distribution of the rash and the presence of burrows. Whenever possible, the diagnosis of scabies should be confirmed by identifying the mite, mite eggs, or mite fecal matter (scybala). This can be done by carefully removing a mite from the end of its burrow using the tip of a needle or by obtaining skin scraping to examine under a microscope. It is important to remember that a person can still be infested even if mites, eggs, or fecal matter cannot be found.

How long can scabies mites live?

On a person, scabies mites can live for as long as one to two months. Off a person, scabies mites usually do not survive more than 48–72 hours. Scabies mites will die if exposed to a temperature of 50° C (122° F) for 10 minutes.

Can scabies be treated?

Yes. Products used to treat scabies are called scabicides because they kill scabies mites; some also kill eggs. Scabicides to treat human scabies are available only with a doctor's prescription; no over-the-counter products have been tested and approved for humans.

Always follow carefully the instructions provided by the doctor and pharmacist, as well as those contained in the box or printed on the label. When treating adults and older children, scabicide cream or lotion is applied to all areas of the body from the neck down to the feet and toes; when treating infants and young children, the cream or lotion also is applied to the head and neck. The medication should be left on the body for the recommended time before it is washed off. Clean clothes should be worn after treatment.

In addition to the infested person, treatment also is recommended for household members and sexual contacts, particularly those who have had prolonged skin-to-skin contact with the infested person. All persons should be treated at the same time in order to prevent reinfestation. Retreatment may be necessary if itching continues more than two to four weeks after treatment or if new burrows or rash continue to appear.

Never use a scabicide intended for veterinary or agricultural use to treat humans!

How soon after treatment will I feel better?

If itching continues more than two to four weeks after initial treatment or if new burrows or rash continue to appear (if initial treatment includes more than one application or dose, then the two-to-four-week time period begins after the last application or dose), retreatment with scabicide may be necessary; seek the advice of a physician.

Did I get scabies from my pet?

No. Animals do not spread human scabies. Pets can become infested with a different kind of scabies mite that does not survive or reproduce on humans but causes "mange" in animals. If an animal with "mange" has close contact with a person, the animal mite can get under the person's skin and cause temporary itching and skin irritation. However, the animal mite cannot reproduce on a person and will die on its own in a couple of days

Can scabies be spread by swimming in a public pool?

Scabies is spread by prolonged skin-to-skin contact with a person who has scabies. Scabies sometimes also can be spread by contact with items such as clothing, bedding, or towels that have been used by a person with scabies, but such spread is very uncommon unless the infested person has crusted scabies. Scabies is very unlikely to be spread by water in a swimming pool.

How can I remove scabies mites from my house, carpet, or clothes?

Scabies mites do not survive more than two to three days away from human skin. Items such as bedding, clothing, and towels used by a person with scabies can be decontaminated by machine-washing in hot water and drying using the hot cycle or by dry-cleaning. Items that cannot be washed or dry-cleaned can be decontaminated by removing from any body contact for at least 72 hours.

Because persons with crusted scabies are considered very infectious, careful vacuuming of furniture and carpets in rooms used by these persons is recommended.

193

If I come in contact with a person who has scabies, should I treat myself?

No. If a person thinks he or she might have scabies, he/she should contact a doctor. The doctor can examine the person, confirm the diagnosis of scabies, and prescribe an appropriate treatment.

Sleeping with or having sex with any scabies-infested person presents a high risk for transmission. The longer a person has skin-to-skin exposure, the greater is the likelihood for transmission to occur. Although briefly shaking hands with a person who has non-crusted scabies could be considered as presenting a relatively low risk, holding the hand of a person with scabies for 5–10 minutes could be considered to present a relatively high risk of transmission. However, transmission can occur even after brief skin-to-skin contact, such as a handshake, with a person who has crusted scabies. In general, a person who has skin-to-skin contact with a person who has crusted scabies would be considered a good candidate for treatment.

To determine when prophylactic treatment should be given to reduce the risk of transmission, early consultation should be sought with a health care provider.

Section 13.9

Cercarial Dermatitis (Swimmer's Itch)

This section excerpted from "Swimmer's Itch FAQs," Centers for Disease Control and Prevention (www.cdc.gov), November 2, 2010.

What is swimmer's itch?

Swimmer's itch, also called cercarial dermatitis, appears as a skin rash caused by an allergic reaction to certain microscopic parasites that infect some birds and mammals. These parasites are released from infected snails into fresh and salt water (such as lakes, ponds, and oceans). While the parasite's preferred host is the specific bird or mammal, if the parasite comes into contact with a swimmer, it burrows into the skin causing an allergic reaction and rash. Swimmer's itch is found throughout the world and is more frequent during summer months.

How does water become infested with the parasite?

The adult parasite lives in the blood of infected animals such as ducks, geese, gulls, swans, and certain mammals such as muskrats and raccoons. The parasites produce eggs that are passed in the feces of infected birds or mammals.

If the eggs land in or are washed into the water, the eggs hatch, releasing small, free-swimming microscopic larvae. These larvae swim in the water in search of a certain species of aquatic snail.

If the larvae find one of these snails, they infect the snail, multiply, and undergo further development. Infected snails release a different type of microscopic larvae (or cercariae, hence the name cercarial dermatitis) into the water. This larval form then swims about searching for a suitable host (bird, muskrat) to continue the lifecycle. Although humans are not suitable hosts, the microscopic larvae burrow into the swimmer's skin and may cause an allergic reaction and rash. Because these larvae cannot develop inside a human, they soon die.

What are the signs and symptoms of swimmer's itch?

Within minutes to days after swimming in contaminated water, you may experience tingling, burning, or itching of the skin. Small reddish pimples appear within 12 hours. Pimples may develop into small blisters. Scratching the areas may result in secondary bacterial infections. Itching may last up to a week or more but will gradually go away.

Because swimmer's itch is caused by an allergic reaction to infection, the more often you swim or wade in contaminated water, the more likely you are to develop more serious symptoms. The greater the number of exposures to contaminated water, the more intense and immediate symptoms of swimmer's itch will be.

Be aware that swimmer's itch is not the only rash that may occur after swimming in fresh or salt water.

Do I need to see my health care provider for treatment?

Most cases of swimmer's itch do not require medical attention. If you have a rash, you may try the following for relief:

- Use corticosteroid cream
- Apply cool compresses to the affected areas
- Bathe in Epsom salts or baking soda
- Soak in colloidal oatmeal baths
- Apply baking soda paste to the rash (made by stirring water into baking soda until it reaches a paste-like consistency)
- Use an anti-itch lotion

Though difficult, try not to scratch. Scratching may cause the rash to become infected. If itching is severe, your health care provider may suggest prescription-strength lotions or creams to lessen your symptoms.

Swimmer's itch is not contagious and cannot be spread from one person to another.

Who is at risk for swimmer's itch?

Anyone who swims or wades in infested water may be at risk. Larvae are more likely to be present in shallow water by the shoreline. Children are most often affected because they tend to swim, wade, and play in the shallow water more than adults. Also, they are less likely to towel dry themselves when leaving the water.

Once an outbreak of swimmer's itch has occurred in water, will the water always be unsafe?

No. Many factors must be present for swimmer's itch to become a problem in water. Since these factors change (sometimes within a swim season), swimmer's itch will not always be a problem. However, there is no way to know how long water may be unsafe. Larvae generally survive for 24 hours once they are released from the snail. However, an infected snail will continue to produce cercariae throughout the remainder of its life. For future snails to become infected, migratory birds or mammals in the area must also be infected so the lifecycle can continue.

What can be done to reduce the risk of swimmer's itch?

Take the following precautions to reduce the likelihood of developing swimmer's itch:

- Do not swim in areas where swimmer's itch is a known problem or where signs have been posted warning of unsafe water.

- Do not swim near or wade in marshy areas where snails are commonly found.

- Towel dry or shower immediately after leaving the water.

- Do not attract birds (e.g., by feeding them) to areas where people are swimming.

- Encourage health officials to post signs on shorelines where swimmer's itch is a current problem.

Section 13.10

Dermatophytes (Tinea and Ringworm)

This section excerpted from "Dermatophytes (Ringworm)," Centers for Disease Control and Prevention (www.cdc.gov), July 17, 2009.

What are dermatophytes?

Dermatophytes are types of fungi that cause common skin, hair, and nail infections. Infections caused by these fungi are also known by the names "tinea" and "ringworm." It is important to emphasize that "ringworm" is not caused by a worm, but rather by a type of fungus called a "dermatophyte." One example of a very common dermatophyte infection is athlete's foot, which is also called tinea pedis. Another common dermatophyte infection affecting the groin area is jock itch, also known as tinea cruris.

Trichophyton rubrum and *Trichophyton tonsurans* are two common dermatophytes. These two species are usually transmitted from person to person. Another common dermatophyte is *Microsporum canis*, which is transmitted from animals such as cats and dogs to people. Dermatophytes like to live on moist areas of the skin, such as places where there are skin folds. They can also contaminate items in the environment, such as clothing, towels, and bedding.

Who gets dermatophyte infections?

Dermatophyte infections are very common. They can affect anyone, including people who are otherwise healthy. Dermatophyte infections may be more common among people with suppressed immune systems, people who use communal baths, and people who are involved in contact sports such as wrestling. Outbreaks of infections can occur in schools, households, and institutional settings.

The dermatophyte infection that affects the scalp and hair is known as tinea capitis. It is especially common among school-aged children. For reasons that are not well understood, tinea capitis does not usually occur after puberty. Other kinds of dermatophyte infections tend to be more common in adolescents and adults.

How are dermatophyte infections spread?

Spread usually occurs through direct contact with an infected person or animal. Clothing, bedding, and towels can also become contaminated and spread the infection.

What are the symptoms of a dermatophyte infection?

Dermatophyte infections can affect the skin on almost any area of the body, such as the scalp, legs, arms, feet, groin, and nails. These infections are usually itchy. Redness, scaling, or fissuring of the skin, or a ring with irregular borders and a cleared central area may occur. If the infection involves the scalp, an area of hair loss may result. More aggressive infections may lead to an abscess or cellulitis. Areas infected by dermatophytes may become secondarily infected by bacteria.

How soon do symptoms appear?

Symptoms typically appear between 4 and 14 days following exposure.

If I have symptoms, should I see my doctor?

Yes. Most of the time these infections can be successfully treated with medication prescribed by your doctor.

How is a dermatophyte infection diagnosed?

Your doctor may make a presumptive diagnosis based on your symptoms and physical examination. To confirm the diagnosis your doctor may obtain scrapings of affected skin or clippings of affected nails. These may be examined under a microscope and may be sent to the laboratory for a fungal culture. Keep in mind that the results of the fungal culture may not be available for two to four weeks.

How can dermatophyte infections be treated?

The particular medication and duration of treatment is based on the location of the infection. Scalp infections usually require treatment with an oral antifungal medication. Infections of other areas of skin are usually treated with topical antifungal medications. Nail infections can be challenging to treat and may be treated with oral and/or topical antifungal medications.

How can dermatophyte infections be prevented?

Good hygiene, such as regular handwashing, is important. People should avoid sharing hairbrushes, hats, and other articles of clothing that may come into contact with infected areas. Pets with signs of skin disease should be evaluated by a veterinarian.

There is a ringworm outbreak in my child's school/day care center. What should I do?

You should contact your local health department. Your local health department may have information about how long children with ringworm should remain out of school/day care. Tell your child not to share personal items, such as clothing, hairbrushes, and hats, with other people. Encourage frequent handwashing. Take your child to the pediatrician if she/he develops symptoms.

My pet has ringworm and I am worried about ringworm in my house. What should I do?

Make sure your pets have been evaluated by a veterinarian. If you develop symptoms, be sure to seek medical attention.

There are no federal guidelines about ringworm and environmental disinfection. Transmission of the infection may occur via direct contact with an infected person or animal or from contact with contaminated environmental surfaces. A reasonable approach is to perform regular cleaning to help remove spores from the environment. For surfaces that are safe to bleach, a quarter cup of bleach in a gallon of water can be used for disinfection. For fabric surfaces or soft items that are washable, a hot water wash and hot air drying may help to remove and kill spores.

Section 13.11

Toxocariasis

"Toxocariasis FAQs," Centers for Disease Control and
Prevention (www.cdc.gov), November 2, 2010.

What is toxocariasis?

Toxocariasis is an infection transmitted from animals to humans
(zoonosis) caused by the parasitic roundworms commonly found in the
intestine of dogs (*Toxocara canis*) and cats (*T. cati*).

What are the clinical manifestations of toxocariasis?

Approximately 13.9% of the U.S. population has antibodies to *Toxo-cara*. This suggests that tens of millions of Americans may have been
exposed to the *Toxocara* parasite.

There are two major forms of toxocariasis:

- **Ocular toxocariasis:** Toxocara infections can cause ocular
  toxocariasis, an eye disease that can cause blindness. Ocular
  toxocariasis occurs when a microscopic worm enters the eye; it
  may cause inflammation and formation of a scar on the retina.

- **Visceral toxocariasis:** Heavier or repeated *Toxocara* infections,
  while rare, can cause visceral toxocariasis, a disease that causes
  abnormalities in the body's organs or central nervous system.
  Symptoms of visceral toxocariasis, which are caused by the movement of the worms through the body, include fever, coughing,
  asthma, or pneumonia.

How serious is infection with Toxocara?

In most cases, *Toxocara* infections are not serious, and many people, especially adults infected by a small number of larvae (immature
worms), may not notice any symptoms. The most severe cases are rare,
but are more likely to occur in young children, who often play in dirt
or eat dirt (pica) contaminated by dog or cat stool.

How is toxocariasis spread?

The most common *Toxocara* parasite of concern to humans is *T. canis*, which puppies usually contract from the mother before birth or from her milk. The larvae mature rapidly in the puppy's intestine; when the pup is three or four weeks old, they begin to produce large numbers of eggs that contaminate the environment through the animal's stool. The eggs soon develop into infective larvae.

How can I get toxocariasis?

You or your children can become infected after accidentally ingesting (swallowing) infective *Toxocara* eggs in soil or other contaminated surfaces.

What is the treatment for toxocariasis?

See your health care provider to discuss the possibility of infection and, if necessary, to be examined. A blood test is available for diagnosis.

Visceral toxocariasis is treated with antiparasitic drugs, usually in combination with anti-inflammatory medications. Treatment of ocular toxocariasis is more difficult and usually consists of measures to prevent progressive damage to the eye.

How can you prevent toxocariasis?

- Have your veterinarian treat your dogs and cats, especially young animals, regularly for worms.

- Wash your hands with soap and warm water after playing with your pets or other animals, after outdoor activities, and before handling food.

- Teach children the importance of washing hands to prevent infection.

- Do not allow children to play in areas that are soiled with pet or other animal stool.

- Clean your pet's living area at least once a week. Feces should be either buried or bagged and disposed of in the trash.

- Teach children that it is dangerous to eat dirt or soil.

Chapter 14

Other Diseases Associated with Infections

Chapter Contents

Section 14.1

Encephalitis

Encephalitis literally means an inflammation of the brain, but it usually refers to brain inflammation caused by a virus. It's a rare disease that occurs in approximately 0.5 per 100,000 individuals—most commonly in children, the elderly, and people with weakened immune systems (e.g., those with HIV/AIDS or cancer).

Although several thousand cases of encephalitis (also called acute viral encephalitis or aseptic encephalitis) are reported to the Centers for Disease Control and Prevention (CDC) every year, experts suspect that many more may go unreported because the symptoms are so mild.

Signs and Symptoms

Symptoms in milder cases of encephalitis usually include:

- fever;

- headache;

- poor appetite;

- loss of energy;

- a general sick feeling.

In more severe cases of encephalitis, a person is more likely to experience high fever and any of a number of symptoms that relate to the central nervous system, including:

- severe headache;

- nausea and vomiting;

- stiff neck;

- confusion;
- disorientation;
- personality changes;
- convulsions (seizures);
- problems with speech or hearing;
- hallucinations;
- memory loss;
- drowsiness;
- coma.

It's harder to detect some of these symptoms in infants, but important signs to look for include:

- vomiting;
- a full or bulging soft spot (fontanel);
- crying that doesn't stop or that seems worse when an infant is picked up or handled in some way;
- body stiffness.

Because encephalitis can follow or accompany common viral illnesses, there sometimes are signs and symptoms of these illnesses beforehand. But often, the encephalitis appears without warning.

Causes

Because encephalitis can be caused by many types of germs, the infection can be spread in several different ways.

One of the most dangerous and most common causes of encephalitis is the herpes simplex virus (HSV). HSV is the same virus that causes cold sores around the mouth, but when it attacks the brain it may occasionally be fatal. Fortunately, HSV encephalitis is very rare.

Encephalitis can be a very rare complication of Lyme disease transmitted by ticks or of rabies spread by rabid animals.

Mosquitoes can also transmit the viruses for several types of encephalitis, including West Nile encephalitis, St. Louis encephalitis, and Western Equine encephalitis. Over the last several years in the United States, there's been concern about the spread of West Nile virus, which is transmitted to humans by mosquitoes that pick up the virus by biting infected birds.

Milder forms of encephalitis can follow or accompany common childhood illnesses, including measles, mumps, chickenpox, rubella (German measles), and mononucleosis. Viruses like chickenpox spread mostly via the fluids of the nose and throat, usually during a cough or sneeze.

Less commonly, encephalitis can result from a bacterial infection, such as bacterial meningitis, or it may be a complication of other infectious diseases like syphilis. Certain parasites, like toxoplasmosis, can also cause encephalitis in people with weakened immune systems.

Contagiousness

Brain inflammation itself is not contagious, but any of the various viruses that cause encephalitis can be. Of course, just because a child gets a certain virus does not mean that he or she will develop encephalitis. Still, to be safe, children should avoid contact with anyone who has encephalitis.

Prevention

Encephalitis cannot be prevented except to try to prevent the illnesses that may lead to it. Encephalitis that may be seen with common childhood illnesses can be largely prevented through proper immunization. Have your kids immunized according to the immunization schedule recommended by your doctor. Kids should also avoid contact with anyone who already has encephalitis.

In areas where encephalitis can be transmitted by insect bites, especially mosquitoes, kids should:

- avoid being outside at dawn and dusk (when mosquitoes are most active);
- wear protective clothing like long sleeves and long pants;
- use insect repellent.

Also, all standing water around your home should be drained, including buckets, birdbaths, flowerpots, and tire swings because these are breeding grounds for mosquitoes.

To avoid tick bites:

- limit kids' contact with soil, leaves, and vegetation;
- have kids wear long-sleeved, light-colored shirts and long pants when outdoors;
- check your kids and your pets frequently for ticks.

Duration

For most forms of encephalitis, the acute phase of the illness (when symptoms are the most severe) usually lasts up to a week. Full recovery can take much longer, often several weeks or months.

Diagnosis

Doctors use several tests to diagnose encephalitis, including:

- imaging tests, such as computed tomography (CT) scans or magnetic resonance imaging (MRI), to check the brain for swelling, bleeding, or other abnormalities;

- electroencephalogram (EEG), which records the electrical signals in the brain, to check for abnormal brain waves;

- blood tests to confirm the presence of bacteria or viruses in the blood, and whether a person is producing antibodies (specific proteins that fight infection) in response to a germ;

- lumbar puncture, or spinal tap, in which cerebrospinal fluid (the fluid that surrounds the brain and spinal cord) is checked for signs of infection.

Treatment

Some children with very mild encephalitis can be monitored at home, but most will need care in a hospital, usually in an intensive care unit. Doctors will carefully monitor their blood pressure, heart rate, and breathing, as well as their body fluids, to prevent further swelling of the brain.

Because antibiotics aren't effective against viruses, they aren't used to treat encephalitis. However, antiviral drugs can be used to treat some forms of encephalitis, especially the type caused by the herpes simplex virus. Corticosteroids may also be used in some cases to reduce brain swelling. If a child is having seizures, anticonvulsants may also be given.

Over-the-counter (OTC) medications, like acetaminophen, can be used to treat fever and headaches.

Many people with encephalitis make a full recovery. In some cases, swelling of the brain can lead to permanent brain damage and lasting complications like learning disabilities, speech problems, memory loss, or lack of muscle control. Speech, physical, or occupational therapy may be necessary in these cases. It's difficult to predict the outcome for each patient at the time the illness begins, but some types of encephalitis are known to cause more serious complications, such as Japanese encephalitis.

Rarely, if the brain damage is severe, encephalitis can lead to death. Infants younger than 1 year and adults older than 55 are at greatest risk of death from encephalitis.

When to Call the Doctor

Call your doctor if your child has a high fever, especially if he or she also has a childhood illness (measles, mumps, chickenpox) or is recovering from one.

Seek immediate medical attention if your child has any of the following symptoms:

- Severe headache
- Convulsions (seizures)
- Stiff neck
- Inability to look at bright lights
- Double vision
- Difficulty walking
- Problems with speech or hearing
- Difficulty moving an arm or leg
- Loss of sensation anywhere in the body
- Sudden personality changes
- Problems with memory
- Extreme drowsiness or lethargy
- Loss of consciousness

If your infant has any of the following symptoms, seek immediate medical care:

- High fever or any fever higher than 100.4° F (38° C) in infants younger than three months old
- Fullness or bulging in the soft spot
- Any stiffness
- Floppiness or decreased tone
- Lethargy
- Poor appetite or reduced feeding
- Vomiting
- Crying that won't stop

Section 14.2

Meningitis

This section excerpted from "Meningitis Questions and Answers," Centers for Disease Control and Prevention (www.cdc.gov), March 11, 2011.

What is meningitis?

Meningitis is an inflammation of the membranes that cover the brain and spinal cord. People sometimes refer to it as spinal meningitis. Meningitis is usually caused by a viral or bacterial infection. Knowing whether meningitis is caused by a virus or bacterium is important because the severity of illness and the treatment differ depending on the cause. Viral meningitis is generally less severe and clears up without specific treatment. But bacterial meningitis can be quite severe and may result in brain damage, hearing loss, or learning disabilities. For bacterial meningitis, it is also important to know which type of bacteria is causing the meningitis because antibiotics can prevent some types from spreading and infecting other people.

What are the signs and symptoms of meningitis?

High fever, headache, and stiff neck are common symptoms of meningitis in anyone over the age of two years. These symptoms can develop over several hours, or they may take one to two days. Other symptoms may include nausea, vomiting, discomfort looking into bright lights, confusion, and sleepiness. In newborns and small infants, the classic symptoms of fever, headache, and neck stiffness may be absent or difficult to detect. Infants with meningitis may appear slow or inactive, have vomiting, be irritable, or be feeding poorly. As the disease progresses, patients of any age may have seizures.

Bacterial Meningitis

How is bacterial meningitis diagnosed?

Early diagnosis and treatment are very important. If symptoms occur, the patient should see a doctor immediately. The diagnosis is usually made by growing bacteria from a sample of spinal fluid.

Can bacterial meningitis be treated?

Bacterial meningitis can be treated with a number of effective antibiotics. It is important, however, that treatment be started early in the course of the disease. Appropriate antibiotic treatment of most common types of bacterial meningitis should reduce the risk of dying from meningitis to below 15%, although the risk is higher among the elderly.

Is bacterial meningitis contagious?

Yes, some forms of bacterial meningitis are contagious. The bacteria can mainly be spread from person to person through the exchange of respiratory and throat secretions. This can occur through coughing, kissing, and sneezing. Fortunately, none of the bacteria that cause meningitis are as contagious as things like the common cold or the flu. Also, the bacteria are not spread by casual contact or by simply breathing the air where a person with meningitis has been.

However, sometimes the bacteria that cause meningitis have spread to other people who have had close or prolonged contact with a patient with meningitis caused by *Neisseria meningitidis* (also called meningococcal meningitis) or *Haemophilus influenzae* type b (Hib). People who qualify as close contacts of a person with meningitis caused by *N. meningitidis* should receive antibiotics to prevent them from getting the disease.

Are there vaccines against bacterial meningitis?

Yes, there are vaccines against Hib, against some serogroups of *N. meningitidis*, and many types of *Streptococcus pneumoniae*. The vaccines are safe and highly effective.

Viral Meningitis

What causes viral meningitis?

Different viral infections can lead to viral meningitis. But most cases in the United States, particularly during the summer and fall months, are caused by enteroviruses (which include enteroviruses, coxsackie viruses, and echoviruses). Most people who are infected with enteroviruses either have no symptoms or only get a cold, rash, or mouth sores with low-grade fever. And, only a small number of people with enterovirus infections develop meningitis.

Other viral infections that can lead to meningitis include mumps, herpesvirus (such as Epstein-Barr virus, herpes simplex viruses, and varicella-zoster virus—the cause of chickenpox and shingles), measles, and influenza.

Arboviruses, which mosquitoes and other insects spread, can also cause infections that can lead to viral meningitis. And lymphocytic choriomeningitis virus, which is spread by rodents, is a rare cause of viral meningitis.

How is viral meningitis diagnosed?

Viral meningitis is usually diagnosed by laboratory tests of a patient's spinal fluid. The test can reveal whether the patient is infected with a virus or a bacterium. The exact cause of viral meningitis can sometimes be found through tests that show which virus has infected a patient; however, identifying the exact virus causing meningitis may be difficult.

Because the symptoms of viral meningitis are similar to those of bacterial meningitis, which is usually more severe and can be fatal, it is important for people suspected of having meningitis to seek medical care and have their spinal fluid tested. A hospital stay may be necessary in more severe cases or for people with weak immune systems.

How is viral meningitis treated?

There is no specific treatment for viral meningitis. Most patients completely recover on their own within two weeks. Antibiotics do not help viral infections, so they are not useful in the treatment of viral meningitis. Doctors often will recommend bed rest, plenty of fluids, and medicine to relieve fever and headache.

How is the virus spread?

Different viruses that cause viral meningitis are spread in different ways. Enteroviruses, the most common cause of viral meningitis, are most often spread through direct contact with an infected person's stool. The virus is spread through this route mainly among small children who are not yet toilet trained. It can also be spread this way to adults changing the diapers of an infected infant.

Enteroviruses and other viruses (such as mumps and varicella-zoster virus) can also be spread through direct or indirect contact with respiratory secretions (saliva, sputum, or nasal mucus) of an infected person. This usually happens through kissing or shaking hands with an infected person or by touching something they have handled and then rubbing your own nose or mouth. The viruses can also stay on surfaces for days and can be transferred from objects. Viruses also can spread directly when infected people cough or sneeze and send droplets containing the virus into the air we breathe.

The time from when a person is infected until they develop symptoms (incubation period) is usually between three and seven days for enteroviruses. An infected person is usually contagious from the time they develop symptoms until the symptoms go away. Young children and people with low immune systems may spread the infection even after symptoms have resolved.

If you are around someone with viral meningitis, you may be at risk of becoming infected with the virus that made them sick. But you have only a small chance of developing meningitis as a complication of the illness.

How can I reduce my chances of becoming infected with viruses that can lead to viral meningitis?

The specific measures for preventing or reducing your risk for viral meningitis depend on the cause.

Following good hygiene practices can reduce the spread of viruses, such as enteroviruses, herpesviruses, and measles and mumps viruses. Preventing the spread of virus can be difficult, especially since sometimes people are infected with a virus (like an enterovirus) but do not appear sick. Thus, it is important to always practice good hygiene to help reduce your chances of becoming infected with a virus or of passing one on to someone else:

- Wash your hands thoroughly and often. This is especially important after changing diapers, using the toilet, or coughing or blowing your nose in a tissue.

- Cleaning contaminated surfaces, such as handles and doorknobs or the TV remote control, with soap and water and then disinfecting them with a dilute solution of chlorine-containing bleach also may decrease the spread of viruses.

- The viruses that cause viral meningitis can be spread by direct and indirect contact with respiratory secretions, so it is important to cover your cough with a tissue or, if you do not have a tissue, to cough into your upper arm. After using a tissue, place it in the trash and wash your hands.

- Avoid kissing or sharing a drinking glass, eating utensil, lipstick, or other such items with sick people or with others when you are sick.

- Receiving vaccinations included in the childhood vaccination schedule can protect children against some diseases that can lead to viral meningitis.

- Avoiding bites from mosquitoes and other insects that carry diseases that can infect humans may help reduce your risk for viral meningitis.

Section 14.3

Pneumonia

This section excerpted from "What Is Pneumonia?" National Heart, Lung, and Blood Institute (www.nhlbi.nih.gov), March 1, 2011.

Pneumonia is an infection in one or both of the lungs. Many germs—such as bacteria, viruses, and fungi—can cause pneumonia.

The infection inflames your lungs' air sacs, which are called alveoli. The air sacs may fill up with fluid or pus, causing symptoms such as a cough with phlegm (a slimy substance), fever, chills, and trouble breathing.

Pneumonia is common in the United States. Treatment for pneumonia depends on its cause, how severe your symptoms are, and your age and overall health. Many people can be treated at home, often with oral antibiotics.

Signs and Symptoms

The signs and symptoms of pneumonia vary from mild to severe. Many factors affect how serious pneumonia is, including the type of germ causing the infection and your age and overall health.

See your doctor promptly if you have these symptoms:

- A high fever

- Shaking chills

- A cough with phlegm (a slimy substance), which doesn't improve or worsens

- Shortness of breath with normal daily activities
- Chest pain when you breathe or cough
- Feel suddenly worse after a cold or the flu

People who have pneumonia may have other symptoms, including nausea (feeling sick to the stomach), vomiting, and diarrhea.

Symptoms may vary in certain populations. Newborns and infants may not show any signs of the infection. Or, they may vomit, have a fever and cough, or appear restless, sick, or tired and without energy.

Diagnosis

Pneumonia can be hard to diagnose because it may seem like a cold or the flu. You may not realize it's more serious until it lasts longer than these other conditions.

Your doctor will diagnose pneumonia based on your medical history, a physical exam, and test results.

Your doctor will listen to your lungs with a stethoscope. If you have pneumonia, your lungs may make crackling, bubbling, and rumbling sounds when you inhale. Your doctor also may hear wheezing. Your doctor may find it hard to hear sounds of breathing in some areas of your chest.

If your doctor thinks you have pneumonia, he or she may recommend a chest X-ray, blood tests, or a blood culture. Your doctor may recommend other tests if you're in the hospital, have serious symptoms, are older, or have other health problems.

Treatment

Treatment for pneumonia depends on the type of pneumonia you have and how severe it is. Most people who have community-acquired pneumonia—the most common type of pneumonia—are treated at home. The goals of treatment are to cure the infection and prevent complications.

If you have pneumonia, follow your treatment plan, take all medicines as prescribed, and get ongoing medical care. Ask your doctor when you should schedule follow-up care. Your doctor may want you to have a chest X-ray to make sure the pneumonia is gone.

Although you may start feeling better after a few days or weeks, fatigue (tiredness) can persist for up to a month or more.

Bacterial Pneumonia

Bacterial pneumonia is treated with medicines called antibiotics. You should take antibiotics as your doctor prescribes. You may start to feel better before you finish the medicine, but you should continue taking it as prescribed. If you stop too soon, the pneumonia may come back.

Most people begin to improve after one to three days of antibiotic treatment. This means that they should feel better and have fewer symptoms, such as cough and fever.

Viral Pneumonia

Antibiotics don't work when the cause of pneumonia is a virus. If you have viral pneumonia, your doctor may prescribe an antiviral medicine to treat it. Viral pneumonia usually improves in one to three weeks.

Prevention

Pneumonia can be very serious and even life threatening. When possible, take steps to prevent the infection, especially if you're in a high-risk group.

Vaccines are available to prevent pneumococcal pneumonia and the flu. Vaccines can't prevent all cases of infection. However, compared to people who don't get vaccinated, those who do and still get pneumonia tend to have the following:

- Milder cases of the infection

- Pneumonia that doesn't last as long

- Fewer serious complications

Section 14.4

Reye Syndrome

What is Reye syndrome?

Reye syndrome is a rare illness that affects all bodily organs but is most harmful to the brain and the liver. It occurs primarily among children who are recovering from a viral infection, such as chicken pox or the flu. It usually develops a week after the onset of the viral illness but can also occur a few days after onset. Liver-related complications of Reye syndrome include fatty deposits, abnormal liver function tests, and poor blood clotting and bleeding caused by liver failure.

What are the symptoms of Reye syndrome?

Reye syndrome is often misdiagnosed as encephalitis, meningitis, diabetes, drug overdose, poisoning, sudden infant death syndrome, or psychiatric illness.

Symptoms include persistent or recurrent vomiting, listlessness, personality changes such as irritability or combativeness, disorientation, delirium, convulsions, and loss of consciousness. If these symptoms are present during or soon after a viral illness, medical attention should be sought immediately. The symptoms of Reye syndrome in infants do not follow a typical pattern; for example, vomiting does not always occur. The onset of Reye syndrome can be rapid, and signs and symptoms may worsen within hours.

What causes Reye syndrome?

The cause of Reye syndrome remains a mystery. However, studies have shown that using aspirin to treat viral illnesses increases the risk of developing Reye syndrome. A physician should be consulted before giving a child any aspirin or anti-nausea medicines during a viral illness, which could hide the symptoms of the condition.

How is Reye syndrome diagnosed?

If your child becomes sick with a possible case of Reye syndrome, doctors will want blood tests to evaluate his or her liver function. They may also evaluate other possible causes of liver problems and make sure your child does not have one of the rare inherited disorders that mimic Reye syndrome. In addition to blood and urine tests, diagnostic procedures may include spinal taps or liver biopsy.

How is Reye syndrome treated?

There is no cure for Reye syndrome. Successful management, which relies on early diagnosis, is aimed primarily at protecting the brain from irreversible damage by reducing brain swelling, preventing complications in the lungs, and anticipating cardiac arrest.

If my child has been diagnosed with Reye syndrome, what should I ask our doctor?

Speak to your doctor about possible long-term complications connected with Reye syndrome. Though rare, Reye syndrome can result in permanent liver or nervous system damage.

Who is at risk for Reye syndrome?

Reye syndrome occurs most commonly in children between the ages of 4 and 12, although it can occur at any age. It usually develops about a week after common viral infections such as influenza or chickenpox. Reye syndrome can also develop after an ordinary upper respiratory infection such as a cold. The precise reason is unknown, but using aspirin to treat a viral illness or infection may trigger the condition in children.

Reye syndrome may be a metabolic condition—one without symptoms (asymptomatic)—that is unmasked by viral illnesses.

What is the best way to prevent Reye syndrome?

To reduce the risk of Reye syndrome, avoid giving aspirin or medications that contain aspirin to your child to treat viral illnesses. Other names for aspirin include: acetylsalicylic acid, acetylsalicylate, salicylic acid, and salicylate. Unless specifically instructed to do so by your child's doctor, do not give aspirin to anyone younger than 19.

If your child or teenager has the flu or chickenpox, use other medications such as acetaminophen, ibuprofen, or naproxen sodium to reduce fever or relieve pain. Check the label on any medication to make sure it does not include aspirin before giving it your child, and be sure to give the correct dose.

Part Three

Medical Conditions Appearing in Childhood

Chapter 15

Allergies in Children

Chapter Contents

Section 15.1

Allergic Reactions in Kids

This section includes "What Are Allergies" and "Allergy Testing for Children," reprinted with permission from the Allergy and Asthma Foundation of America (www.aafa.org), © 2005; reviewed by David A. Cooke, MD, FACP, April 2012. It also includes "What Causes Allergies" and "Treatment" reprinted with permission from the Allergy and Asthma Foundation of America (www.aafa.org), © 2011.

What Are Allergies

Allergies reflect an overreaction of the immune system to substances that usually cause no reaction in most individuals. These substances can trigger sneezing, wheezing, coughing, and itching. Allergies are not only bothersome, but many have been linked to a variety of common and serious chronic respiratory illnesses (such as sinusitis and asthma). Additionally, allergic reactions can be severe and even fatal. However, with proper management and patient education, allergic diseases can be controlled, and people with allergies can lead normal and productive lives.

Common Allergic Diseases

- **Allergic rhinitis (hay fever or "indoor/outdoor," "seasonal," "perennial," or "nasal" allergies):** Characterized by nasal stuffiness, sneezing, nasal itching, clear nasal discharge, and itching of the roof of the mouth and/or ears.

- **Allergic asthma (asthma symptoms triggered by an allergic reaction):** Characterized by airway obstruction that is at least partially reversible with medication and is always associated with allergy. Symptoms include coughing, wheezing, shortness of breath or rapid breathing, chest tightness, and occasional fatigue and slight chest pain.

- **Food allergy:** Most prevalent in very young children and frequently outgrown, food allergies are characterized by a broad range of allergic reactions. Symptoms may include itching or swelling of lips or tongue; tightness of the throat with hoarseness; nausea and vomiting; diarrhea; occasionally chest tightness and wheezing; itching of the eyes; decreased blood pressure or loss of consciousness and anaphylaxis.

- **Drug allergy:** Is characterized by a variety of allergic responses affecting any tissue or organ. Drug allergies can cause anaphylaxis; even those patients who do not have life-threatening symptoms initially may progress to a life-threatening reaction.

- **Anaphylaxis (extreme response to a food or drug allergy):** Characterized by life-threatening symptoms. This is a medical emergency and the most severe form of allergic reaction. Symptoms include a sense of impending doom; generalized warmth or flush; tingling of palms, soles of feet, or lips; light-headedness; bloating; and chest tightness. These can progress into seizures, cardiac arrhythmia, shock, and respiratory distress. Possible causes can be medications, vaccines, food, latex, and insect stings and bites.

- **Latex allergy:** An allergic response to the proteins in natural, latex rubber characterized by a range of allergic reactions. Persons at risk include health care workers, patients having multiple surgeries, and rubber-industry workers. Symptoms include hand dermatitis, eczema, and urticaria; sneezing and other respiratory distress; and lower respiratory problems including coughing, wheezing, and shortness of breath.

- **Insect sting/bite allergy:** Characterized by a variety of allergic reactions; stings cannot always be avoided and can happen to anyone. Symptoms include pain, itching, and swelling at the sting site or over a larger area and can cause anaphylaxis. Insects that sting include bees, hornets, wasps, yellow jackets, and fire and harvest ants.

- **Urticaria (hives, skin allergy):** A reaction of the skin, or a skin condition commonly known as hives. Characterized by the development of itchy, raised white bumps on the skin surrounded by an area of red inflammation. Acute urticaria is often caused by an allergy to foods or medication.

- **Atopic dermatitis (eczema, skin allergy):** A chronic or recurrent inflammatory skin disease characterized by lesions, scaling, and flaking; it is sometimes called eczema. In children, it may be aggravated by an allergy or irritant.

- **Contact dermatitis (skin allergy):** Characterized by skin inflammation; this is the most common occupational disease representing up to 40% of all occupational illnesses. Contact dermatitis is one of the most common skin diseases in adults. It results from the direct contact with an outside substance with the skin. There are currently about 3,000 known contact allergens.

- **Allergic conjunctivitis (eye allergy):** Characterized by inflammation of the eyes; it is the most common form of allergic eye disease. Symptoms can include itchy and watery eyes and lid distress. Allergic conjunctivitis is also commonly associated with the presence of other allergic diseases such as atopic dermatitis, allergic rhinitis, and asthma.

What Causes Allergies

The substances that cause allergic disease in people are known as allergens. "Antigens," or protein particles like pollen, food, or dander, enter our bodies through a variety of ways. If the antigen causes an allergic reaction, that particle is considered an "allergen"—an antigen that triggers an allergic reaction. These allergens can get into our body in several ways:

- Inhaled into the nose and the lungs (examples are airborne pollens of certain trees, grasses, and weeds; house dust that include dust mite particles, mold spores, cat and dog dander, and latex dust)

- Ingested by mouth (frequent culprits include shrimp, peanuts, and other nuts)

- Injected (such as medications delivered by needle like penicillin or other injectable drugs, and venom from insect stings and bites)

- Absorbed through the skin (plants such as poison ivy, sumac, and oak and latex are examples)

What makes some pollen cause allergies, and not others?

Plant pollens that are carried by the wind cause most allergies of the nose, eyes, and lungs. These plants (including certain weeds, trees, and grasses) are natural pollutants produced at various times of the year when their small, inconspicuous flowers discharge literally billions of pollen particles.

Because the particles can be carried significant distances, it is important for you not only to understand local environmental conditions, but also conditions over the broader area of the state or region in which you live. Unlike the wind-pollinated plants, conspicuous wild flowers or flowers used in most residential gardens are pollinated by bees, wasps, and other insects and therefore are not widely capable of producing allergic disease.

What is the role of heredity in allergy?

Like baldness, height, and eye color, the capacity to become allergic is an inherited characteristic. Yet, although you may be born with the genetic capability to become allergic, you are not automatically allergic to specific allergens. Several factors must be present for allergic sensitivity to be developed:

* The specific genes acquired from parents
* The exposure to one or more allergens to which you have a genetically programmed response
* The degree and length of exposure

A baby born with the tendency to become allergic to cow's milk, for example, may show allergic symptoms several months after birth. A genetic capability to become allergic to cat dander may take three to four years of cat exposure before the person shows symptoms. These people may also become allergic to other environmental substances with age.

On the other hand, poison ivy allergy (contact dermatitis) is an example of an allergy in which hereditary background does not play a part. The person with poison ivy allergy first has to be exposed to the oil from the plant. This usually occurs during youth, when a rash does not always appear. However, the first exposure may sensitize or cause the person to become allergic, and, when subsequent exposure takes place, a contact dermatitis rash appears and can be quite severe. Many plants are capable of producing this type of rash. Substances other than plants, such as dyes, metals, and chemicals in deodorants and cosmetics, can also cause a similar dermatitis.

Allergy Testing for Children

What is an allergy?

An allergy is the body's immune system response to specific elements in the environment. Children with allergies react to certain substances in their everyday environment, which usually don't cause reactions in other children.

About 20% of Americans—one in every five adults and children—have allergies, including allergic asthma. About 80% of children with asthma have allergies. Food allergies occur in 8% of children younger than age six.

How do allergies affect children and how do they get them?

Children seem to be more vulnerable to allergies than adults. Allergies to food, house dust mites, animal dander, and pollen are most common. These allergies show up as allergic rhinitis (hay fever), asthma, and atopic dermatitis (eczema). Also, frequent ear infections may be related to allergy.

If both parents have allergies, their (biological) child has a 75% chance of having allergies. If one parent is allergic, or if relatives on one side of the family have allergies, then the child has about a 50% chance of developing allergies.

There is some evidence that breast-feeding helps prevent children from developing food allergies and eczema.

What are signs or symptoms of allergy in a child?

Symptoms develop as the body releases special antibodies called IgE (immunoglobin E), which are the key players in allergic reaction. These special antibodies can trigger the release of chemicals that can cause the physical symptoms and changes associated with allergies such as:

- hives;
- runny nose;
- itching or swelling of the lips, tongue, or throat;
- upset stomach, cramps, bloating, or diarrhea;
- wheezing or difficulty breathing;
- anaphylactic shock—a life-threatening body reaction requiring emergency care.

What tests are generally used to diagnose allergies?

First, keep in mind that allergy tests are not the sole basis for diagnosing or treating an allergy. Health care providers make an allergy diagnosis based on several factors:

- History of the child's experiences and family history of allergy/asthma

- Physical exam of the child to detect signs of allergy

- Allergy testing for sensitivity to specific allergens

Allergy tests help your physician confirm allergies your child may have. When an allergy test pinpoints a reaction to a specific allergen(s), your health care provider also can use this information in developing "immunotherapy"—allergy shots—specifically for your child, if appropriate.

Skin tests for allergies: Skin prick tests are the most common tests for allergy. Small amounts of suspect allergy triggers are introduced through the skin of the arm or back by pricking or puncturing the skin with a needle or similar device. If your child is allergic to a substance, you will see a raised, red itchy bump, also called a "wheal." Reactions usually appear within 15 minutes. This positive result indicates that the IgE antibody is present when your child comes in contact with the specific allergen. The size of the wheal is important: the bigger it is, the more sensitive your child is to that particular substance. This test is the least time consuming and expensive. You may have to discontinue certain medications, especially antihistamines, several days prior to testing.

There are four kinds of skin tests: scratch, puncture, prick, and intradermal. Your allergist may use one or more skin tests to analyze your child's response to various substances. Keep in mind that you may see a false-positive or a false-negative skin test. Results often depend on how well the test is performed.

Skin prick, puncture, and intradermal tests may be difficult with young children afraid of needles. There is some possibility of a life-threatening anaphylactic response if a person is extremely sensitive to a substance. Your health care provider will be prepared to react swiftly to this kind of response.

Blood tests for allergies: The RAST (radioallergosorbent test) and related blood tests use radioactive or enzyme markers to detect levels of IgE antibodies. These tests are useful when a skin test is difficult due to a widespread skin rash, anxiety about skin pricks, or if the child has the potential for a sudden and severe allergic response to test allergens.

Skin tests and these blood tests are very comparable in their ability to diagnose sensitivity to specific allergens. Both kinds of tests are considered to be about 90% accurate.

Elimination diet: An elimination diet is often used to help isolate sensitivity to specific foods. Your health care provider sets up a diet without foods that you suspect may affect your child. Because milk, soybeans, eggs, wheat, peanuts, nuts, shellfish, and corn are the main culprits for more than 80% of people who have food allergies, these foods are usually not included in the starting diet.

Your child will stay on the prescribed diet for four to seven days. If the symptoms do not subside, additional foods are eliminated until the allergy symptoms stop. Once the symptoms disappear, new foods are added to the basic diet, one at a time, until symptoms reappear.

The chief drawback to an elimination diet is making sure your child is eating "pure" foods. Common food allergens are "hidden ingredients" in hundreds of packaged or processed foods. In order for an elimination diet to be successful, check ingredients for foods you give your child to eat. If your child is a fussy or picky eater, an elimination diet can be difficult. Your health care provider can suggest helpful approaches.

Fasting is a radical way to identify food allergies. Although very effective for detecting problem foods, this kind of elimination diet is hard to do with children. Fasting is best done under medical supervision and often is used for "extreme" cases where a child is suspected to have allergies to many types of food.

Are there other allergy tests?

These tests are considered the most effective and usual way to help diagnose allergies to specific substances. You also may hear of other allergy tests. These tests may work, but as yet, they are unproven or not universally accepted allergy testing methods. If your health care provider suggests one of these tests, consider getting a second opinion about allergy testing for your child:

- Cytotoxicity blood test
- Electroacupuncture biofeedback
- Urine autoinjection
- Skin titration
- Sublingual provocative testing
- Candidiasis allergy theory
- Basophil histamine release

What kind of doctor does allergy testing?

Allergy testing usually is done by an allergist. An allergist specializes in diagnosing and treating allergies. Some allergists specialize in treating children. To find a board-certified allergist or pediatric allergist near you, contact:

- American Academy of Allergy, Asthma & Immunology at 414-272-6071 or http://www.aaaai.org;

- American College of Allergy, Asthma & Immunology at 800-842-7777 or http://www.acaai.org.

What can parents do if their child has a positive allergy test?

A positive allergy test helps your physician figure out the best treatment plan for your child. The doctor may prescribe specific medicine for the allergy(s) and suggest ways to cut down or eliminate substances in your child's environment that can trigger an allergic response. Many allergies are mild to moderate. Most allergies are easily managed with the right treatment plan.

Treatment

Good allergy treatment is based on the results of your allergy tests, your medical history, and the severity of your symptoms. It can include three different treatment strategies: avoidance of allergens, medication options, and/or immunotherapy (allergy shots).

Avoiding your allergens: The best way to prevent allergy symptoms and minimize your need for allergy medicine is to avoid your allergens as much as possible and to eliminate the source of allergens from your home and other environments. For important tips, talk to your doctor.

Medication: Some people don't take allergy medicines because they don't take their symptoms seriously ("Oh, it's only my allergies."). The result may be painful complications such as sinus or ear infections. Don't take the risk. There are so many safe prescription and non-prescription medicines to relieve allergy symptoms! Following is a brief list of medications taken for allergies. They are available in non-prescription and prescription form:

- **Antihistamines and decongestants** are the most common medicines used for allergies. Antihistamines help relieve rashes and hives, as well as sneezing, itching, and runny nose. Prescription antihistamines are similar to their non-prescription counterparts, but many of them do not cause drowsiness. Decongestant pills, sprays, and nose drops reduce stuffiness by shrinking swollen membranes in the nose.

It is important to remember that using a non-prescription nasal decongestant spray more than three days in a row may cause the swelling and stuffiness in your nose to become worse, even after you stop using the medicine. This is called a "rebound" reaction. Some non-prescription "cold" medicines combine an antihistamine, a pain reliever like aspirin or acetaminophen, and a decongestant. Aspirin can cause asthma attacks in some people. Don't take a chance: if you have asthma, talk with your doctor before taking any non-prescription allergy medicine.

- **Eye drops** may provide temporary relief from burning or bloodshot eyes. However, only prescription allergy eye drops contain antihistamines that can reduce itching, tearing, and swelling.

- **Corticosteroid creams or ointments** relieve itchiness and halt the spread of rashes. Corticosteroids are not the same as anabolic steroids that are used illegally by some athletes to build muscles. If your rash does not go away after using a nonprescription corticosteroid for a week, see your doctor.

- **Corticosteroid nasal sprays** help reduce the inflammation that causes nasal congestion without the chance of the "rebound" effect found in non-prescription nose sprays.

- **Cromolyn sodium** prevents the inflammation which causes nasal congestion. Because it has few, if any, side effects, cromolyn can be safely used over long periods of time.

- **Oral corticosteroids** may be prescribed to reduce swelling and stop severe allergic reactions. Because these medications can cause serious side effects, you should expect your doctor to carefully monitor you.

- **Epinephrine** comes in pre-measured, self-injectable containers and is the only medication which can help during a life-threatening anaphylactic attack. To be effective, epinephrine must be given within minutes of the first sign of serious allergic reaction.

New prescription and non-prescription drugs are approved periodically. If the prescription you are taking is not on this list, ask your doctor which category it falls into, so that you can refer to this list.

Immunotherapy (allergy shots): When it is not possible to avoid your allergens and treatment with medications alone does not solve the problem, immunotherapy can often prevent allergy symptoms. It involves giving a person increasingly higher doses of their allergen over time. For reasons that we do not completely understand, the person gradually becomes less sensitive to that allergen. This can be effective for some people with hay fever, certain animal allergies, and insect stings. It is usually not effective for allergies to food, drugs, or feathers, nor is it effective for hives or eczema.

Section 15.2

Food Allergies

"Food Allergies," reprinted with permission from the Allergy and Asthma Foundation of America (www.aafa.org), © 2005. Reviewed by David A. Cooke, MD, FACP, April 2012.

Reactions to food are common. These reactions range from mild to severe and may result from your body's negative response to certain foods or from a true food allergy. Any food can cause an allergic reaction, but only eight foods cause 9 out of 10 reactions. They are milk, soy, eggs, wheat, peanuts, tree nuts, fish, and shellfish.

What is a food allergy?

The job of immune system cells is to find foreign substances such as viruses and bacteria and get rid of them. Normally, this response protects us from dangerous diseases. People with food allergies have super-sensitive immune systems that react to harmless substances found in food and drink. These substances are called allergens. When people have an allergy, there are antibodies to the allergens in their blood and throughout their body. When that person eats a food to which they are allergic, the food allergens react to antibodies on cells releasing chemicals.

Who gets a food allergy?

From 3% to 8% of children have reactions to some foods. Only 1% to 2% have true food allergies. Some children seem to grow out of their sensitivity to certain foods, often by age four. Allergies to peanuts, tree nuts, and shellfish usually do not go away, though.

From 1% to 2% of adults have true food allergies. But people of any age can have sudden allergic reactions to a food that had previously not been a problem for them.

If you have an allergy, a reaction is triggered within minutes to two hours after you consume the allergen. How soon and how severe the reaction is depends on how sensitive you are to the food, the amount of the food consumed, other food consumed, the manner in which it is prepared (i.e., cooked or uncooked, seasoned or unseasoned), and any other medical problems you have.

Severe, life-threatening reactions are more common with allergies to peanuts, tree nuts, shellfish, fish, and eggs. These life-threatening reactions are more common in people who also have asthma.

What are the symptoms?

Reactions can affect different body systems:

- **The digestive tract, which first comes into contact with food:** Some symptoms, such as swelling and itching of the lips, the lining of the mouth as well as throat tightness and hoarseness may occur quickly. When the food enters the stomach and then the intestines, nausea, cramping, pain, vomiting, and diarrhea may occur.

- **Body systems, such as the skin, lungs, and blood vessels, that are affected after the food leaves the digestive tract:** These reactions can occur in minutes or within two hours. Often, hives and swelling of the skin occur. Anaphylaxis, the most dangerous and life-threatening result of a food allergy, usually occurs within minutes after consuming the food. When this happens, blood vessels widen so much that blood pressure falls. Symptoms include wheezing, difficulty breathing, throat tightness, nausea, rapid pulse, flushing, faintness, itching of the palms and sole of the feet, and even passing out. Without speedy treatment, this intense allergic reaction can cause death. (See the *Asthma and Allergy Answers* factsheet "What Is Anaphylaxis" at http://www.aafa.org/display.cfm?id=9&sub=20&cont=281).

The first severe reaction to a food may be unexpected. Sometimes the patient may at first have minor symptoms such as stomach cramping or hives.

How is a food allergy diagnosed?

If your doctor suspects you may have a food allergy, the first step is to take a detailed medical history and physical exam. Other tests are used to confirm that you are allergic to certain foods. Some tests use extracts of the suspected foods:

- **The skin test involves scratching or pricking your skin with one or more extracts.** If your body makes an antibody to the food, redness, itching, and minor swelling will occur at the test site. However, the tests are not 100% accurate. A positive skin test supports the diagnosis of food allergy, but still does not guarantee that the symptoms are caused by the allergy. In fact, many people regularly eat foods that they have tested positive but have never experienced a reaction. A negative test does not completely rule out the possibility that allergy is the problem. The accuracy of the skin tests for food allergies varies greatly with the particular food being tested.

- **RAST is a blood test done in a laboratory.** It is used to test a sample of blood for antibody to a specific food. While more costly and less sensitive than skin testing, RAST is particularly useful when eczema and other skin conditions make skin testing difficult. It also may be used to confirm a diagnosis when there is a risk of an anaphylactic reaction to skin tests.

- **Another test is the oral food challenge.** This test provides the most convincing results. It is required if the relationship between the eating a specific food and symptoms is still unclear after skin tests. Your doctor will explain that all oral challenges—giving patients the suspected foods—carry a risk of causing an allergic reaction. They should be done with a specialist physician present and in a setting where allergic reactions can be treated promptly.

- **If the diagnosis is still unclear, you may be put on an elimination diet.** The first step is to follow the usual diet for 10 to 14 days. You keep a record of what and how much you eat, when a reaction occurred, and what the reaction was. The foods suspected of causing the reaction are then removed from your diet. Make sure that the foods are not in other foods you eat. For example, egg or milk may be in mayonnaise or salad dressings. Elimination diet should only be used for a limited period of time such as 10–14 days. If you have symptoms, or if multiple food sensitivities are suspected, you will be referred to a specialist for further evaluation and treatment.

If you still have symptoms, or if multiple food sensitivities are suspected, the doctor may put you on a strict commercial diet preparation to eliminate most foods. Food may then be put back in your diet. If your symptoms are significant, this is done only with a doctor present.

Are there other concerns in diagnosing a food allergy?

Several factors make diagnosis difficult. The reaction may depend on the amount of food consumed, the presence of other foods that can slow digestion, and medications such as antihistamines that may hide reactions. The proteins—the antigens within the food or drink that cause the allergy—may be altered by cooking or processing in some way. The antigens may be in only part of the food, such as the skin of an apple. Some are present only at a particular stage of ripeness.

Reaction apparently due to a food or food additive may in reality be due to another food that was accidentally added to the mixture during preparation.

Toxins and food poisoning can cause symptoms that can be confused with food allergy. Some foods upset the stomach and resemble food allergy. Examples are prunes, soybeans, and onions.

Some medical conditions such as hiatal hernia, ulcers, and diverticulosis are associated with acute symptoms after eating.

Some people can't digest lactose, because they don't produce enough lactase, and may have symptoms after drinking milk. The reactions may be confused with food allergy.

What can be done to avoid developing food allergies?

To prevent or modify the development of food allergy, identify early in life people who are most at risk:

- Those with a family history of allergy
- Babies with allergy antibodies in their umbilical cord blood or serum
- Infants less than 12 months old with antibodies to egg and other foods including peanut, codfish, and milk

Consult a doctor about whether to test an infant for allergy antibodies. If positive, talk with the doctor about how to decrease the incidence and severity of the food allergy.

Allergic reactions to cow's milk or soy formula can appear within days or months after birth. There is evidence that infants who are breast-fed exclusively during their first 6 to 12 months of life develop fewer allergies by age one or two than infants fed with formula. The American Academy of Pediatrics (AAP) recommends exclusive breast-feeding as ideal nutrition for about the first six months of life. Furthermore, a maternal diet that avoids eggs, cow milk, peanuts, and fish while nursing may help reduce eczema in infants.

What are some tips to follow to prevent an allergic reaction?

- Do not consume foods that cause a reaction. People with a severe allergy can go into anaphylactic shock from trace amounts of the food to which they are allergic. Touching foods cause some people to have a severe reaction.

- Read the ingredients lists on food labels to make sure allergy-causing foods are not mixed in. Read the list even if you have had the product before. Ingredients may change.

- If you are traveling, send special foods ahead. Stay in hotels with kitchenettes so you can prepare your own food.

- When eating out, always ask restaurant staff about ingredients in food and how it was prepared. Cooking oils can have allergens. Peanut oil is often used in cooking, particularly in Thai cuisine.

- For infants, elemental formulas or formulas with altered protein should prevent food reactions. Discuss the various formula options with your doctor. Do not assume products labeled "hypoallergenic" will not cause a reaction.

What can I do if I have a reaction?

If you have a severe reaction, take medication and seek medical care promptly. Injectable epinephrine, such as EpiPen or Ana-Kit, should always be at hand for treating anaphylactic shock. Get medical care promptly after using epinephrine, even if you feel better. Symptoms may reoccur in a few hours.

Antihistamines and steroids also may be taken to lessen symptoms. Prompt treatment often can limit the severity of the reaction. If you have life-threatening allergies, wear a Medic-Alert bracelet to let health care workers know of your allergy in an emergency.

Chapter 16

Blood and Circulatory Disorders in Children

Chapter Contents

Section 16.1

Anemia

This section excerpted from "What Is Anemia?," National Heart,
Lung, and Blood Institute (www.nhlbi.nih.gov), August 1, 2010.

Anemia is a condition in which your blood has a lower than normal
number of red blood cells. Anemia also can occur if your red blood cells
don't contain enough hemoglobin, an iron-rich protein that gives blood
its red color.

If you have anemia, your body doesn't get enough oxygen-rich blood.
As a result, you may feel tired and have other symptoms. Severe or
long-lasting anemia can damage the heart, brain, and other organs of
the body.

Causes

The three main causes of anemia are blood loss, lack of red blood cell
production, and high rates of red blood cell destruction. Some people
have anemia due to more than one of these factors.

Blood Loss

Blood loss is the most common cause of anemia, especially iron-
deficiency anemia. Blood loss can be short term or persist over time.
Heavy menstrual periods or bleeding in the digestive or urinary
tract can cause blood loss. Surgery, trauma, or cancer also can cause
blood loss.

Lack of Red Blood Cell Production

Both acquired and inherited conditions and factors can prevent
your body from making enough red blood cells.

Diet: A diet that lacks iron, folic acid (folate), or vitamin B12 can
prevent your body from making enough red blood cells. Your body also
needs small amounts of vitamin C, riboflavin, and copper to make red
blood cells.

Hormones: Your body needs the hormone erythropoietin to make red blood cells. This hormone stimulates the bone marrow to make these cells. A low level of this hormone can lead to anemia.

Diseases and disease treatments: Chronic diseases, like kidney disease and cancer, can make it hard for your body to make enough red blood cells. Some cancer treatments may damage the bone marrow or damage the red blood cells' ability to carry oxygen. People who have HIV/AIDS may develop anemia due to infections or medicines used to treat their diseases.

Pregnancy: Anemia can occur during pregnancy due to low levels of iron and folic acid and changes in the blood.

Aplastic anemia: Some infants are born without the ability to make enough red blood cells. This condition is called aplastic anemia. Infants and children who have aplastic anemia often need blood transfusions to increase the number of red blood cells in their blood.

High Rates of Red Blood Cell Destruction

Both acquired and inherited conditions and factors can cause your body to destroy too many red blood cells.

One example of an acquired condition that can do this is an enlarged or diseased spleen. The spleen is an organ that removes worn-out red blood cells from the body. If the spleen is enlarged or diseased, it may remove more red blood cells than normal, causing anemia.

Examples of inherited conditions that can cause your body to destroy too many red blood cells include sickle cell anemia, thalassemias, and lack of certain enzymes.

Signs and Symptoms

The most common symptom of anemia is fatigue (feeling tired or weak). If you have anemia, it may seem hard to find the energy to do normal activities.

Other signs and symptoms of anemia include the following:

- Shortness of breath

- Dizziness

- Headache

- Coldness in the hands and feet

- Pale skin

• Chest pain

These signs and symptoms can occur because your heart has to work harder to pump oxygen-rich blood through your body. Mild to moderate anemia may cause very mild symptoms or none at all.

Diagnosis

Your doctor will diagnose anemia based on your medical and family histories, a physical exam, and results from tests and procedures. Because anemia doesn't always cause symptoms, your doctor may find out you have it while checking for another condition.

Your doctor may ask whether you have any of the common signs or symptoms of anemia. He or she also may ask whether you've had an illness or condition that could cause anemia. You also may be asked about the medicines you take, your diet, and whether you have family members who have anemia or a history of it.

Your doctor will do a physical exam to find out how severe your anemia is and to check for possible causes.

Often, the first test used to diagnose anemia is a complete blood count (CBC). The CBC measures many parts of your blood. If the CBC results show that you have anemia, you may need other tests.

If your doctor thinks that you have anemia due to internal bleeding, he or she may suggest several tests to look for the source of the bleeding. A test to check the stool for blood may be done in your doctor's office or at home.

Your doctor also may want to do bone marrow tests. These tests show whether your bone marrow is healthy and making enough blood cells.

Treatment

Treatment for anemia depends on the type, cause, and severity of the condition. Treatments may include dietary changes or supplements, medicines, or procedures.

The goal of treatment is to increase the amount of oxygen that your blood can carry. This is done by raising the red blood cell count and/or hemoglobin level. Another goal is to treat the underlying condition or cause of the anemia.

Dietary Changes and Supplements

To raise your vitamin or iron level, your doctor may ask you to change your diet or take vitamin or iron supplements. Common vitamin supplements are vitamin B12 and folic acid (folate). Vitamin C some-times is given to help the body absorb iron.

Medicines

Your doctor may prescribe medicines to increase the number of red blood cells your body makes or to treat an underlying cause of anemia. Some of these medicines include the following:

- Antibiotics to treat infections
- Hormones to treat heavy menstrual bleeding in teenaged and adult women
- A man-made version of erythropoietin to stimulate your body to make more red blood cells
- Medicines to prevent the body's immune system from destroying its own red blood cells
- Chelation therapy for lead poisoning

Procedures

If your anemia is severe, you may need a medical procedure to treat it. Procedures include blood transfusions and blood and marrow stem cell transplants.

Blood transfusion: A blood transfusion is a safe, common proce-dure in which blood is given to you through an intravenous (IV) line in one of your blood vessels.

Blood and marrow stem cell transplant: A blood and marrow stem cell transplant replaces your faulty stem cells with healthy ones from another person (a donor). Stem cells are found in the bone mar-row. They develop into red and white blood cells and platelets.

Surgery

If you have serious or life-threatening bleeding that's causing ane-mia, you may need surgery. For example, you may need surgery to control ongoing bleeding due to a stomach ulcer or colon cancer. If your body is destroying red blood cells at a high rate, you may need to have your spleen removed.

Prevention

You may be able to prevent repeat episodes of some types of ane-mia, especially those caused by lack of iron or vitamins. Dietary changes or supplements can prevent these types of anemia from occurring again.

Treating anemia's underlying cause may prevent the condition (or prevent repeat episodes). For example, if medicine is causing your anemia, your doctor may prescribe another type of medicine.

You can't prevent some types of inherited anemia, such as sickle cell anemia. If you have an inherited anemia, talk with your doctor about treatment and ongoing care.

Anemia and Children/Teens

Infants and young children have a greater need for iron because of their rapid growth. Not enough iron can lead to anemia. Preterm and low-birth-weight babies often are watched closely for anemia.

Most of the iron your child needs comes from food. Talk with your child's doctor about a healthy diet and good sources of iron, vitamins B12 and C, and folic acid (folate). Only give your child iron supplements if the doctor prescribes them. You should carefully follow instructions on how to give your child these supplements.

If your child has anemia, his or her doctor may ask whether the child has been exposed to lead. Lead poisoning in children has been linked to iron-deficiency anemia.

Teenagers are at risk for anemia, especially iron-deficiency anemia, because of their growth spurts. Routine screenings for anemia often are started in the teen years.

Older children and teens who have certain types of severe anemia may be at higher risk for injuries or infections. Talk with your child's doctor about whether your child needs to avoid high-risk activities, such as contact sports.

Girls begin to menstruate and lose iron with each monthly period. Some girls and women are at higher risk for anemia due to excessive blood loss from menstruation or other causes, low iron intake, or a history of anemia. These girls and women may need regular screenings and follow-up for anemia.

Section 16.2

Sickle Cell Anemia

This section excerpted from "What Is Sickle Cell
Anemia?," National Heart, Lung, and Blood Institute
(www.nhlbi.nih.gov), February 1, 2011.

Sickle cell anemia is the most common form of sickle cell disease
(SCD). SCD is a serious disorder in which the body makes sickle-
shaped red blood cells.

Normal red blood cells are disc-shaped and look like doughnuts
without holes in the center. They move easily through your blood
vessels. Sickle cells contain abnormal hemoglobin called sickle hemoglobin or hemoglobin S. Sickle cells are stiff and sticky. They tend to
block blood flow in the blood vessels of the limbs and organs. Blocked
blood flow can cause pain, serious infections, and organ damage.

In sickle cell anemia, the number of red blood cells is low because
sickle cells don't last very long. Sickle cells usually die after only
about 10 to 20 days. The bone marrow can't make new red blood cells
fast enough to replace the dying ones.

Sickle cell anemia has no widely available cure. Blood and marrow stem cell transplants may offer a cure for a small number of
people. With proper care and treatment, many people who have the
disease can have improved quality of life and reasonable health
much of the time.

Causes

Sickle cell anemia is an inherited disease. People who have the
disease inherit two genes for sickle hemoglobin—one from each parent.

People who inherit a sickle hemoglobin gene from one parent
and a normal gene from the other parent have a condition called
sickle cell trait. Their bodies make sickle hemoglobin and normal
hemoglobin.

People who have sickle cell trait usually have few, if any, symptoms
and lead normal lives. However, people who have sickle cell trait can
pass the sickle hemoglobin gene to their children.

Signs and Symptoms

The signs and symptoms of sickle cell anemia vary. Some people have mild symptoms. Others have very severe symptoms and often are hospitalized for treatment.

Sickle cell anemia is present at birth, but many infants don't show any signs until after four months of age. The most common signs and symptoms are linked to anemia and pain. Other signs and symptoms are linked to the disease's complications.

Signs and Symptoms Related to Anemia

The most common symptom of anemia is fatigue (feeling tired or weak). Other signs and symptoms of anemia may include the following:

- Shortness of breath

- Dizziness

- Headaches

- Coldness in the hands and feet

- Paler than normal skin or mucous membranes (the tissue that lines your nose, mouth, and other organs and body cavities)

- Jaundice (a yellowish color of the skin or whites of the eyes)

Signs and Symptoms Related to Pain

Sudden pain throughout the body is a common symptom of sickle cell anemia. This pain is called a sickle cell crisis. Sickle cell crises often affect the bones, lungs, abdomen, and joints. These crises occur when sickled red blood cells block blood flow to the limbs and organs.

The pain from sickle cell anemia can be acute or chronic, but acute pain is more common. Acute pain is sudden and can range from mild to very severe. The pain usually lasts from hours to as long as a week or more.

Many people who have sickle cell anemia also have chronic pain, especially in their bones. Chronic pain often lasts for weeks or months and can be hard to bear and mentally draining. Chronic pain may limit your daily activities.

Many factors can play a role in sickle cell crises. Often, more than one factor is involved and the exact cause isn't known. For example, the risk of a sickle cell crisis increases if you're dehydrated. You can't control other factors, such as infections.

Complications

Sickle cell crises can affect many parts of the body and cause many complications.

Hand-foot syndrome: Sickle cells can block the small blood vessels in the hands and feet in children (usually those younger than four years of age). It can lead to pain, swelling, and fever.

Splenic crisis: Normally, the spleen filters out abnormal red blood cells and helps fight infections. In some cases, the spleen may trap red blood cells that should be in the bloodstream. This causes the spleen to grow large and leads to anemia.

Infections: Both children and adults who have sickle cell anemia may get infections easily and have a hard time fighting them. This is because sickle cell anemia can damage the spleen, an organ that helps fight infections.

Infants and young children who have damaged spleens are more likely to get serious infections that can kill them within hours or days.

Acute chest syndrome: Acute chest syndrome is a life-threatening condition linked to sickle cell anemia. This syndrome is similar to pneumonia. An infection or sickle cells trapped in the lungs cause acute chest syndrome.

Pulmonary hypertension: Damage to the small blood vessels in the lungs makes it hard for the heart to pump blood through the lungs. This causes blood pressure in the lungs to rise. Shortness of breath and fatigue are the main symptoms.

Delayed growth and puberty in children: Children who have sickle cell anemia often grow more slowly than other children. They may reach puberty later.

Stroke: Two forms of stroke can occur in people who have sickle cell anemia. One form occurs if a blood vessel in the brain is damaged and blocked. This type of stroke occurs more often in children than adults. The other form of stroke occurs if a blood vessel in the brain bursts.

Eye problems: Sickle cells also can affect the small blood vessels that deliver oxygen-rich blood to the eyes. Sickle cells can block these vessels or cause them to break open and bleed. This can damage the retinas—thin layers of tissue at the back of the eyes.

Priapism: Males who have sickle cell anemia may have painful, unwanted erections because the sickle cells block blood flow out of an erect penis. Over time, priapism can damage the penis and lead to impotence.

Gallstones: When red blood cells die, they release their hemoglobin. The body breaks down this protein into a compound called bilirubin. Too much bilirubin in the body can cause stones to form in the gallbladder, called gallstones.

Ulcers on the legs: Sickle cell ulcers (sores) usually begin as small, raised, crusted sores on the lower third of the leg. Leg sores may occur more often in males than in females. These sores usually develop in people who are aged 10 years or older.

Multiple organ failure: Multiple organ failure is rare, but serious. It happens if you have a sickle cell crisis that causes two out of three major organs (lungs, liver, or kidneys) to fail. Often, multiple organ failure occurs during an unusually severe pain crisis.

Diagnosis

A simple blood test, done at any time during a person's lifespan, can detect whether he or she has sickle hemoglobin. However, early diagnosis is very important.

In the United States, all states mandate testing for sickle cell anemia as part of their newborn screening programs. Doctors also can diagnose sickle cell disease before birth. This is done using a sample of amniotic fluid or tissue taken from the placenta.

Treatment

Sickle cell anemia has no widely available cure. However, treatments can help relieve symptoms and treat complications. Infants who have been diagnosed with sickle cell anemia through newborn screening are treated with antibiotics to prevent infections. Their parents are educated about the disease and how to manage it. These initial treatment steps have greatly improved the outcome for children who have sickle cell anemia.

Mild pain often is treated at home with over-the-counter pain medicines, heating pads, rest, and plenty of fluids. More severe pain may need to be treated in a day clinic, emergency room, or hospital.

Severe sickle cell anemia can be treated with a medicine called hydroxyurea. This medicine prompts your body to make fetal hemoglobin, the type of hemoglobin that newborns have.

Preventing Complications

Blood transfusions are commonly used to treat worsening anemia and sickle cell complications. A sudden worsening of anemia due to an infection or enlarged spleen is a common reason for a blood transfusion.

Infections can be a major complication of sickle cell anemia throughout life, but especially during childhood. To prevent infections in babies and young children, treatments include daily doses of antibiotics and all routine vaccinations. Doctors also give many children a vitamin called folic acid (folate) to help boost red blood cell production.

Stroke prevention and treatment are now possible for children and adults who have sickle cell anemia. Starting at age two, children who have sickle cell anemia can have routine ultrasound scans of their heads.

Prevention

Sickle cell anemia is an inherited disease. If a person is born with it, steps should be taken to reduce its complications.

People who are at high risk of having a child with sickle cell anemia and are planning to have children may want to consider genetic counseling. You can find information about genetic counseling from health departments, neighborhood health centers, medical centers, and clinics that care for people who have sickle cell anemia.

Section 16.3

Thalassemia

This section excerpted from "What Are Thalassemias?," National Heart, Lung, and Blood Institute (www.nhlbi.nih.gov), August 1, 2010.

Thalassemias are inherited blood disorders. They cause the body to make fewer healthy red blood cells and less hemoglobin than normal. People who have thalassemias can have mild or severe anemia.

Treatments for thalassemias have improved greatly in recent years. People who have moderate or severe thalassemias are now living longer and have better quality of life. However, complications from thalassemias and their treatments are frequent. People who have moderate or severe thalassemias must closely follow their treatment plans.

Causes

Genes control how the body makes hemoglobin protein chains. When these genes are missing or altered, thalassemias occur.

Thalassemias are inherited disorders—that is, they're passed from parents to children through the genes.

Normal hemoglobin, also called hemoglobin A, has four protein chains—two alpha globin and two beta globin. The two major types of thalassemia, alpha and beta, are named after defects in these protein chains.

People who get faulty hemoglobin genes from one parent but normal genes from the other are called carriers. Carriers often have no signs of illness other than mild anemia. However, they can pass the faulty genes on to their children. People who have moderate to severe forms of thalassemia have inherited faulty genes from both parents.

Signs and Symptoms

A lack of oxygen in the bloodstream causes the signs and symptoms of thalassemias. The severity of symptoms depends on the severity of the disorder.

No symptoms: Alpha thalassemia silent carriers generally have no signs or symptoms of the disorder. This is because the lack of alpha globin protein is so minor that the body's hemoglobin works normally.

Mild anemia: People who have alpha or beta thalassemia trait can have mild anemia. However, many people who have these types of thalassemia have no signs or symptoms. Mild anemia can make you feel fatigued. Mild anemia caused by alpha or beta thalassemia trait often is mistaken for iron-deficiency anemia.

Mild to moderate anemia and other signs and symptoms: People who have beta thalassemia intermedia have mild to moderate anemia. They also may have other health problems, such as slowed growth and delayed puberty, bone problems, and an enlarged spleen.

Severe anemia and other signs and symptoms: People who have hemoglobin H disease or beta thalassemia major (also called Cooley anemia) have severe thalassemia. Signs and symptoms occur within the first two years of life. They may include severe anemia and other health problems, such as the following:

- A pale and listless appearance

- Poor appetite

- Dark urine (a sign that red blood cells are breaking down)

- Slowed growth and delayed puberty

- Jaundice (a yellowish color of the skin or whites of the eyes)

- An enlarged spleen, liver, and heart

- Bone problems (especially bones in the face)

Diagnosis and Prevention

Doctors diagnose thalassemias using blood tests, including a CBC and special hemoglobin tests. Moderate and severe thalassemias usually are diagnosed in early childhood. This is because signs and symptoms, including severe anemia, occur within the first two years of life. People who have milder forms of thalassemia may be diagnosed after a routine blood test shows they have anemia.

Because thalassemias are passed from parents to children through genes, family genetic studies also can help diagnose the disorder. If you know of family members who have thalassemias and you're thinking of having children, consider talking with your doctor and/or a genetic counselor. They can help determine your risk for passing the disorder to your children.

Treatment

Treatments for thalassemias depend on the type and severity of the disorder. People who are carriers or who have alpha or beta thalassemia trait have mild or no symptoms. They need little or no treatment.

Doctors use three standard treatments for moderate and severe forms of thalassemia. These include blood transfusions, iron chelation therapy, and folic acid supplements. Other treatments have been developed or are being tested, but they're used much less often.

Section 16.4

Hemophilia

This section excerpted from "What Is Hemophilia?," National Heart, Lung, and Blood Institute (www.nhlbi.nih.gov), July 1, 2011.

Hemophilia is a rare bleeding disorder in which the blood doesn't clot normally. If you have hemophilia, you may bleed for a longer time than others after an injury. You also may bleed inside your body (internally), especially in your knees, ankles, and elbows. This bleeding can damage your organs and tissues and may be life threatening.

Hemophilia usually is inherited. People born with hemophilia have little or no clotting factor. Clotting factor is a protein needed for normal blood clotting.

The two main types of hemophilia are A and B. If you have hemophilia A, you're missing or have low levels of clotting factor VIII. About 9 out of 10 people who have hemophilia have type A. If you have hemophilia B, you're missing or have low levels of clotting factor IX.

Rarely, hemophilia can be acquired. This can happen if your body forms antibodies (proteins) that attack the clotting factors in your bloodstream.

Hemophilia can be mild, moderate, or severe, depending on how much clotting factor is in your blood. About 7 out of 10 people who have hemophilia A have the severe form of the disorder.

Hemophilia usually occurs in males (with rare exceptions). About 1 in 5,000 males are born with hemophilia each year.

Causes

If you have inherited hemophilia, you're born with the disorder. It's caused by a defect in one of the genes that determine how the body makes blood clotting factor VIII or IX. These genes are located on the X chromosomes.

A male who has a faulty hemophilia gene on his X chromosome will have hemophilia. A female must have the faulty gene on both of her X chromosomes to have hemophilia, which is very rare. If a female has the faulty gene on only one of her X chromosomes, she is a "hemophilia carrier." Carriers don't have hemophilia, but they can pass the faulty gene to their children.

Some males who have the disorder are born to mothers who aren't carriers. In these cases, a mutation (random change) occurs in the gene as it is passed to the child.

Signs and Symptoms

The major signs and symptoms of hemophilia are excessive bleeding and easy bruising. The extent of bleeding depends on how severe the hemophilia is. Children who have mild hemophilia may not have signs unless they have excessive bleeding from a dental procedure, an accident, or surgery.

Signs of external bleeding may include these symptoms:

- Bleeding in the mouth from a cut or bite or from cutting or losing a tooth

- Nosebleeds for no obvious reason

- Heavy bleeding from a minor cut

- Bleeding from a cut that resumes after stopping for a short time

Signs of internal bleeding may include the following:

- Blood in the urine (from bleeding in the kidneys or bladder)

- Blood in the stool (from bleeding in the intestines or stomach)

- Large bruises (from bleeding into the large muscles of the body)

Bleeding in the knees, elbows, or other joints is another common form of internal bleeding in people who have hemophilia. This bleeding can occur without obvious injury. At first, the bleeding causes tightness in the joint with no real pain or any visible signs of bleeding. The joint then becomes swollen, hot to touch, and painful to bend.

Internal bleeding in the brain is a very serious complication of hemophilia. It can happen after a simple bump on the head or a more serious injury. The signs and symptoms of bleeding in the brain include the following:

- Long-lasting, painful headaches or neck pain or stiffness

- Repeated vomiting

- Sleepiness or changes in behavior

- Sudden weakness or clumsiness of the arms or legs or problems walking

- Double vision

- Convulsions or seizures

Diagnosis

If you or your child appears to have a bleeding problem, your doctor will ask about your personal and family medical histories. You or your child also will likely have a physical exam and blood tests to diagnose hemophilia.

Severe hemophilia can cause serious bleeding problems in babies. Thus, children who have severe hemophilia usually are diagnosed during the first year of life. People who have milder forms of hemophilia may not be diagnosed until they're adults.

The bleeding problems of hemophilia A and hemophilia B are the same. Only special blood tests can tell which type of the disorder you or your child has. Knowing which type is important because the treatments are different.

Pregnant women who are known hemophilia carriers can have the disorder diagnosed in their unborn babies as early as 10 weeks into their pregnancies.

Treatment

The main treatment for hemophilia is called replacement therapy. Concentrates of clotting factor VIII or IX are slowly dripped or injected into a vein. These infusions help replace the clotting factor that's missing or low.

Clotting factor concentrates can be made from human blood. With the current methods of screening and treating donated blood, the risk of getting an infectious disease from human clotting factors is very small.

To further reduce the risk, you or your child can take clotting factor concentrates that aren't made from human blood. These are called recombinant clotting factors. Clotting factors are easy to store, mix, and use at home—it only takes about 15 minutes to receive the factor.

You may have replacement therapy on a regular basis to prevent bleeding. This is called preventive or prophylactic therapy. Or, you may only need replacement therapy to stop bleeding when it occurs. This use of the treatment, on an as-needed basis, is called demand therapy. Demand therapy is less intensive and expensive than preventive therapy. However, there's a risk that bleeding will cause damage before you receive the demand therapy.

Section 16.5

Thrombocytopenia

This section excerpted from "What Is Thrombocytopenia?" National Heart, Lung, and Blood Institute (www.nhlbi.nih.gov), August 1, 2010.

Thrombocytopenia is a condition in which your blood has a lower than normal number of blood cell fragments called platelets.

Platelets are made in your bone marrow. They travel through your blood vessels and stick together (clot) to stop any bleeding that may happen if a blood vessel is damaged. Platelets also are called thrombocytes because a clot also is called a thrombus.

When your blood has too few platelets, mild to serious bleeding can occur. How long thrombocytopenia lasts depends on its cause. It can range from days to years.

Causes

Many factors can cause thrombocytopenia. The condition can be inherited, or it can develop at any age. Sometimes the cause of thrombocytopenia isn't known. Many factors can cause a low platelet count, such as the following:

- The body's bone marrow doesn't make enough platelets.

- The bone marrow makes enough platelets, but the body destroys them or uses them up.

- The spleen holds on to too many platelets. The spleen is an organ that normally stores about one-third of the body's platelets. It also helps your body fight infection and remove unwanted cell material.

- A combination of these factors.

Signs and Symptoms

Mild to serious bleeding are the main signs and symptoms of thrombocytopenia. Bleeding can occur inside the body (internal bleeding) or underneath or from the skin (external bleeding). Mild thrombocytopenia often has no signs or symptoms. Many times, it's found during a routine blood test.

Check with your doctor if you have any signs of bleeding. Severe thrombocytopenia can cause bleeding in almost any part of the body. This can lead to a medical emergency and should be treated right away.

External bleeding usually is the first sign of a low platelet count. External bleeding may cause purpura or petechiae. Purpura are purple, brown, and red bruises. This bruising may happen easily and often. Petechiae are small red or purple dots on your skin.

Other signs of external bleeding include the following:

- Prolonged bleeding, even from minor cuts

- Bleeding or oozing from the mouth or nose, especially nosebleeds or bleeding from brushing your teeth

- Abnormal vaginal bleeding (especially heavy menstrual flow)

A lot of bleeding after surgery or dental work also may mean you have a bleeding problem.

Heavy bleeding into the intestines or the brain (internal bleeding) is serious and can be fatal. Signs and symptoms include the following:

- Blood in the urine or stool or bleeding from the rectum. Blood in the stool can appear as red blood or as a dark, tarry color. (Taking iron supplements also can cause dark, tarry stools.)

- Headaches and other neurological symptoms. These problems are very rare, but you should discuss them with your doctor.

Diagnosis

Your doctor will diagnose thrombocytopenia based on your medical history, a physical exam, and test results. Your doctor may ask about factors that can affect your platelets, such as the medicines you take, your eating habits, your risk for AIDS, and a family history of low platelet counts.

Your doctor will also do a physical exam to look for signs and symptoms of bleeding, such as bruises or spots on the skin. He or she will check your abdomen for signs of an enlarged spleen or liver.

Your doctor may recommend one or more of the following tests to help diagnose a low platelet count:

- Complete blood count

- Blood smear

- Bone marrow tests

Treatment

If your condition is mild, you may not need treatment. A fully normal platelet count isn't necessary to prevent bleeding, even with severe cuts or accidents.

Thrombocytopenia often improves when its underlying cause is treated. People who inherit the condition usually don't need treatment.

If a reaction to a medicine is causing a low platelet count, your doctor may prescribe another medicine. If your immune system is causing a low platelet count, your doctor may prescribe medicines to suppress the immune system.

If your thrombocytopenia is severe, your doctor may prescribe treatments such as medicines, blood or platelet transfusions, or splenectomy.

Medicines: Your doctor may prescribe corticosteroids to slow platelet destruction or immunoglobulin to help your body make more platelets. He or she also may prescribe other medicines to help your body make more platelets.

Blood or platelet transfusions: Blood or platelet transfusions are used to treat people who have active bleeding or are at a high risk of bleeding.

Splenectomy: A splenectomy is surgery to remove the spleen. This surgery may be used if treatment with medicines doesn't work.

Prevention

Whether you can prevent thrombocytopenia depends on its specific cause. Usually the condition can't be prevented. However, you can take steps to prevent health problems associated with the condition.

- Avoid heavy drinking. Alcohol slows the production of platelets.

- Try to avoid contact with toxic chemicals. Chemicals such as pesticides, arsenic, and benzene can slow the production of platelets.

- Avoid medicines that you know have decreased your platelet count in the past.

- Be aware of medicines that may affect your platelets and raise your risk of bleeding. Two examples of such medicines are aspirin and ibuprofen.

- Talk with your doctor about getting vaccinated for viruses that can affect your platelets. You may need vaccines for mumps, measles, rubella, and chickenpox.

Section 16.6

Thrombophilia
(Excessive Blood Clotting)

This section excerpted from "What Causes Excessive Blood Clotting?"
National Heart, Lung, and Blood Institute (www.nhlbi.nih.gov),
August 1, 2010.

Excessive blood clotting is a condition in which blood clots form too easily or don't dissolve properly. Normally, blood clots form to seal small cuts or breaks on blood vessel walls and stop bleeding. Slow blood flow in the blood vessels also can cause blood clots to form.

Excessive blood clotting has many causes. Regardless of the cause, problem blood clots can limit or block blood flow. This can damage the body's organs and may even cause death. Excessive blood clotting can be acquired or genetic. Acquired causes of excessive blood clotting are more common than genetic causes.

"Acquired" means that another disease, condition, or factor triggers the condition. For example, atherosclerosis can damage the blood vessels, which can cause blood clots to form. Other acquired causes of excessive blood clotting include smoking, overweight and obesity, and hospitalization.

"Genetic" means the condition is caused by a faulty gene. Most genetic defects that cause excessive blood clotting occur in the proteins needed for blood clotting. Defects also can occur with the substances that delay or dissolve blood clots.

Although the acquired and genetic causes of the condition aren't related, a person can have both. People at highest risk for excessive blood clotting have both causes.

Signs and Symptoms

Signs and symptoms of excessive blood clotting depend on where the clots form. For example, symptoms of a blood clot in the heart or lungs may include chest pain, shortness of breath, and upper body discomfort in the arms, back, neck, or jaw. These symptoms may suggest a heart attack or pulmonary embolism (PE).

Signs and symptoms of a blood clot in the deep veins of the leg may include pain, redness, warmth, and swelling in the lower leg. These signs and symptoms may suggest deep vein thrombosis (DVT).

Signs and symptoms of a blood clot in the brain may include headaches, speech changes, paralysis (an inability to move), dizziness, and trouble speaking or understanding speech. These signs and symptoms may suggest a stroke.

If you have any of these signs or symptoms, call your doctor right away. The cause of the blood clot needs to be found and treated as soon as possible. You may need emergency care.

Complications of Blood Clots

Blood clots can form in, or travel to, the arteries or veins in the brain, heart, kidneys, lungs, and limbs. Blood clots can limit or block blood flow. This can damage the body's organs and cause many problems, including stroke, heart attack, kidney problems and kidney failure, pulmonary embolism, deep vein thrombosis, and pregnancy-related problems. In some cases, blood clots can be fatal.

Diagnosis

If your doctor thinks that you have excessive blood clotting based on your signs and symptoms, he or she will look for the cause of the condition.

Your doctor may ask you detailed questions about your medical history and your family's medical history. Your doctor will also do a physical exam to see how severe your blood clotting problem is and to look for its possible causes.

Your doctor may recommend blood tests to look at your blood cells and the clotting process. If he or she thinks you may have a genetic condition, you may need more blood tests. Tests to find the cause of excessive blood clotting may be delayed for weeks or even months while you receive treatment for a problem blood clot.

Treatment

Excessive blood clotting is treated with medicines. Depending on the size and location of the clot(s), you may need emergency treatment and/or routine treatment.

Emergency treatment: Blood clots can be dangerous. They can damage the body and lead to serious problems, such as stroke, heart attack, kidney failure, deep vein thrombosis, or pulmonary embolism. Blood clots also can cause miscarriages, stillbirths, or pregnancy-related problems.

Emergency treatment to prevent these problems often consists of medicines that can quickly break up clots. These medicines, called thrombolytics or "clot busters," are used to treat large clots that cause severe symptoms. These medicines can cause sudden bleeding. Thus, they're used only in life-threatening situations.

Routine treatment: Anticoagulants, or "blood thinners," are used as routine treatment for excessive blood clotting. These medicines prevent blood clots from forming. They also keep existing blood clots from getting larger.

Blood thinners are taken as either a pill, an injection under the skin, or through a needle or tube inserted into a vein (called intravenous, or IV, injection).

Some people must take blood thinners for the rest of their lives if their risk of forming blood clots remains high.

The most common side effect of blood thinners is bleeding. This happens if the medicine thins your blood too much. This side effect can be life threatening. Bleeding can occur inside your body (internal bleeding) or underneath or from the skin (external bleeding).

Know the warning signs of bleeding, so you can get help right away:

- Unexplained bleeding from the gums and nose
- Increased menstrual flow
- Bright red vomit or vomit that looks like coffee grounds
- Bright red blood in your stools or black, tarry stools
- Pain in your abdomen or severe pain in your head
- Sudden changes in vision
- Sudden loss of movement in your arms and legs
- Memory loss or confusion

A lot of bleeding after a fall or injury or easy bruising or bleeding also may mean that your blood is too thin. Call your doctor right away if you have any of these signs.

Prevention

You can't prevent genetic causes of excessive blood clotting. However, you can take steps to control or avoid some acquired risk factors.

- Treat conditions that can lead to excessive blood clotting, such as diabetes or heart and vascular diseases.

- Make lifestyle changes, such as quitting smoking or losing weight.

- Avoid medicines that contain the female hormone estrogen if you have risk factors for excessive blood clotting. Ask your doctor about other, safer options.

- Stay active if you can. Move your legs, flex, and stretch during long trips. This helps keep blood flowing in your calves.

- Talk with your doctor about ways to lower your homocysteine level if it's high. You may need more vitamin B6, vitamin B12, or folate.

Your doctor may give you blood thinners before, during, and/or after surgery or medical procedures to prevent excessive blood clotting.

Section 16.7

von Willebrand Disease

This section excerpted from "What Is von Willebrand Disease?," National Heart, Lung, and Blood Institute (www.nhlbi.nih.gov), June 1, 2011.

Von Willebrand disease (VWD) is a bleeding disorder. It affects your blood's ability to clot. If your blood doesn't clot, you can have heavy, hard-to-stop bleeding after an injury. The bleeding can damage your internal organs. Rarely, the bleeding may even cause death.

In VWD, you either have low levels of a certain protein in your blood or the protein doesn't work well. The protein is called von Willebrand factor, and it helps your blood clot.

Von Willebrand factor also carries clotting factor VIII, another important protein that helps your blood clot. Factor VIII is the protein that's missing or doesn't work well in people who have hemophilia, another bleeding disorder.

VWD is more common and usually milder than hemophilia. In fact, VWD is the most common inherited bleeding disorder. It occurs in about 1 out of every 100 to 1,000 people. VWD affects both males and females, while hemophilia mainly affects males.

The three major types of VWD are called type 1, type 2, and type 3. Most people who have VWD have type 1, a mild form. This type usually doesn't cause life-threatening bleeding. You may need treatment only if you have surgery, tooth extraction, or trauma. Treatment includes medicines and medical therapies.

Some people who have severe forms of VWD need emergency treatment to stop bleeding before it becomes life threatening.

Early diagnosis is important. With the proper treatment plan, even people who have type 3 VWD can live normal, active lives.

Causes

VWD is almost always inherited. You can inherit type 1 or type 2 VWD if only one of your parents passes the gene on to you. You usually inherit type 3 VWD only if both of your parents pass the gene on to you.

Some people have the genes for the disorder but don't have symptoms. However, they still can pass the genes on to their children.

Some people get VWD later in life as a result of other medical conditions. This type of VWD is called acquired von Willebrand syndrome.

Signs and Symptoms

If you have type 1 or type 2 VWD, you may have the following mild-to-moderate bleeding symptoms:

- Frequent, large bruises from minor bumps or injuries

- Frequent or hard-to-stop nosebleeds

- Prolonged bleeding from the gums after a dental procedure

- Heavy or prolonged menstrual bleeding in women

- Blood in your stools from bleeding in your intestines or stomach

- Blood in your urine from bleeding in your kidneys or bladder

- Heavy bleeding after a cut or other accident

- Heavy bleeding after surgery

People who have type 3 VWD may have all of the aforementioned symptoms and severe bleeding episodes for no reason. These bleeding episodes can be fatal if not treated right away. People who have type 3

VWD also may have bleeding into soft tissues or joints, causing severe pain and swelling.

Heavy menstrual bleeding often is the main symptom of VWD in women. Doctors call this menorrhagia. They define it as the following:

- Bleeding with clots larger than about one inch in diameter

- Anemia (low red blood cell count) or low blood iron

- The need to change pads or tampons more than every hour

However, just because a woman has heavy menstrual bleeding doesn't mean she has VWD.

Diagnosis

Early diagnosis of VWD is important to make sure that you're treated and can live a normal, active life.

People who have type 1 or type 2 VWD may not have major bleeding problems. Thus, they may not be diagnosed unless they have heavy bleeding after surgery or some other trauma.

On the other hand, type 3 VWD can cause major bleeding problems during infancy and childhood. So children who have type 3 VWD usually are diagnosed during their first year of life.

To find out whether you have VWD, your doctor will likely ask questions about your medical history and your family's medical history. Your doctor will also do a physical exam to look for unusual bruising or other signs of recent bleeding. He or she also will look for signs of liver disease or anemia (a low red blood cell count).

Your doctor may recommend one or more blood tests to diagnose the disorder:

- **Von Willebrand factor antigen:** This test measures the amount of von Willebrand factor in your blood.

- **Von Willebrand factor ristocetin cofactor activity:** This test shows how well your von Willebrand factor works.

- **Factor VIII clotting activity:** This test checks the clotting activity of factor VIII. Some people who have VWD have low levels of factor VIII activity, while others have normal levels.

- **Von Willebrand factor multimers:** This test is done if one or more of the first three tests are abnormal. It helps your doctor diagnose what type of VWD you have.

- **Platelet function test:** This test measures how well your platelets are working.

Treatment

Treatment for VWD is based on the type of VWD you have and how severe it is. Most cases of VWD are mild, and you may need treatment only if you have surgery, tooth extraction, or an accident.

Medicines are used to accomplish the following:

- Increase the amount of von Willebrand factor and factor VIII released into the bloodstream

- Replace von Willebrand factor

- Prevent the breakdown of blood clots

- Control heavy menstrual bleeding in women

Chapter 17

Cancer in Children

Chapter Contents

Section 17.1

Leukemia

About Leukemia

The term leukemia refers to cancers of the white blood cells (also called leukocytes or WBCs). When a child has leukemia, large numbers of abnormal white blood cells are produced in the bone marrow. These abnormal white cells crowd the bone marrow and flood the bloodstream, but they cannot perform their proper role of protecting the body against disease because they are defective.

As leukemia progresses, the cancer interferes with the body's production of other types of blood cells, including red blood cells and platelets. This results in anemia (low numbers of red cells) and bleeding problems, in addition to the increased risk of infection caused by white cell abnormalities.

As a group, leukemias account for about 25% of all childhood cancers and affect about 2,200 American young people each year. Luckily, the chances for a cure are very good with leukemia. With treatment, most children with leukemia will be free of the disease without it coming back.

Types of Leukemia

In general, leukemias are classified into acute (rapidly developing) and chronic (slowly developing) forms. In children, about 98% of leukemias are acute.

Acute childhood leukemias are also divided into acute lymphocytic leukemia (ALL) and acute myelogenous leukemia (AML), depending on whether specific white blood cells called lymphocytes (or myelocytes), which are linked to immune defenses, are involved.

Approximately 60% of children with leukemia have ALL, and about 38% have AML. Although slow-growing chronic myelogenous leukemia (CML) may also be seen in children, it is very rare, accounting for fewer than 50 cases of childhood leukemia each year in the United States.

Causes

The ALL form of the disease most commonly occurs in younger children ages two to eight, with a peak incidence at age four. But it can affect all age groups.

Kids have a 20% to 25% chance of developing ALL or AML if they have an identical twin who was diagnosed with the illness before age six. In general, nonidentical twins and other siblings of children with leukemia have two to four times the average risk of developing this illness.

Children who have inherited certain genetic problems—such as Li-Fraumeni syndrome, Down syndrome, Klinefelter syndrome, neurofibromatosis, ataxia telangiectasia, or Fanconi's anemia—have a higher risk of developing leukemia, as do kids who are receiving medical drugs to suppress their immune systems after organ transplants.

Children who have received prior radiation or chemotherapy for other types of cancer also have a higher risk for leukemia, usually within the first eight years after treatment.

In most cases, neither parents nor kids have control over the factors that trigger leukemia, although current studies are investigating the possibility that some environmental factors may increase the risk that a child will develop the disease. Most leukemias arise from noninherited mutations (changes) in the genes of growing blood cells. Because these errors occur randomly and unpredictably, there is currently no effective way to prevent most types of leukemia.

To limit the risk of prenatal radiation exposure as a trigger for leukemia (especially ALL), women who are pregnant or who suspect that they might be pregnant should always inform their doctors before undergoing tests or medical procedures that involve radiation (such as X-rays).

Regular checkups can spot early symptoms of leukemia in the relatively rare cases where this cancer is linked to an inherited genetic problem, to prior cancer treatment, or to use of immunosuppressive drugs for organ transplants.

Symptoms

Because their infection-fighting white blood cells are defective, kids with leukemia may experience increased episodes of fevers and infections. They also may become anemic, because leukemia affects the bone marrow's production of oxygen-carrying red blood cells. This makes them appear pale, and they may become abnormally tired and short of breath while playing.

Children with leukemia might bruise and bleed very easily, experience frequent nosebleeds, or bleed for an unusually long time after even a minor cut because leukemia destroys the bone marrow's ability to produce clot-forming platelets.

Other symptoms of leukemia can include:

- pain in the bones or joints, sometimes causing a limp;

- swollen lymph nodes (sometimes called swollen glands) in the neck, groin, or elsewhere;

- an abnormally tired feeling;

- poor appetite.

In about 12% of kids with AML and 6% of those with ALL, spread of leukemia to the brain causes headaches, seizures, balance problems, or abnormal vision. If ALL spreads to the lymph nodes inside the chest, the enlarged gland can crowd the trachea (windpipe) and important blood vessels, leading to breathing problems and interference with blood flow to and from the heart.

Diagnosis

Your child's doctor will perform a physical examination to check for signs of infection, anemia, abnormal bleeding, and swollen lymph nodes. The doctor will also feel your child's abdomen to see if there is an enlarged liver or spleen because they can become enlarged with some cancers in children.

In addition to doing a physical exam, the doctor will take a medical history by asking you about symptoms, past health, your family's health history, medications your child is taking, allergies, and other issues.

After this exam, the doctor will order a CBC (complete blood count) to measure the numbers of white cells, red cells, and platelets in your child's blood. A blood smear will be examined under a microscope to check for certain specific types of abnormal blood cells usually seen in patients with leukemia. Blood chemistries will also be checked.

Then, depending on the results of the physical exam and preliminary blood tests, your child may need:

- a bone marrow biopsy and aspiration, in which marrow samples are removed (usually from the back of the hip) for testing;

- a lymph node biopsy, in which lymph nodes are removed and examined under a microscope to look for abnormal cells;

- a lumbar puncture (spinal tap), where a sample of spinal fluid is removed from the lower back and examined for evidence of abnormal cells—this will show whether the leukemia has spread to the central nervous system (brain and spinal cord).

Bone marrow or lymph node samples will be examined and additional testing done to determine the specific type of leukemia. In addition to these basic lab tests, cell evaluations might be done, including genetic studies to distinguish between specific types of leukemia and certain features of the leukemia cells. Kids will receive anesthesia or sedative medications for any painful procedures.

Treatment

Certain features of a child's leukemia, such as age and initial white blood cell count, are used in determining the intensity of treatment needed to achieve the best chance for cure. Although all kids with ALL are treated with chemotherapy, the dosages and drug combinations may differ.

To decrease the chance that leukemia will invade the child's central nervous system, patients receive intrathecal chemotherapy, the administration of cancer-killing drugs into the cerebrospinal fluid around the brain and spinal cord.

Radiation treatments, which use high-energy rays to shrink tumors and keep cancer cells from growing, may be used in addition to intrathecal chemotherapy for certain high-risk patients. Children then require continued close monitoring by a pediatric oncologist, a specialist in childhood cancer.

After treatment begins, the goal is remission of the leukemia (when there is no longer evidence of cancer cells in the body). Once remission has occurred, maintenance chemotherapy is usually used to keep the child in remission. Maintenance chemotherapy is given in cycles over a period of two to three years to keep the cancer from returning. Leukemia will almost always relapse (reoccur) if this additional chemotherapy isn't given. Sometimes the cancer will return in spite of maintenance chemotherapy, and other forms of chemotherapy will then be necessary.

Sometimes a bone marrow transplant may be necessary in addition to—or instead of—chemotherapy, depending on the type of leukemia a child has. During a bone marrow transplant, healthy bone marrow is introduced into a child's body.

Intensive leukemia chemotherapy has certain side effects, including hair loss, nausea and vomiting, and increased risk for infection or bleeding in the short term, as well as other potential health problems down the line. As your child is treated for leukemia, the cancer treatment team will watch closely for those side effects.

But with the proper treatment, the outlook for kids who are diagnosed with leukemia is quite good. Some forms of childhood leukemia have a remission rate of up to 90%; all kids then require regular maintenance chemotherapy and other treatment to continue to be cancer-free. Overall cure rates differ depending on the specific features of a child's disease. Most childhood leukemias have very high remission rates. And the majority of kids can be cured (meaning that they are in permanent remission) of the disease.

Section 17.2

Lymphoma

"Lymphoma," August 2010, reprinted with permission from www.kidshealth .org. Copyright © 2010 The Nemours Foundation. This information was provided by KidsHealth, one of the largest resources online for medically reviewed health information written for parents, kids, and teens. For more articles like this one, visit www.KidsHealth.org, or www.TeensHealth.org.

The term lymphoma refers to cancers that originate in the body's lymphatic tissues. Lymphatic tissues include the lymph nodes (also called lymph glands), thymus, spleen, tonsils, adenoids, and bone marrow, as well as the channels (called lymphatics or lymph vessels) that connect them. Although many types of cancer eventually spread to parts of the lymphatic system, lymphomas are distinct because they actually originate there.

About 1,700 kids younger than 20 years old are diagnosed with lymphoma each year in the United States. Lymphomas are divided into two broad categories, depending on the appearance of their cancerous (malignant) cells. These are known as Hodgkin's lymphoma and non-Hodgkin lymphoma (NHL). Together, they are the third most common type of cancer in children.

Hodgkin's Lymphoma

This type of lymphoma is defined by the presence of specific malignant cells, called Reed-Sternberg cells, in the lymph nodes or in some other lymphatic tissue. Hodgkin's lymphoma affects about 3 out of every 100,000 Americans, most commonly during early and late adulthood (between ages 15 and 40 and after age 55).

The most common first symptom of Hodgkin's lymphoma is a painless enlargement of the lymph nodes (a condition known as swollen glands) located in the neck, above the collarbone, in the underarm area, or in the groin.

If cancer involves the lymph nodes in the center of the chest, pressure from this swelling may trigger an unexplained cough, shortness of breath, or problems in blood flow to and from the heart.

About a third of patients have other nonspecific symptoms, including fatigue, poor appetite, itching, or hives. Unexplained fever, night sweats, and weight loss are also common.

Non-Hodgkin Lymphoma (NHL)

There are about 500 new cases of non-Hodgkin lymphoma diagnosed each year in kids in the United States. It may occur at any age during childhood, but is rare before age 3. NHL is slightly more common than Hodgkin disease in kids younger than 15 years old.

In non-Hodgkin lymphoma, there is malignant growth of specific types of lymphocytes (a kind of white blood cell that collects in the lymph nodes). Malignant growth of lymphocytes is also seen in one of the forms of leukemia (acute lymphoblastic leukemia, or ALL), which sometimes makes it difficult to distinguish between lymphoma and leukemia in children. In general, people with lymphoma have no or only minimal bone marrow involvement, whereas those with leukemia have extensive bone marrow involvement.

Risk for Childhood Lymphoma

Both Hodgkin disease and NHL tend to occur more often in people with certain severe immune deficiencies—including people with inherited immune defects, adults with human immunodeficiency virus (HIV) infection, or those who have been treated with immunosuppressive drugs after organ transplants.

Although no lifestyle factors have been definitely linked to childhood lymphomas, kids who have received either radiation treatments or chemotherapy for other types of cancer seem to have a higher risk of developing lymphoma later in life.

In most cases, neither parents nor kids have control over the factors that cause lymphomas. Most lymphomas come from noninherited mutations (errors) in the genes of growing blood cells. Regular pediatric checkups can sometimes spot early symptoms of lymphoma in the relatively rare cases where this cancer is linked to an inherited immune problem, HIV infection, prior cancer treatment, or treatment of immunosuppressive drugs for organ transplants.

Diagnosis

The doctor will check your child's weight and perform a physical examination to look for enlarged lymph nodes and signs of local infection. He or she will also examine your child's chest using a stethoscope and will feel the abdomen to check for pain, organ enlargement, or fluid accumulation.

In addition to doing a physical exam, the doctor will take a medical history by asking you about your child's past health, your family's health, and other issues.

Sometimes, when a child is found to have an enlarged lymph node for no apparent reason, the doctor will watch the node closely to see if it continues to grow. The doctor may prescribe antibiotics if the gland is believed to be infected by bacteria, or do blood tests for certain types of infection. If the lymph node remains enlarged, the next step is a biopsy (the removal and examination of tissue, cells, or fluids from the body). Biopsies are also necessary for lymphomas that involve the bone marrow or structures within the chest or abdomen.

Depending on the location of the tissue to be sampled, the biopsy may be done using a thin hollow needle (known as needle aspiration) or a small surgical incision made under general anesthesia. Sometimes, a biopsy may require a surgical excision under anesthesia, where a piece of the lymph node or the entire lymph node is removed.

In the laboratory, tissue samples obtained from the biopsy are examined to determine the specific type of lymphoma. In addition to these basic lab tests, more sophisticated tests are also generally done, including genetic studies, to distinguish between specific types of lymphoma.

To identify which areas of the body are affected by lymphoma, the following tests are also commonly used:

- Blood tests, including complete blood count

- Blood chemistry, including tests of liver and kidney function

- Bone marrow biopsy or aspiration
- Lumbar puncture (spinal tap) to check for cancer spread to the central nervous system (brain and spinal cord)
- Ultrasound
- Computed tomography (CT) of the chest and abdomen, and sometimes X-rays
- Magnetic resonance imaging (MRI)
- Bone scan, gallium scan, and/or positron emission tomography (PET) scan (when a radioactive material is injected into the bloodstream to look for evidence of tumors throughout the body)

These tests are important for determining the spread of the lymphoma within the body to guide which type of treatment should be used.

Treatment

Treatment of childhood lymphoma is largely determined by staging. Staging is a way to categorize or classify patients according to how extensive the disease is at the time of diagnosis.

Chemotherapy (the use of highly potent medical drugs to kill cancer cells) is the primary form of treatment for all types of lymphoma. In certain cases, radiation (the use of high-energy rays to shrink tumors and keep cancer cells from growing) may also be used.

Short-Term and Long-Term Side Effects

Intensive lymphoma chemotherapy affects the bone marrow, causing anemia and bleeding problems, and increasing the risk for serious infections. Chemotherapy and radiation treatments have many other side effects—some short-term (such as hair loss, changes in skin color, increased infection risk, and nausea and vomiting) and some long-term (such heart and kidney damage, reproductive problems, thyroid problems, or the development of another cancer later in life)—that parents should discuss with their doctor.

Relapses

Although most kids do recover from lymphoma, some with severe disease will have a relapse (reoccurrence of the cancer). For these children, bone marrow transplants and stem cell transplants are often among the newest treatment options.

During a bone marrow/stem cell transplant, intensive chemotherapy with or without radiation therapy is given to kill residual cancerous cells. Then, healthy bone marrow/stem cells are introduced into the body in the hopes that it will begin producing white blood cells that will help the child fight infections.

New Treatments

Promising new treatments being developed for childhood lymphomas include several different types of immune therapy, specifically the use of antibodies to deliver chemotherapy medicines or radioactive chemicals directly to lymphoma cells. This direct targeting of lymphoma cells may avoid the toxic side effects that occur when today's chemotherapy and radiation treatments damage normal, noncancerous body tissues.

Section 17.3

Neuroblastoma

Most people have never heard of neuroblastoma, a rare type of cancer that almost always occurs in infants and young children. It's actually the most common type of cancer in infants, but it's still rare enough that many doctors have never cared for a child with neuroblastoma.

Although neuroblastoma sometimes forms before a child is born, it usually isn't found until later, when the tumor begins to grow and affect the body. When neuroblastoma is diagnosed in infancy, the chance of recovery is good.

About Neuroblastoma

Neuroblastoma is a rare disease in which a solid tumor (a lump or mass caused by uncontrolled or abnormal cell growth) is formed by special nerve cells called neuroblasts. Normally, these immature cells grow and mature into functioning nerve cells. But in neuroblastoma, they become cancer cells instead.

Neuroblastoma most commonly starts in the tissue of the adrenal glands, the triangular glands on top of the kidneys that produce hormones responsible for controlling heart rate, blood pressure, and other important functions. Like other cancers, neuroblastoma can spread (metastasize) to other parts of the body, such as the lymph nodes, skin, liver, and bones.

In a few cases, the tendency to get this type of cancer can be passed down from a parent to a child (familial type), but most cases of neuroblastoma (98%) aren't inherited (sporadic type). It occurs almost exclusively in infants and children and is slightly more common in boys than in girls.

Children diagnosed with neuroblastoma are usually younger than five years old, with the majority of new cases occurring among those younger than one year old. Only about 700 new cases of neuroblastoma are diagnosed each year in the United States.

Causes

Neuroblastoma occurs when neuroblasts grow and divide uncontrollably instead of developing into nerve cells. The exact cause of this abnormal growth is unknown, but scientists believe it's related to a defect in the genes of a neuroblast that allows it to divide uncontrollably.

Signs and Symptoms

The effects of neuroblastoma can vary widely depending on where the disease first started and how much it has spread to other parts of the body. The first symptoms are often vague and may include irritability, fatigue, loss of appetite, and fever. But because these early warning signs can develop gradually and mimic those of other common childhood illnesses, neuroblastoma can be difficult to diagnose.

In young children, neuroblastoma often is discovered when a parent or doctor feels an unusual lump or mass somewhere in the child's body—most often in the abdomen, though tumors also can appear in the neck, chest, and elsewhere.

The most common signs of neuroblastoma are caused by the tumor pressing on nearby tissues as it grows or by the cancer spreading to other areas. These signs vary depending on how much the cancer has grown and where it has spread.

For example, a child may have:

- a swollen stomach, abdominal pain, and decreased appetite (if the tumor is in the abdomen);

- bone pain or soreness, black eyes, bruises, and pale skin (if the cancer has spread to the bones);

- weakness, numbness, inability to move a body part, or difficulty walking (if the cancer presses on the spinal cord);

- drooping eyelid, unequal pupils, sweating, and red skin, which are signs of nerve damage in the neck known as Horner's syndrome (if the tumor is in the neck);

- difficulty breathing (if the cancer is in the chest).

Diagnosis

If a doctor suspects neuroblastoma, your child may undergo a variety of tests to confirm the diagnosis and rule out other causes of symptoms. These tests may include simple urine and blood tests, imaging studies (such as X-rays, a CT scan, an MRI, an ultrasound, and a bone scan), and a biopsy (removal and examination of a tissue sample).

These tests help to determine the location and size of the original (primary) tumor and determine whether it has spread to other areas of the body, a process called staging. Additional tests, such as bone marrow aspiration and biopsy, also may be performed.

The doctor also might order a MIBG scintiscan. In this imaging test, MIBG (iodine-131-meta-iodobenzyl-guanidine, a type of radioactive material) is injected into the blood and attaches to neuroblastoma cells. This allows the doctor to see whether the neuroblastoma has spread to other parts of the body. MIBG is also used at higher doses to treat neuroblastoma and may be used for scanning after treatment to determine if any cancer cells remain.

In rare cases, neuroblastoma may be detected by ultrasound before birth.

Treatment

Most cases of neuroblastoma require treatment. The type will depend on several factors—including the child's age, the characteristics of the tumor, and whether the cancer has spread—that determine risk.

The three risk groups are: low risk, intermediate risk, and high risk. Children with low-risk or intermediate-risk neuroblastoma have a good chance of being cured. However, about one-half of all children with neuroblastoma have the high-risk type, which can be difficult to cure.

Because some cases of neuroblastoma disappear on their own without treatment, doctors also sometimes use "watchful waiting" before trying other treatments.

Typical treatments for neuroblastoma include surgery to remove the tumor, radiation therapy, and chemotherapy. If the tumor hasn't spread to other parts of the body, surgery is usually enough.

Unfortunately, in most cases the neuroblastoma has spread by the time it's diagnosed. In these cases, chemotherapy and surgery are the primary treatments and may be performed in conjunction with radiation therapy and stem cell or bone marrow transplantation.

Another treatment the doctor might suggest is retinoid therapy. Scientists believe that retinoids (a class of substances chemically related to vitamin A) can help cure neuroblastoma by encouraging cancer cells to turn into mature nerve cells. Retinoids are often used after other treatments to help prevent the cancer from growing back.

Newer treatment options include tumor vaccines and immunotherapy using monoclonal antibodies, special substances that can be injected into the body to seek out and attach to cancer cells. They're sometimes used to deliver drugs or other treatments directly to cancer cells, helping to improve treatment.

Prognosis

With treatment, many children with neuroblastoma have a good chance of surviving. In general, neuroblastoma has a more favorable outcome if the cancer hasn't spread or if the child is younger than one year old when it's diagnosed. High-risk neuroblastoma is harder to cure and is more likely to become resistant to standard therapies or come back (recur) after initially successful treatment.

Late Effects

"Late effects" are problems that patients can develop after cancer treatments have ended. Some late effects of neuroblastoma include growth and developmental delays and loss of function in involved organs.

Children treated for neuroblastoma may also be at higher risk for other cancers.

The risk of developing these late effects depends on various factors, such as the specific treatments used and the child's age during treatment.

Although rare, some kids with neuroblastoma develop opsoclonus-myoclonus syndrome, a condition in which their immune system attacks normal nerve tissue. As a result, some might experience learning disabilities, delays in muscle and movement development, language problems, and behavioral problems.

Caring for Your Child

Being told that your child has cancer can be a terrifying and overwhelming experience, and treatment of neuroblastoma can take a tremendous toll on your child and family. At times, you might feel helpless.

But you play a vital role in your child's treatment. During this difficult time, it's important to stay informed and learn as much as you can about neuroblastoma and its treatment. Being knowledgeable will help you make informed decisions and better help your child cope with the tests and treatments. Don't be afraid to ask the doctors questions.

Although you might feel like it at times, you're not alone. You might find it helpful to find a support group for parents whose kids are coping with cancer (several are groups specifically for parents of children with neuroblastoma).

Parents often struggle with how much to tell a child who's diagnosed with cancer. While there's no one-size-fits-all answer, experts do agree that it's best to be honest—but to tailor the details to your child's degree of understanding and emotional maturity. Give as much information as your child requires, but not more.

And when explaining treatment, try to break it down into steps. Addressing each part as it comes—visiting various doctors, having a special machine take pictures of the body, needing an operation—can make the big picture less overwhelming. Be sure to explain to your child that the disease is not the result of anything that he or she did.

Also remember that it's common for siblings to feel neglected, jealous, and angry when a child is seriously ill. Explain as much as they can understand, and enlist family members, teachers, and friends to help keep some sense of normalcy for them.

And finally, as hard as it may be, try to take care of yourself. Parents who get the support they need are better able to support their children.

Section 17.4

Sarcoma and Bone Tumors

What Are Bone Tumors and Sarcoma?

Tumors are lumps of tissue that form when cells divide uncontrollably.

When tumors start inside the skeleton, such as in the leg bones, the arm bones, or the ribs, they are called bone tumors. When they start inside other tissues, such as muscles, fat, or blood vessels, they are called soft tissue tumors.

Tumors can be either benign or malignant.

Benign tumors are not cancerous and do not spread from their original (primary) site. They can, however, come back (recur) at their original site.

Malignant tumors are cancerous and have the potential to spread cancer cells to other parts of the body (metastasis).

Both bone tumors and soft tissue tumors can be either benign or malignant. When these tumors are cancerous, they are called sarcomas.

Types of Sarcoma

Ewing Sarcoma

Ewing sarcoma can start in any bone in the body. This includes the leg bones, the ribs, the pelvis, and the arm bones. Other tumors in the Ewing sarcoma family can develop in soft tissue.

Osteosarcoma

Osteosarcoma starts in cells that are supposed to build new bone. Instead, these cells destroy bone and weaken it. This can happen in any bone.

In children, it most often starts near the knee, either in the thigh-bone (femur) or the shin bone (tibia). Sometimes it spreads to other bones or the lungs. Very rarely, it begins outside the bone.

Soft Tissue Sarcomas

Soft tissue sarcomas can start in any of the soft tissues that connect or support other structures. These include muscles, tendons, fat, blood vessels, lymph vessels, nerves, and the soft tissues in and around joints.

Most often soft tissue sarcomas affect the muscles that attach to bones and allow us to bend our joints (skeletal muscles). This type is called rhabdomyosarcoma. It can start in any muscle in the body, including around the head, next to the brain, in the bladder, or in an arm or leg.

Rarely, children get other kinds of soft tissue sarcomas.

Bone Tumors and Sarcoma in Children

Any child may get a bone tumor (benign or malignant) or sarcoma. Doctors do not know what causes the disease. Some factors may increase a child's risk for sarcoma, but most children who have sarcoma have none of these risk factors.

For example, children with certain uncommon inherited conditions have a greater risk of developing soft tissue sarcoma. Most children with sarcoma don't have this risk factor. They developed the disease for unknown reasons.

Age may affect risk. Adolescents and young adults develop osteosarcoma more often than any other age group. The Ewing family of tumors is most common in adolescents. Soft tissue sarcoma is rare in children at any age.

Bone Tumors and Sarcoma Stages

Staging refers to the way doctors classify cancer. They may consider where it is in the body, whether it has spread, its size, and several other factors.

The staging system is different for each type of cancer and sarcoma. Some cancer is staged only after surgery. The cancer's stage, along with your child's health and other factors, helps doctors choose treatments.

Osteosarcoma and Ewing tumors of the bone may be localized (in only one part of the body) or metastatic (spread to another part of the body).

Soft tissue sarcomas, including rhabdomyosarcoma, may be divided into four stages based on these factors:

- Whether the tumor is more than two inches across
- Whether the tumor has spread to lymph nodes
- Whether the tumor has spread to other areas of the body
- How much the tumor resembles normal tissue and how fast it is growing

Symptoms of Bone Tumors and Sarcoma

The signs and symptoms of bone tumors and sarcoma depend on the type of disease, where it is, and how much it has grown or spread. The symptoms listed here can also be caused by other health problems that are not cancer.

Symptoms by Disease

Symptoms of bone tumors and sarcoma vary by disease.

Ewing Sarcoma Symptoms

Ewing sarcoma may cause these symptoms:

- Unexplained lump with pain and swelling
- Pain in a bone or in the pelvis, back, or chest wall

Osteosarcoma Symptoms

Osteosarcoma may cause these symptoms:

- Bone or joint pain that gets worse
- Unexplained lump or swelling in the arm or leg
- Broken bone for no known reason

Soft Tissue Sarcoma Symptoms

Symptoms of soft tissue sarcoma can vary based on the location of the tumor. Children with rhabdomyosarcoma (sarcoma in a skeletal muscle) most often have a lump that grows quickly in their arm or leg. A tumor in or around the urinary tract can cause problems with urination. A tumor at the base of the skull can compress nerves, causing weakness or pain in the head.

Bone Tumor and Sarcoma Diagnosis

Your child's doctor will start with a thorough exam to look for signs of cancer and will ask about your child's health background. Then the doctor may suggest a number of tests to help tell the type of cancer and see whether it has spread.

If the doctor thinks that your child may have sarcoma, he will perform a biopsy to confirm the diagnosis.

Your child's doctor may also want your child to have pictures taken of the inside of her body, such as an X-ray, ultrasound, CT (computed tomography) scan, MRI (magnetic resonance imaging), or positron emission tomography (PET) scan.

These are called imaging studies, and they allow the doctor to look for tumors or areas of cancer activity.

Treatment

More than two-thirds of young patients with sarcoma survive without a return of their cancer (recurrence) for more than five years after their diagnosis. Most live much longer.

The cure rate ranges from 20% to 90%. It depends on the type of sarcoma, the extent of disease at the time of diagnosis, and how quickly the sarcoma responds to the first treatment.

Your child's doctor and health care team will suggest a treatment plan for your child based on many factors, such as:

- the type of sarcoma your child has;

- the location, size, and stage of the bone tumor or sarcoma;

- your child's age and overall health.

After the first round of treatment, your doctor will check to see how the cancer is responding and may change the treatment plan.

Treatment Basics by Disease

Many children receive more than one type of treatment.

Ewing Sarcoma Treatment

For this disease, doctors use chemotherapy. Many children also have surgery to remove tumors. Doctors may also suggest radiation because it tends to work well against this form of cancer.

Osteosarcoma Treatment

Children with this disease almost always have chemotherapy, then surgery to remove as much of the cancer as possible.

Soft Tissue Sarcoma Treatment

Treatment for this disease may depend on the location of the cancer. Most children have surgery to remove tumors. Doctors most often use chemotherapy and radiation as well to control the cancer or kill cancer that remains after surgery.

Many patients with sarcoma or other types of cancer take part in clinical trials.

These research studies give children the chance to get the very latest treatment options being studied—options that are not offered at all treatment centers.

Treatment Options for Bone Tumors and Sarcoma

Surgery

Surgery is common for some types of sarcoma. But it may not be the right choice in all cases. The first step may be a biopsy, a procedure used to check for cancer.

In some cases of soft tissue sarcoma, doctors use surgery to remove as much of the tumor as they can, along with some of the healthy tissue around it, before giving chemotherapy.

More often, doctors give chemotherapy first, before surgery. This is most common with osteosarcoma and Ewing sarcoma.

When doctors must remove bone, they may replace it with bone from somewhere else in the body or with a device, such as a metal implant. This helps support the bone that remains. Doctors add the device at the same time the tumor is taken out.

In rare cases of osteosarcoma or Ewing sarcoma in a child's arm or leg, doctors need to remove the whole limb. Our surgeons are leaders in operations called "limb sparing," which means removing areas of cancer in bone without having to amputate.

Fewer and fewer children need amputation as doctors learn more about how to use other treatments well along with less extensive surgery.

Chemotherapy

Chemotherapy means giving medicines that go throughout your child's body to kill cancer cells. These medicines spread around the body through the bloodstream.

Doctors can give these medicines through a vein, as a shot in the skin or muscle, or by mouth. The method depends on the medicine, and the type and location of the cancer.

The exact mix of medicines and how long they are given depend on the type of cancer or sarcoma your child has. Researchers are studying new mixes of medicines to find the most effective combination for each type of the disease.

This may be your child's main treatment. Doctors may also use chemotherapy before surgery to shrink a tumor and/or after surgery to kill any cancer cells that may still be in your child's body.

Radiation

Radiation uses high-energy X-rays to kill cancer cells and reduce the size of tumors.

Some types of sarcoma, such as Ewing sarcoma, tend to respond very well to this treatment. Others, such as osteosarcoma, do not respond as well.

Most often doctors give radiation using a machine outside the body to send rays to the right spot. In some cases, doctors give radiation by putting a small device inside the child's body.

Doctors sometimes use radiation before or after surgery. Before surgery, radiation is used to shrink a tumor so that it's easier to remove.

Even when doctors are able to remove the entire tumor, they may suspect or know that cancer cells are still in the child's body. They may use radiation after surgery to kill any remaining cancer cells.

New Treatments for Bone Tumors and Sarcoma

Researchers are doing studies to find more effective treatments for children with sarcoma.

They are looking for the best mixes of chemotherapy medicines and ways to use radiation with better results. They are also looking for new types of cancer treatments. Their main goals are to improve cure rates and reduce the risk of long-term effects from the disease and treatment.

One current line of research for Ewing sarcoma is in the area of stem cell transplant.

In this treatment, the child receives high-dose chemotherapy designed to kill cancer cells. Such high doses damage the child's bone marrow, which makes stem cells—cells that grow to become red blood cells, white blood cells, and platelets.

After the high-dose chemotherapy, doctors give the child an infusion of bone marrow or stem cells to create new bone marrow.

Your child's doctor will talk with you in detail about any new treatment that might be a match for your child. Then you can decide whether you want to try this option.

Section 17.5

Wilms Tumor (Nephroblastoma)

Most parents can't think of anything more frightening than being told their child has cancer. Fortunately, most kids with Wilms tumor, a rare kidney cancer, survive and go on to live normal, healthy lives due to the highly treatable nature of the disease.

Also known as nephroblastoma, Wilms tumor can affect both kidneys but usually develops in just one. Doctors believe that the tumor begins to grow as a fetus develops in the womb, with some cells that are destined to form into the kidneys malfunctioning and forming a tumor.

Signs and Symptoms

Before being diagnosed with Wilms tumor, most children do not show any signs of having cancer, and usually act and play normally. Often, a parent may discover a firm, smooth lump in the child's abdomen. It is not uncommon for the mass to grow quite large before it is discovered—the average Wilms tumor is one pound at diagnosis.

Some children also may have nausea, stomach pain, high blood pressure (hypertension), blood in the urine, loss of appetite, or fever.

Even though Wilms tumors often are large when found, most have not spread to other areas of the body. This makes it easier to successfully treat than if the cancer cells have spread (metastasized) to other parts of the body.

Diagnosis

Several tests are used to confirm a Wilms tumor diagnosis and determine the stage of the disease. Tests that might be used include:

- **Ultrasonography (ultrasound or US)**, usually the first tool used to diagnose the condition, uses sound waves instead of X-rays to generate an image of the area doctors wish to view.

- **CT or CAT scan** produces a detailed cross-sectional view of an organ through X-rays. It is extremely useful in detecting tumors and determining whether cancer has spread to other areas.

- **MRI** uses radio waves and strong magnets to produce detailed pictures of the internal parts of the body. This provides more intricate images that allow doctors to see if the cancer has invaded any major blood vessels near the kidney.

- **X-rays** are used to look for any metastasized areas, especially in the lungs.

- **Bone scans** use small amounts of radioactive material to highlight areas of diseased bone, if any exist.

- **Laboratory tests** such as blood tests and urinalysis check the general health of a patient and to detect any adverse side effects (such as low red or white blood cell counts) of the treatment.

The chance of Wilms tumor being hereditary ("running in the family") is so rare that there is no test to screen those who may pass the disease onto their offspring. However, certain genetic factors like birth defect syndromes can increase the likelihood of developing the disease. Those with a family history or personal history of Beckwith-Wiedemann syndrome (a condition associated with larger-than-normal internal organs), WAGR (marked by defects of the iris, kidneys, urinary tract, or genitalia), or Denys-Drash syndrome (a defect of the genitalia) are at risk.

Kids with risk factors for Wilms tumor should be screened for the disease through an ultrasound every three months until about age six or seven. Those at high risk may undergo screening until they're a little older.

Treatment

Treatment is determined by many factors, the most important being the stage of the cancer at diagnosis, and the condition, or histology, of the cancer cells when observed under a microscope. "Favorable" histology is associated with a good chance of a cure; tumors with "unfavorable" histology are more aggressive and difficult to cure. About 95% of Wilms tumors have favorable histology.

Doctors use a staging system to describe the extent of a metastasized tumor. It is extremely useful in determining prognosis (possibility for a cure) and the best course of treatment. For example, a child with very aggressive disease should be given an intensive regimen of medication to achieve the best chance for a cure. A child with less-invasive disease should be given the least amount needed to reduce long-term side effects from toxicity.

The stages are:

- **Stage I:** Cancer is found in one kidney only and can be completely removed by surgery. About 41% of all Wilms tumors are stage I.

- **Stage II:** Cancer has spread beyond the kidney to the surrounding area, but can be completely removed by surgery. About 23% are stage II.

- **Stage III:** Cancer has not spread beyond the abdomen, but cannot be completely removed by surgery. About 23% are stage III.

- **Stage IV:** Cancer has spread to distant parts of the body; most commonly, the lungs, liver, bone, and/or brain. About 10% are stage IV.

- **Stage V:** Cancer is found in both kidneys at diagnosis (also called bilateral tumors). About 5% are stage V.

Surgery is most often used to treat Wilms tumor. For stages I through IV, a radical nephrectomy removal of the cancer along with the entire kidney, ureter (tube that carries urine from the kidney to the bladder), adrenal gland (hormone-producing gland that sits on top of the kidney), and surrounding fatty tissue is done.

Since stage V patients have cancer involvement in both kidneys, removing both kidneys would result in kidney failure and the need for a kidney transplant. As a result, surgeons usually take out as much of the cancer as possible and preserve as much healthy kidney tissue as they can to avoid an organ transplant.

Regardless of the stage and histology, all treatment plans usually include both surgery and chemotherapy, and the more advanced stages also may require radiation therapy. Chemotherapy uses drugs (administered either orally or intravenously) to enter the bloodstream, circulate throughout the body, and kill cancerous cells wherever they may be. Radiation uses high-energy X-ray beams to kill specific cells in different areas of the body.

Both treatments have short-term and long-term risks. Temporary or short-term discomfort may include nausea and vomiting, loss of appetite, mouth sores, fatigue, loss of hair, weakened immune system (leaving a patient vulnerable to infection), and bleeding or bruising.

Long-term effects may include the development of secondary cancers (like leukemia) or the weakening of some internal organs, such as the heart. However, these risks are minimal the benefits of treatment far outweighs potential risks.

Caring for Your Child

As much as parents long to have their child out of the hospital, they often feel unsure of whether they can provide appropriate care after their child comes home. The doctors, nurses, and home health services should provide all the information and support needed to help a parent care for a child between hospital visits.

Depending on the treatment regimen (and a child's general health and the doctor's recommendations), appropriate at-home care can vary. Treatment for most children with Wilms tumor is not as intensive as treatment for other cancers (except for more advanced stages) so most kids won't have tremendous restrictions on them.

Most kids undergoing treatment for Wilms don't have special nutritional requirements or need medication for low blood cell counts, as most other cancer patients do. However, parents must watch for signs of distress, like fever, nausea, vomiting, or diarrhea. A child with a high fever should see a doctor right away.

Once a child is finished with therapy, the care team will provide a schedule of follow-up tests. Chest X-rays or CT scans may be taken every several months. Stage and histology of the cancer will determine the ultrasound schedule. Blood work and a physical exam may be required to check for adverse effects of the treatment.

For kids who relapse (the cancer returns), prognosis and treatment depend on their prior therapy, the cancer's histology, and how long it's been since the last treatment. The longer it's been, the better. There are few late recurrences of Wilms tumor, so remaining cancer-free for at least two years after treatment is generally a very good sign.

Chapter 18

Cardiovascular Disorders in Children

Chapter Contents

Section 18.1

Arrhythmia

"Children and Arrhythmia," "Types of Arrhythmia in Children," and
"Treating Arrhythmias in Children," reprinted with permission from
www.heart.org. © 2012 American Heart Association, Inc.

Children and Arrhythmia

If your child has been diagnosed with an abnormal heart rate, you're
probably alarmed. That's understandable. But by learning more about
your child's condition, you'll be less afraid. You'll also be better able to
care for your child.

About Heart Rhythms

The heart rate is the number of times the heart beats each minute.
In an older child or teenager who's resting, the heart beats about 70
times a minute. In a newborn it beats about 140 times a minute. Usually the heart rhythm is regular. This means the heart beats evenly
(at regular intervals). The heart rate changes easily. Exercise makes
the heart beat faster. During sleep it slows down.

An irregular heartbeat is an arrhythmia. The most common irregu-
larity occurs during breathing. When a child breathes in, the heart
rate normally speeds up for a few beats. When the child breathes out,
it slows down again. This variation with breathing is called sinus arrhythmia. It's completely normal.

Sometimes a doctor may find other kinds of arrhythmia. Then he or
she may want to perform some tests. The doctor may also recommend
that a pediatric cardiologist (a doctor specializing in children's heart
problems) examine your child.

Knowing Your Child's History

Arrhythmias (also called dysrhythmias) may occur at any age. Many
times they have no symptoms. Often parents and children never suspect an arrhythmia and are surprised when a doctor finds one during
a routine physical exam. Rhythm abnormalities are usually evaluated

much like other health problems. Your child's history—or what you and your child report about the problem—is very important. You may be asked questions like:

- Is your child aware of unusual heartbeats?
- Does anything bring on the arrhythmia? Is there anything your child or the family can do to make it stop?
- If it's a fast rate, how fast?
- Does your child feel weak, lightheaded, or dizzy?
- Has your child ever fainted?

Some medicines may make arrhythmias worse. Be sure to tell your doctor about all the prescribed and over-the-counter medications that your child takes. If your child has an arrhythmia, discuss this with the doctor and ask what to look for.

Types of Arrhythmia in Children

There are many different kinds of abnormal heart rhythms that may occur in children and adults. Learn about the types of arrhythmias that may occur and how they might manifest in children. If an abnormal rhythm occurs, it's important to find out what kind it is. Treatment recommendations depend on its type. Arrhythmias can cause the heart rate to be irregular, fast or slow. Fast rhythms are called tachycardia. Slow ones are called bradycardia.

Abnormal Heart Rhythms

Long Q-T Syndrome (LQTS)

LQTS is an infrequent, hereditary disorder of the heart's electrical rhythm that can occur in otherwise healthy people. It usually affects children or young adults. Studies of otherwise healthy people with LQTS indicate that they had at least one episode of fainting by the age of 10. The majority also had a family member with a long Q-T interval.

When the heart contracts, it emits an electrical signal. This signal can be recorded on an electrocardiogram (ECG) and produces a characteristic waveform. The different parts of this waveform are designated by letters—P, Q, R, S, and T. The Q-T interval represents the time for electrical activation and inactivation of the ventricles, the lower chambers of the heart. A doctor can measure the time it takes for the Q-T interval to occur (in fractions of a second), and can tell if it occurs in a normal amount of time. If it takes longer than normal, it's called a prolonged Q-T interval.

What are the symptoms of LQTS? People with LQTS may not have any symptoms. People who do have symptoms often exhibit fainting (syncope) and abnormal rate and/or rhythm of the heartbeat (arrhythmia). People with this syndrome may show prolongation of the Q-T interval during physical exercise, intense emotion (such as fright, anger, or pain), or when startled by a noise. Some arrhythmias are potentially fatal, causing sudden death. In one type of inherited LQTS, the person may also become deaf.

People with LQTS don't necessarily have a prolonged Q-T interval all the time. At the time that they have an electrocardiogram (such as during a routine physical examination), the Q-T interval may actually be normal. Alternatively, some healthy young people may not have a routine ECG, and LQTS may be suspected because of their family history or because of unexplained fainting episodes. In any family where repeated episodes of fainting or a history of sudden death exists, an investigation of the cause, including LQTS, should be undertaken.

How is LQTS treated? There are treatments for LQTS, including medications such as beta blockers. Sometimes a surgical procedure is performed, and some people may benefit from an implantable defibrillator.

Premature Atrial Contraction (PAC) and Premature Ventricular Contraction (PVC)

Premature beats or extra beats most often cause irregular heart rhythms. Those that start in the upper chambers (atria) are called premature atrial contractions or PACs. Premature ventricular contractions or PVCs start in the ventricles. If you've ever had the feeling that your heart "skipped a beat," it was probably from this type of arrhythmia. The heart really doesn't skip a beat. Instead, an extra beat comes sooner than normal. Then there's usually a pause that causes the next beat to be more forceful. You felt this more-forceful beat.

Premature beats are very common in normal children and teenagers— most people have them at some time. Usually no cause can be found and no special treatment is needed. The premature beats may disappear later. Even if they continue, your child will stay well and won't need any restrictions. Occasionally premature beats may be caused by disease or injury to the heart. Your child's doctor may recommend more tests to make sure your child's heart is okay.

Tachycardia

A fast heart rate is called tachycardia. The definition of "too fast" usually depends on the person's age and physical activity. A newborn has tachycardia if the resting rate is more than 160 beats per minute. A teenager is considered to have tachycardia if the resting heart rate is more than 90 beats per minute. An exercising teenager may have a normal heart rate of up to 200 beats per minute.

Sinus Tachycardia

Sinus tachycardia is a normal increase in the heart rate. It occurs with fever, excitement, and exercise. No treatment is needed. Rarely, disease, such as anemia (low blood counts) or increased thyroid activity, can cause this fast heart rate. In these cases, when the disease is treated, the tachycardia goes away.

Supraventricular Tachycardia (SVT)

The most common abnormal tachycardia in children is supraventricular tachycardia. It's also called paroxysmal atrial tachycardia (PAT) or paroxysmal supraventricular tachycardia (PSVT). The fast heart rate involves both the heart's upper and lower chambers. This isn't a life-threatening problem for most children and adolescents. Treatment is only considered if episodes are prolonged or frequent. For many infants, SVT is a time-limited problem. Treatment with medications often stops after 6 to 12 months.

SVT may occur in very young infants with otherwise-normal hearts. The heart rate is usually more than 220 beats a minute. Infants with an SVT episode may breathe faster than normal and seem fussy or sleepier than usual. This situation must be diagnosed and treated to return the heart rate to normal. Once the rhythm is normal, medication usually can prevent future episodes.

Sometimes SVT can be detected while a baby is still in the womb. Then the mother may take medications to slow her baby's heart rate. If an older infant or child has SVT, the child may be aware of the rapid heart rate. This may be associated with palpitations, dizziness, lightheadedness, chest discomfort, upset stomach, or weakness. Some children can learn ways to slow down their heart rate. Straining—such as closing the nose and mouth and trying to breathe out—may be successful. This is called a Valsalva maneuver.

Older children are more likely to have more episodes of tachycardia. They're more likely to need prolonged treatment. They also may need more diagnostic tests. It's unusual for episodes of SVT to keep a child from enjoying normal activities. Most children who have episodes of tachycardia stay well even though they may need to keep taking medicine. Your child will probably need periodic check-ups but will be able to enjoy unrestricted normal activities.

Treating SVT usually has two parts. The first is stopping a current episode; the second is preventing recurrences. The approach to preventing recurrences depends on the child's age. In some cases—especially those of infants—the child may need to enter the hospital for treatment and special studies.

Sometimes simple procedures can stop a fast heart rhythm. Gagging or putting ice on the face are examples. Your child's doctor can explain this to you in more detail. At other times intravenous medications may be needed to control or stop the tachycardia. Another way to stop SVT is to place a small catheter (a thin, flexible tube) through the nostril into the esophagus. A small amount of electricity is sent through this catheter to stop the SVT. On rare occasions doctors stop SVT by giving a small electrical shock to the chest wall. This is called electrical countershock or cardioversion. A sedative or anesthetic is given before this procedure.

Wolff-Parkinson-White Syndrome

If an abnormal conduction pathway runs between the atria and ventricles, the electrical signal may arrive at the ventricles sooner than normal. This condition is called Wolff-Parkinson-White syndrome (WPW syndrome). It's named after the three people who first described it. WPW syndrome is recognized by certain changes on the ECG. Many people with WPW syndrome don't have symptoms but are at risk of sudden cardiac arrest.

Often medication can improve this condition. Sometimes, though, such treatment doesn't work. Then your child will need more tests. Eliminating the abnormal pathway by passing energy through a catheter may be needed. Surgery is another option.

Ventricular Tachycardia (VT)

Ventricular tachycardia is a fast heart rate that starts in the lower chambers (ventricles). This uncommon but potentially serious condition can threaten a child's life. VT may result from serious heart disease; it usually requires prompt treatment. VT occasionally occurs in children with otherwise normal hearts. Often specialized tests, including an intracardiac electrophysiologic procedure, may be needed to evaluate the tachycardia and the effect of drug treatment. Some forms of VT may not need treatment.

If treatment is required, it includes medicines and addressing the cause, if possible. The type and length of treatment depends on what's causing the problem. In some people radiofrequency ablation or surgery may be needed to control the tachycardia.

Bradycardia

A heart rate that's too slow is called bradycardia. What's "too slow" depends on a person's age and activity. A newborn usually won't have a heart rate of less than 80 beats a minute. An athletically trained teenager may have a normal resting heart rate of 50 beats a minute.

Sick Sinus Syndrome

Sometimes the sinus node doesn't work properly. Some children who've had open-heart surgery have this problem. When the sinus node's work is seriously disturbed, it's called sick sinus syndrome. A child with this syndrome may not have any symptoms or may be tired, dizzy, or faint. Children with sick sinus syndrome have episodes of tachycardia and bradycardia. Fortunately, sick sinus syndrome is unusual in children. If it does occur, an artificial pacemaker, medications, or both may be needed.

Complete Heart Block

Heart block means that the heart's electrical signal can't pass normally from the upper to the lower chambers. The electrical signal within the heart is blocked, not the blood flow. When this occurs, another "natural" pacemaker in the lower chambers takes over, but at a slower rate.

Heart block may be present at—or even before—birth. (This is congenital heart block.) Disease or an injury to the electrical conduction system during heart surgery can also cause it. When the natural pacemaker in the lower chambers isn't fast enough or reliable enough, an artificial pacemaker is put in.

Treating Arrhythmias in Children

Many options are available to treat rhythm abnormalities in children. Most treatment is directed at a specific problem. A detailed discussion of all the options isn't possible here.

Medications

Many rhythm disorders, especially tachycardias, respond to medications. Several drugs are now available and more are being developed. These drugs can't cure the arrhythmia, but they can improve symptoms. They do this by preventing the episodes from starting, decreasing the heart rate during the episode, or shortening how long the episode lasts.

Sometimes it's hard to find the best medication for a child. Several drugs may need to be tried before the right one is found. Some children must take medication every day; others need medications only when they have a tachycardia episode. It's very important to take the medication as prescribed.

All medications have side effects, including drugs to treat arrhythmias. Most of the side effects aren't serious and disappear when the dose is changed or the medication is stopped. But some side effects are very serious. That's why some children are admitted to the hospital to begin the medication. If your child is prescribed medication, it's very important that your child take the medication just the way the doctor prescribes it.

It's often necessary to monitor how much of a drug is in your child's blood. The goal is to make sure there's enough of the drug to be effective, but not so much that harmful side effects occur. These blood tests require taking a small amount of blood from a vein or the finger. It's a good idea to talk to your child about this before the doctor visit.

Other Treatments

Radiofrequency ablation: Some tachycardias are life-threatening or significantly interfere with a child's normal activities. These problems may warrant more permanent treatment. One procedure, called radiofrequency catheter ablation, is done with several catheters in the heart. One is positioned right over the area that's causing the tachycardia. Then its tip is heated and that small area of the heart is altered so electrical current won't pass through the tissue.

Surgery: Sometimes surgery that interrupts the abnormal connection in the heart is required to permanently stop the tachycardia.

Artificial pacemaker: A variety of rhythm disorders can be controlled with an artificial pacemaker. Slow heart rates, such as heart block, are the most common reason to use a pacemaker. But new technology now let's doctors treat some fast heart rates with a pacemaker, too. An artificial pacemaker is a small device (one to two ounces, 1.5 by 1.5 inches). It's put inside the body and connected to the heart with a thin wire. It works by sending small, painless amounts of electricity to the heart to make it beat.

Inserting a pacemaker is a simple operation. The wires are attached to the heart, and the pacemaker is placed in the abdomen (belly) or under the skin of the chest wall. Sometimes only one wire is attached to the heart. In other cases two wires are used. Many different models and brands of pacemakers exist. Some can sense when your child is active and increase the heart's beating to keep up with exercise.

If your child has a pacemaker, he or she will need regular checkups. It's important to check the pacemaker's battery and make sure the wires are working properly. Pacemaker batteries usually last for years, but the pacemaker will still need to be replaced periodically throughout the user's lifetime. Sometimes the wires also need to be replaced. Regular checkups can show if anything needs replacing.

Most children with pacemakers can engage in normal activities. Your doctor may advise against participating in some contact sports, however. Talk to your child's cardiologist about this.

Section 18.2

Heart Murmurs

"Heart Murmurs," reprinted with permission from www.heart.org. © 2012 American Heart Association, Inc.

What causes heart murmurs?

Heart murmurs are most often caused by defective heart valves. A stenotic heart valve has a smaller-than-normal opening and can't open completely. A valve may also be unable to close completely. This leads to regurgitation, which is blood leaking backward through the valve when it should be closed.

Murmurs also can be caused by conditions such as pregnancy, fever, thyrotoxicosis (a diseased condition resulting from an overactive thyroid gland), or anemia.

A diastolic murmur occurs when the heart muscle relaxes between beats. A systolic murmur occurs when the heart muscle contracts.

Systolic murmurs are graded by intensity (loudness) from one to six. A grade 1/6 is very faint, heard only with a special effort. A grade 6/6 is extremely loud. It's heard with a stethoscope slightly removed from the chest.

What are innocent heart murmurs?

Innocent heart murmurs are sounds made by the blood circulating through the heart's chambers and valves or through blood vessels near the heart. They're sometimes called other names such as "functional" or "physiologic" murmurs.

Are innocent heart murmurs normal?

Innocent murmurs are common in children and are quite harmless. In any group of children, a large percentage is likely to have had one at some time. Innocent murmurs also may disappear and then reappear. Most innocent murmurs disappear when a child reaches adulthood, but some adults still have them. When a child's heart rate changes, such as during excitement or fear, the innocent murmurs may become louder or softer. This still doesn't mean that the murmur is abnormal.

Sometimes, when a doctor first hears the murmur through a stethoscope, he or she may want to have other tests done to be sure the murmur is innocent. After that, there's no need for a cardiac reevaluation unless the patient or doctor has more questions. The child doesn't need medication, won't have cardiac symptoms, and doesn't have a heart problem or heart disease. A parent doesn't need to pamper the child or restrict his or her diet or activities. The child can be as active as any other normal, healthy child.

Section 18.3

Hyperlipidemia (High Cholesterol)

Adults are not the only people affected by high cholesterol. Children also might have high levels of cholesterol, which can result in health concerns when the child gets older. Too much cholesterol leads to a build-up of a material, called plaque, on the walls of the arteries that supply blood to the heart and other organs. Plaque can narrow the arteries and block the blood flow to the heart, causing heart problems. Cholesterol also is related to other health problems including stroke.

What Causes High Cholesterol in Children?

Cholesterol levels in children are linked to three factors: heredity, diet, and obesity. In most cases, kids with high cholesterol have a parent who also has elevated cholesterol.

How Is High Cholesterol in Children Diagnosed?

Health care professionals can check cholesterol in school-age children with a simple blood test. Conducting such a test is especially important if there is a strong family history of heart disease or if a parent of the child has high cholesterol. The blood test results will reveal whether a child's cholesterol is too high.

Updated guidelines and recommendations for the treatment of high cholesterol in children eight years of age and older were issued by the American Academy of Pediatrics in July 2008. These guidelines recommend medical treatment of elevated LDL ([low-density lipoprotein] bad cholesterol) if the value is greater than 190 mg/dL in patients with no risk factors for cardiovascular disease if diet modification has been unsuccessful. Medical treatment is recommended for patients with an LDL greater than 160 mg/dL who have a family history of premature onset of cardiovascular disease or other risk factors, including obesity, hypertension, or cigarette smoking. Medical treatment is recommended for patients with an LDL greater than 130 mg/dL who have diabetes.

How Is High Cholesterol in Children Treated?

The best way to treat cholesterol in children is with a diet and exercise program that involves the entire family. If changes in diet and exercise do not have the desired effect, medicine might be considered for children older than eight years. Some drugs used to treat cholesterol in children include cholestyramine, colestipol, and colesevelam. Recent studies in children with very high cholesterol have supported the safe use of drugs in the statin class. A child's cholesterol levels should be retested after three months of dietary changes and/or medicines.

Help Lower Your Child's Cholesterol

You can help lower your child's cholesterol levels by encouraging your child to do the following:

- Eat foods low in total fat, saturated fat, and cholesterol. The amount of fat a child consumes should be 30% or less of daily total calories (45 to 65 grams of fat or less per day). This suggestion does *not* apply to children under the age of two.

- The American Academy of Pediatrics currently recommends that children two years and older follow a healthy diet according to the current Dietary Guidelines for Americans This should include low-fat dairy products. For children 12 months to two years of age who are overweight or obese, or who have a family history of obesity, high cholesterol, or cardiovascular disease, the use of reduced-fat milk is recommended.

- Exercise regularly. Regular aerobic exercise—such as biking, running, walking, and swimming—can help raise HDL [high-density lipoprotein] levels and lower your family's risk for cardiovascular disease.

- Maintain a healthy weight.

- Substitute unsaturated fat for saturated fat. Saturated fat is usually solid at room temperature and comes from animal fats, coconut, and palm oils. Unsaturated fat is liquid at room temperature and comes from plants. Olive oil, canola oil, and peanut oil are examples of unsaturated fat.

- Select a variety of foods so your child can get all the nutrients he or she needs.

- Children and adolescents at higher risk for cardiovascular disease with elevated LDL values above their target goals are advised to undergo nutritional counseling and engage in regular physical activity.

What Are Some Examples of Good Foods?

- **For breakfast:** Fruit, cereal, oatmeal, and yogurt are among the good choices for breakfast foods. Use skim or low-fat milk rather than whole or 2% milk.

- **For lunch and dinner:** Bake or grill foods instead of frying them. Use whole-grain breads and rolls to make a healthier sandwich. Also, give your child whole-grain crackers with soups, chili, and stew. Prepare pasta, beans, rice, fish, skinless poultry, or other dishes. Always serve fresh fruit (with the skin) with meals.

- **For snacks:** Fruits, vegetables, breads, and cereals make great snacks for children. Children should avoid soda and fruit drinks.

Section 18.4

Hypertension (High Blood Pressure)

Can children develop high blood pressure?

Despite popular belief, teens, children, and even babies can have high blood pressure. It's not just a disease for the middle-aged and elderly. As with adults, early diagnosis and treatment can reduce or prevent the harmful consequences of this disease.

AHA recommendation: The American Heart Association recommends that all children have yearly blood pressure measurements. Detecting high blood pressure early will improve a child's health.

What is considered "normal" blood pressure in children?

When it comes to blood pressure in children, "normal" is relative. It depends on three factors:

- Gender
- Age
- Height

Your child's doctor can tell you what's right for your child, because "normal" is a complicated calculation based on these factors.

What leads to HBP in children?

- **Diseases including heart and kidney disease:** Certain diseases can cause high blood pressure in children as well as adults. As with all types of secondary hypertension, once the underlying problem is fixed, blood pressure usually returns to normal.

- **Some medications:** Certain medicines can cause high blood pressure, but when they're discontinued, blood pressure usually returns to normal. This is another example of secondary hypertension.

- **Contributing factors:** In a lot of cases, doctors cannot determine the direct cause of HBP in the child. This type of HBP is known as primary or "essential" hypertension. Even though the exact cause is not diagnosed, doctors realize a variety of factors can contribute to the disease, including:

  - family history;
  - excess weight or obesity;
  - race, particularly African-Americans are at increased risk.

What is the treatment for children with high blood pressure?

As in adults, HBP in children is typically managed with lifestyle changes, including:

- enjoying a heart-healthy diet;
- participating in regular physical activity;
- managing weight.

Children and teens should also be taught the dangers of tobacco use and protected from secondhand smoke. While cigarettes aren't directly related to high blood pressure, they do cause a number of health risks. Parents should set a good example by not smoking and educating their children about the hazards of smoking.

The doctor may also prescribe medication if an appropriate diet and regular physical activity don't bring the high blood pressure under control.

Give your kids the best possible start by helping them develop heart-healthy habits early.

A note about adolescents and teenagers: Age, body size, and the degree of sexual maturation determine blood pressure levels in adolescence. Heavier and more sexually mature teenagers tend to have higher blood pressure.

According to research, teenagers who are obese and have high blood pressure may develop thicker arteries by age 30. Fatty buildups in artery walls can lead to a variety of health problems including heart disease and stroke. To help manage children's health risks, parents should partner with the family doctor to:

- help boys and girls manage their own weight and make healthy choices as adolescents;

- discover ways to support and build new habits if the child is already overweight.

Section 18.5

Kawasaki Disease

"Kawasaki Disease," "Kawasaki Disease: Signs, Symptoms, and Diagnosis," and "Kawasaki Disease: Complications, Treatment and Prevention," reprinted with permission from www.heart.org. © 2012 American Heart Association, Inc.

Kawasaki Disease

Kawasaki disease (mucocutaneous lymph node syndrome) is a children's illness characterized by fever, rash, swelling of the hands and feet, irritation and redness of the whites of the eyes, swollen lymph glands in the neck, and irritation and inflammation of the mouth, lips, and throat. These immediate effects of Kawasaki disease are rarely serious; however, long-term heart complications result in some cases and can be seen as early as two weeks after onset of the disease.

Named after Dr. Tomisaku Kawasaki, a Japanese pediatrician, the disease has probably been in existence for a long time but was not recognized as a separate entity until 1967. The incidence is higher in Japan than in any other country. In the United States it is more frequent among children of Asian-American background but can occur in any racial or ethnic group. The disease is relatively common, and in the United States it is a major cause of heart disease in children. In recent years, it has tended to occur in localized outbreaks, most often in the late winter or spring, but is seen year-round. Kawasaki disease almost always affects children; most patients are under five years old, and the average age is about two. Boys develop the illness almost twice as often as girls.

The heart may be affected in as many as one of five children who develop Kawasaki disease. Damage sometimes occurs to the blood vessels that supply the heart muscle (the coronary arteries) and to the heart muscle itself. A weakening of a coronary artery can result in an enlargement or swelling of the blood vessel wall (an aneurysm). Infants less than one year old are usually the most seriously ill and are at greatest risk for heart involvement. The acute phase of Kawasaki disease commonly lasts 10 to 14 days or more. Most children recover fully. The likelihood of developing coronary artery disease later in life is not known and remains the subject of medical investigation.

Cause

The cause of Kawasaki disease is unknown. It does not appear to be hereditary or contagious. Because the illness frequently occurs in outbreaks, an infectious agent (such as a virus) is the likely cause. It is very rare for more than one child in a family to develop Kawasaki disease.

Signs, Symptoms, and Diagnosis

Fever and irritability are often the first indications of the disease. Fever ranges from moderate (101° to 103° F) to high (above 104° F). The lymph glands in the neck may become swollen. A rash usually appears on the back, chest, and abdomen early in the illness; in infants it may develop in the groin. In some cases, the rash may spread to the face. The rash appears as poorly defined spots of various sizes, often bright red. Fever continues to rise and fall, sometimes for as long as three weeks. Bloodshot eyes may develop, and the eyes can become sensitive to light.

The child's tongue may be coated, slightly swollen, and resemble the surface of a strawberry, sometimes referred to as "strawberry tongue." The lips may become red, dry, and cracked; the inside of the mouth may turn darker red than usual.

The palms of the hands and soles of the feet often become red, and hands and feet may swell. Occasionally, a stiff neck will develop. Some children have abdominal pain and diarrhea.

When the fever subsides, the rash and swollen lymph glands usually disappear. The skin around the toenails and fingernails often peels painlessly, usually during the second or third week of illness. The skin on the hands or feet may peel in large pieces.

The knees, hips, and ankles may become swollen and painful. Occasionally joint pain and swelling persist after other symptoms have disappeared, but permanent joint damage doesn't occur. Lines or ridges on fingernails and toenails, formed during the illness, may be seen for weeks or months.

Diagnosis

The diagnosis of Kawasaki disease cannot be made by a single laboratory test or combination of tests. Physicians make the diagnosis after carefully examining a child, observing signs and symptoms and eliminating the possibility of other, similar diseases. Blood tests are used to detect mild anemia, an elevated white blood cell count, and an elevated sedimentation rate, indicating inflammation. A sharp increase in the number of platelets, a major clotting element in blood, also may be found. Urine tests may reveal the presence of protein (albumin) and white blood cells. An echocardiogram (or echo) is used to look for possible damage to the heart or to the coronary arteries that supply blood to the heart muscle. Other blood tests or diagnostic studies may be requested by the physician.

Complications, Treatment and Prevention

Complications

The possibility of heart and coronary artery involvement makes Kawasaki disease unpredictable, but these problems usually are not serious and disappear with time. However, on occasion aneurysm of coronary or other arteries of the body can occur, and some may require medical or surgical treatment. Very rarely, complications may include heart attacks, which can be fatal.

Treatment

Kawasaki disease is frequently treated in the hospital, with a stay from a few days to a few weeks. Some children may receive care at home without hospitalization.

Even though the cause of Kawasaki disease is unknown, specific medications are known to be beneficial. Aspirin is used to reduce fever, rash, joint inflammation, and pain, and to prevent formation of blood clots. Recent studies from Japan, the United States, and other countries indicate that another medication, intravenous gamma globulin, decreases the risk of developing heart disease when given early in the illness. A major goal of treatment both in the hospital and at home is to make a child as comfortable as possible while the illness runs its course.

If tests reveal an aneurysm or other heart or blood vessel abnormality, repeated echocardiograms or other tests may be necessary for several years following recovery from Kawasaki disease. Almost all children return to completely normal activity after the acute phase of the illness. Even if there is no evidence of a heart abnormality when your child recovers from the acute phase of Kawasaki disease, it is important to bring your child in for a follow-up visit with your doctor to be sure that there aren't heart problems that did not show up right away.

Prevention

There is no known prevention for Kawasaki disease. Approximately one child in a hundred may develop the disease a second time. Parents should know that nothing they could have done would have prevented the disease.

Chapter 19

Diabetes in Children

Diabetes mellitus is a group of diseases characterized by high levels of glucose in the blood resulting from defects in insulin production, insulin action, or both. Diabetes is associated with serious complications and premature death, but timely diagnosis and treatment of diabetes can prevent or delay the onset of long-term complications (damage to the cardiovascular system, kidneys, eyes, nerves, blood vessels, skin, gums, and teeth). New management strategies are helping children with diabetes live long and healthy lives.

Type 1 diabetes in U.S. children and adolescents is increasing and more new cases of type 2 diabetes are being reported in young people.

Statistics

Diabetes is one of the most common diseases in school-aged children. According to the 2011 National Diabetes Fact Sheet, about 215,000 young people in the United States under age 20 had diabetes in 2010. This represents 0.26% of all people in this age group.

Based on data from 2002 to 2005, the SEARCH for Diabetes in Youth study reported that approximately 15,600 U.S. youth less than 20 years of age were diagnosed annually with type 1 diabetes, while 3,600 were newly diagnosed with type 2 diabetes. Type 2 diabetes was

This chapter excerpted from "Overview of Diabetes in Children and Adolescents," National Diabetes Education Program (ndep.nih.gov), June 2011.

rare in children younger than 10 years of age, regardless of race or ethnicity. In youth aged 10 to 19 years, type 2 diabetes became increasingly common, especially in minority populations.

Type 1 Diabetes

Type 1 diabetes accounts for 5% to 10% of all diagnosed cases of diabetes but is the leading cause of diabetes in children of all ages. Type 1 diabetes accounts for almost all diabetes in children less than 10 years of age. Type 1 diabetes is an autoimmune disease in which the immune system destroys the insulin-producing beta cells of the pancreas that help regulate blood glucose levels.

Onset: Type 1 diabetes mostly has an acute onset, with children and adolescents usually able to pinpoint when symptoms began. Onset can occur at any age, but it most often occurs in children and young adults. Children and adolescents may present with ketoacidosis as the first indication of type 1 diabetes. Others may have post-meal hyperglycemia, or modest fasting hyperglycemia that rapidly progresses to severe hyperglycemia and/or ketoacidosis in the presence of infection or other stress.

Symptoms: The immunologic process that leads to type 1 diabetes can begin years before the symptoms of type 1 diabetes develop. Symptoms become apparent when most of the beta-cell population is destroyed and usually develop over a short period of time. Early symptoms, which are mainly due to hyperglycemia, include increased thirst and urination, constant hunger, weight loss, and blurred vision. Children also may feel very tired.

As insulin deficiency worsens, ketoacids, formed from the breakdown of fat, build up in the blood and are excreted in the urine and breath. Ketoacids cause shortness of breath and abdominal pain, vomiting, and worsening dehydration. Elevation of blood glucose, acidosis, and dehydration comprise the condition known as diabetic ketoacidosis or DKA. If diabetes is not diagnosed and treated with insulin at this point, the individual can lapse into a life-threatening coma. Often, children with vomiting are mistakenly diagnosed as having gastroenteritis.

Risk factors: A combination of genetic and environmental factors put people at increased risk for type 1 diabetes. Researchers are working to identify these factors so that targeted treatments can be designed to stop the autoimmune process that destroys the pancreatic beta-cells.

Co-morbidities: Children with type 1 diabetes are at risk for the long-term complications of diabetes. Autoimmune diseases such as celiac disease and autoimmune thyroiditis are also associated with type 1 diabetes.

Management: The basic elements of type 1 diabetes management are insulin administration (either by injection or insulin pump), nutrition management, physical activity, blood glucose testing, the avoidance of severe hypoglycemia, and the avoidance of prolonged hyperglycemia or DKA.

All people with diabetes are advised to avoid "liquid carbs (carbohydrates)" such as sugar-containing soda and juices (including 100% fruit juice) and regular pancake syrup. The liquid carbs raise blood glucose rapidly, contain large amounts of carbs in small volumes, are hard to balance with insulin, and provide little or no nutrition.

Children receiving fixed insulin doses of intermediate- and rapid-acting insulins must have food given at the time of peak action of the insulin. They need a consistent carb meal plan that aims for a set amount of carb grams at each meal (e.g., 60 grams of carbs at lunch) and snack since they do not adjust their mealtime insulin for the amount of carb intake.

Children receiving a long-acting insulin analogue or using an insulin pump receive a rapid-acting insulin analogue just before meals, with the amount of pre-meal insulin based on carb content of the meal using an insulin to carb ratio and a correction scale for hyperglycemia. Sources of carbs include starches (breads, crackers, cereal, pasta, rice), fruits and vegetables, dried beans and peas, milk, yogurt, and sweets. In addition to the amount of insulin needed to cover the carbs, extra insulin might be needed if the youth's blood glucose is above the target range before a meal or snack. Further adjustment of insulin or food intake may be made based on anticipation of special circumstances such as increased exercise and intercurrent illness. Children on these regimens are expected to check their blood glucose levels routinely before meals and at bedtime.

Physical activity is a critical element of effective diabetes management. In addition to maintaining cardiovascular fitness and controlling weight, physical activity can help to lower blood glucose levels. To maintain blood glucose levels within the target range during extra physical activity, students will need to adjust their insulin and food intake.

Helping Children and Adolescents Manage Diabetes

The health care professional team, in partnership with the young person with diabetes and parents or other caregivers, needs to develop a personal diabetes management plan and daily schedule. The plan helps the child or teen to follow a healthy meal plan, get regular physical activity, check blood glucose levels, take insulin or oral medication as prescribed, and manage hyperglycemia and hypoglycemia.

Follow a healthy meal plan: Young people with diabetes need to follow a meal plan developed by a registered dietitian, diabetes educator, or physician. For children with type 1 diabetes, the meal plan must ensure proper nutrition for growth. For children with type 2, the meal plan should outline appropriate changes in eating habits that lead to better energy balance and reduce or prevent obesity. A meal plan also helps keep blood glucose levels in the target range.

Children or adolescents and their families can learn how different types of food can affect blood glucose levels. Portion sizes, the right amount of calories for the child's age and activity level, and ideas for healthy food choices at meal and snack time also should be discussed, including reduction in soda and juice intake. Family support for following the meal plan and setting up regular meal times are keys to success, especially if the child or teen is taking insulin.

Get regular physical activity: Children with diabetes need regular physical activity, ideally a total of 60 minutes each day. Physical activity helps to lower blood glucose levels and increase insulin sensitivity, especially in children and adolescents with type 2 diabetes. Physical activity is also a good way to help children control their weight. In children with type 1 diabetes, the most common problem encountered during physical activity is hypoglycemia. If possible, a child or a teen should check blood glucose levels before beginning a game or a sport. If blood glucose levels are too low, the child should not be physically active until the low blood glucose level has been treated.

Check blood glucose levels regularly: Young people with diabetes should know the acceptable range for their blood glucose. Children, particularly those using insulin, should check blood glucose values regularly with a blood glucose meter, preferably one with a built-in memory. A health care team member can teach the child or teen how to use a blood glucose meter properly and how often to use it. Children should keep a journal or other records such as downloaded computer files of their glucose meter results to discuss with their health care team. This information helps providers make any needed changes to the child's or teen's personal diabetes plan.

Take all diabetes medication as prescribed: Parents, caregivers, school nurses, and others can help a child or teen learn how to take medications as prescribed. For type 1 diabetes, a child or teen takes insulin at prescribed times each day via multiple injections or an insulin pump. Some young people with type 2 diabetes need oral medication or insulin or both. In any case, it is important to stress that all medication should be balanced with food and activity every day.

Special Issues

Care of children and teens with diabetes requires integration of diabetes management with the complicated physical and emotional growth needs of children, adolescents, and their families, as well as consideration of teens' emerging autonomy and independence.

Diabetes presents unique issues for young people with the disease. Simple things, such as going to a birthday party, playing sports, or staying overnight with friends, need careful planning. Checking blood glucose, making correct food choices, and taking insulin or oral medication can make school-age children feel "different" from their classmates, and this can be particularly bothersome for teens.

For any child or teen with diabetes, learning to cope with the disease is a big task. Dealing with a chronic illness such as diabetes may cause emotional and behavioral challenges, sometimes leading to depression. Talking to a social worker or psychologist may help young people and their families learn to adjust to the lifestyle changes needed to stay healthy.

Family support: Managing diabetes in children and adolescents is most effective when the entire family gets involved. Families can be encouraged to share concerns with physicians, diabetes educators, dietitians, and other health care team members to get their help in the day-to-day management of diabetes. Extended family members, teachers, school nurses, counselors, coaches, day care providers, and others in the community can provide information, support, guidance, and help with coping skills. These individuals also may be knowledgeable about resources for health education, financial services, social services, mental health counseling, transportation, and home visits.

Diabetes is stressful for both children and their families. Parents should be alert for signs of depression or eating disorders or insulin omission to lose weight and seek appropriate treatment. While all parents should talk to their children about avoiding tobacco, alcohol, and other drugs, this is particularly important for children with diabetes. People with diabetes who smoke have a greatly increased risk of heart disease and circulatory problems. Binge drinking can cause

313

hyperglycemia acutely, followed by an increased risk of hypoglycemia. The symptoms of intoxication are very similar to the symptoms of hypoglycemia and thus may result in delay of treatment of hypoglycemia with potentially disastrous consequences.

Chapter 20

Ear, Nose, and Throat Disorders in Children

Chapter Contents

Section 20.1

Ear Infection (Otitis Media)

This section excerpted from "Ear Infections in Children,"
National Institute on Deafness and Other Communication Disorders
(www.nidcd.nih.gov), October 2010.

What is an ear infection?

An ear infection is an inflammation of the middle ear, usually caused by bacteria, that occurs when fluid builds up behind the eardrum. Anyone can get an ear infection, but children get them more often than adults. Three out of four children will have at least one ear infection by their third birthday. In fact, ear infections are the most common reason parents bring their child to a doctor. The scientific name for an ear infection is otitis media (OM).

What are the symptoms of an ear infection?

There are three main types of ear infections. Each has a different combination of symptoms.

- **Acute otitis media (AOM)** is the most common ear infection. Parts of the middle ear are infected and swollen and fluid is trapped behind the eardrum. This causes pain in the ear—commonly called an earache. Your child might also have a fever.

- **Otitis media with effusion (OME)** sometimes happens after an ear infection has run its course and fluid stays trapped behind the eardrum. A child with OME may have no symptoms, but a doctor will be able to see the fluid behind the eardrum with a special instrument.

- **Chronic otitis media with effusion (COME)** happens when fluid remains in the middle ear for a long time or returns over and over again, even though there is no infection. COME makes it harder for children to fight new infections and also can affect their hearing.

How can I tell if my child has an ear infection?

Most ear infections happen to children before they've learned how to talk. If your child isn't old enough to say "My ear hurts," here are a few things to look for:

- Tugging or pulling at the ear(s)
- Fussiness and crying
- Trouble sleeping
- Fever (especially in infants and younger children)
- Fluid draining from the ear
- Clumsiness or problems with balance
- Trouble hearing or responding to quiet sounds

What causes an ear infection?

An ear infection usually is caused by bacteria and often begins after a child has a sore throat, cold, or other upper respiratory infection. If the upper respiratory infection is bacterial, these same bacteria may spread to the middle ear; if the upper respiratory infection is caused by a virus, such as a cold, bacteria may be drawn to the microbe-friendly environment and move into the middle ear as a secondary infection. Because of the infection, fluid builds up behind the eardrum.

Why are children more likely than adults to get ear infections?

There are several reasons why children are more likely than adults to get ear infections.

Eustachian tubes are smaller and more level in children than they are in adults. This makes it difficult for fluid to drain out of the ear, even under normal conditions. If the eustachian tubes are swollen or blocked with mucus due to a cold or other respiratory illness, fluid may not be able to drain.

A child's immune system isn't as effective as an adult's because it's still developing. This makes it harder for children to fight infections.

As part of the immune system, the adenoids respond to bacteria passing through the nose and mouth. Sometimes bacteria get trapped in the adenoids, causing a chronic infection that can then pass on to the eustachian tubes and the middle ear.

How does a doctor diagnose a middle ear infection?

The first thing a doctor will do is ask you about your child's health. Has your child had a head cold or sore throat recently? Is he having trouble sleeping? Is she pulling at her ears? If an ear infection seems likely, the simplest way for a doctor to tell is to use a lighted instrument, called an otoscope, to look at the eardrum. A red, bulging eardrum indicates an infection.

A doctor also may use a pneumatic otoscope, which blows a puff of air into the ear canal, to check for fluid behind the eardrum. A normal eardrum will move back and forth more easily than an eardrum with fluid behind it.

Tympanometry, which uses sound tones and air pressure, is a diagnostic test a doctor might use if the diagnosis still isn't clear. It measures how flexible the eardrum is at different pressures.

How is an acute middle ear infection treated?

Many doctors will prescribe an antibiotic, such as amoxicillin, to be taken over 7 to 10 days. Your doctor also may recommend over-the-counter pain relievers or eardrops to help with fever and pain.

If your doctor isn't able to make a definite diagnosis of OM and your child doesn't have severe ear pain or a fever, your doctor might ask you to wait a day to see if the earache goes away. Sometimes ear pain isn't caused by infection, and some ear infections may get better without antibiotics. Using antibiotics cautiously and with good reason helps prevent the development of bacteria that become resistant to antibiotics.

If your doctor prescribes an antibiotic, it's important to make sure your child takes it exactly as prescribed and for the full amount of time. Even though your child may seem better in a few days, the infection still hasn't completely cleared from the ear. Stopping the medicine too soon could allow the infection to come back. It's also important to return for your child's follow-up visit, so that the doctor can check if the infection is gone.

How long will it take my child to get better?

Your child should start feeling better within a few days after visiting the doctor. If it's been several days and your child still seems sick, call your doctor. Your child might need a different antibiotic. Once the infection clears, fluid may still remain in the middle ear but usually disappears within three to six weeks.

What happens if my child keeps getting ear infections?

To keep a middle ear infection from coming back, it helps to limit some of the factors that might put your child at risk, such as not being around people who smoke and not going to bed with a bottle. In spite of these precautions, some children may continue to have middle ear infections, sometimes as many as five or six a year. Your doctor may want to wait for several months to see if things get better on their own, but, if the infections keep coming back and antibiotics aren't helping, many doctors will recommend a surgical procedure that places a small ventilation tube in the eardrum to improve air flow and prevent fluid backup in the middle ear. The most commonly used tubes stay in place for six to nine months and require follow-up visits until they fall out.

If placement of the tubes still doesn't prevent infections, a doctor may consider removing the adenoids to prevent infection from spreading to the eustachian tubes.

Can ear infections be prevented?

Currently, the best way to prevent ear infections is to reduce the risk factors associated with them. Here are some things you might want to do to lower your child's risk for ear infections.

- Vaccinate your child against the flu. Make sure your child gets the influenza, or flu, vaccine every year.

- It is recommended that you vaccinate your child with the 13-valent pneumococcal conjugate vaccine (PCV13). The PCV13 protects against more types of infection-causing bacteria than the previous vaccine, the PCV7. If your child already has begun PCV7 vaccination, consult your physician about how to transition to PCV13.

- Wash hands frequently.

- Avoid exposing your baby to cigarette smoke.

- Never put your baby down for a nap, or for the night, with a bottle.

- Don't allow sick children to spend time together. As much as possible, limit your child's exposure to other children when your child or your child's playmates are sick.

Section 20.2

Enlarged Adenoids

"Enlarged Adenoids," November 2010, reprinted with permission from www
.kidshealth.org. Copyright © 2010 The Nemours Foundation. This information
was provided by KidsHealth, one of the largest resources online for medically
reviewed health information written for parents, kids, and teens. For more
articles like this one, visit www.KidsHealth.org, or www.TeensHealth.org.

Often, tonsils and adenoids are surgically removed at the same time.
Although you can see the tonsils at the back of the throat, adenoids
aren't directly visible. A doctor has to use a telescope to get a peek at
them. As an alternative, an X-ray of the head can give the doctor an
idea of the size of someone's adenoids.

So, what are adenoids anyway? They're a mass of tissue in the
passage that connects the back of the nasal cavity to the throat. By
producing antibodies to help the body fight infections, adenoids help
to control bacteria and viruses that enter through the nose.

In kids, adenoids usually shrink after about five years of age and
often practically disappear by the teen years.

Symptoms of Enlarged Adenoids

Because adenoids trap germs that enter the body, adenoid tissue can
temporarily swell as it tries to fight off an infection. These symptoms
are often associated with enlarged adenoids:

- Difficulty breathing through the nose
- Breathing through the mouth
- Talking as if the nostrils are pinched
- Noisy breathing
- Snoring
- Stopped breathing for a few seconds during sleep (sleep apnea)
- Frequent "sinus" symptoms
- Ongoing middle ear infections or middle ear fluid in a school-aged child

If enlarged adenoids are suspected, the doctor may ask about and then check your child's ears, nose, and throat, and feel the neck along the jaw. To get a really close look, the doctor might order one or more X-rays. For a suspected infection, the doctor may prescribe oral antibiotics.

When Is Surgery Necessary?

If enlarged or infected adenoids keep bothering your child and are not controlled by medication, the doctor may recommend surgically removing them with an adenoidectomy. This may be recommended if your child has one or more of the following:

- Difficulty breathing

- Sleep apnea

- Recurrent infections

- Ear infections, middle ear fluid, and hearing loss requiring a second or third set of ear tubes

Having your child's adenoids removed is especially important when repeated infections lead to sinus and ear infections. Badly swollen adenoids can interfere with the ability of the middle ear space to stay ventilated. This can sometimes lead to infections or middle ear fluid causing a temporary hearing loss. So kids whose infected adenoids cause frequent earaches and fluid buildup might also need an adenoidectomy at the time of their ear tube surgery.

And although adenoids can be taken out without the tonsils, if your child is having tonsil problems, they may be removed at the same time. A tonsillectomy with an adenoidectomy is the most common pediatric operation.

What Happens during Surgery

Surgery, no matter how common or simple the procedure, can be frightening for both kids and parents. You can help prepare your child for surgery by talking about what to expect. During the adenoidectomy:

- Your child will receive general anesthesia. This means the surgery will be performed in an operating room so that an anesthesiologist can monitor your child.

- Your child will be asleep for about 20 minutes.

- The surgeon can get to the tonsils and/or the adenoids through your child's open mouth—there's no need to cut through skin.

- The surgeon removes the adenoids and then cauterizes (or seals) the blood vessels.

Your child will wake up in the recovery area. In most cases, the total time in the hospital is less than five hours. Very young children and those who are significantly overweight, or have a chronic disease such as seizure disorders or cerebral palsy, may need to stay overnight for observation.

The typical recuperation after an adenoidectomy often involves several days of moderate pain and discomfort.

In less than a week after surgery, everything should return to normal. The adenoid area will heal naturally, which means there are no stitches to worry about. There's a small chance any tissue that's left behind can swell, but it rarely causes new problems.

After surgery, a child's symptoms usually disappear immediately, unless there's a lot of swelling that could lead to some temporary symptoms.

Even though some kids need surgery, remember that enlarged adenoids are normal in others. If your child's adenoids aren't infected, the doctor may choose to wait to operate because the adenoids may eventually shrink on their own as adolescence approaches.

Section 20.3

Facial Nerve Injuries and Paralysis

What is the facial nerve?

There are actually two facial nerves, one on each side of the head. The facial nerve or seventh cranial nerve is known as a "cranial nerve" since it starts in the brain. It sends branches out to the face, neck, tongue, salivary glands (secrete saliva into the mouth), and the outer ear. A normal functioning nerve allows us to move our face (smile, frown, pout), purse our lips to whistle, and move the neck to make "scary faces." Some nerves that travel with the facial nerve, or "piggyback," allow us to taste with the front of our tongue, make saliva in the mouth, and let us feel the outside of our ear canal.

What problems can develop with the facial nerve?

Problems with the facial nerve result in weakness or paralysis of the face muscles and possibly a loss of taste on the affected side. This nerve loss is one of the most disfiguring since it involves facial movement. Without the nerve connection (innervation) intact, the eye does not close, there is loss of facial muscle tone, and movement on the affected side is reduced or lost.

What causes paralysis of the facial nerve?

It is important to understand the location or pathway the facial nerve takes in the head and face. This understanding makes it easier to see how the nerve is damaged and how this damage may affect function.

The facial nerve starts in the brain and then tracks through a narrow space located inside the ear (internal auditory canal). The nerve then passes through the middle ear (behind the ear drum) and leaves through another narrow passage located under the ear area (stylomastoid foramen). It then branches out to provide muscle movement and sensation to various parts of the face and neck. The branches start

323

inside the parotid gland (in front of the ear) and travel to the forehead, cheek, nose, mouth, and neck.

Anything that may cause swelling or pressure on the nerve can result abnormal function.

Some of the general causes of problems along the pathway of the facial nerve include: congenital (birth) abnormalities, infections of the middle ear (otitis media), cholesteatoma, infections or tumors of the parotid gland, facial and neck trauma, and, uncommonly, as a complication after an operation in the ear area (for example, after a mastoidectomy). One of the most common causes of facial nerve paralysis a viral infection called Bell's palsy.

How is facial paralysis evaluated?

Evaluation begins with thorough history to help determine the cause. A physical examination will help to determine whether the nerve damage is at the brain level (central) or closer to the ear and face area (peripheral).

Usually various tests are performed as part of the evaluation. The nerve (eighth cranial nerve) that allows us to hear is located close to the facial nerve, so it may also be affected (sensorineural hearing loss) when the facial nerve is paralyzed. In addition, problems with the middle ear may also be associated with a hearing loss similar to having the sensation of earplugs in the ears (conductive hearing loss). The type of hearing loss, if present, helps with diagnosis and treatment of the condition.

A thorough examination is performed to determine the level of the paralysis. The extent of facial nerve paralysis can involve all of the nerve (complete) or just a part of the nerve (incomplete).

An X-ray is usually performed after the history and physical examination of the patient. A computed tomography (CT) scan or magnetic resonance imaging (MRI) scan is very useful in making the diagnosis. It can help to determine exactly where swelling, infection, trauma, or tumor may be that is causing the facial nerve abnormality.

More specialized tests involve the use of electrical impulses. A commonly used technique called electromyography (EMG) sends electrical impulses to muscle (as a nerve would do). This is a painless technique that helps to determine whether the problem is with the nerve or the muscle itself.

Another study is known as the nerve excitability test (NET). This study uses electrical impulses to compare the normal facial nerve on one side of the face with the abnormal one on the other. Electroneurobility testing (ENoG) goes further than NET, by giving actual numbers to help with the comparison.

Finally, a group of tests checking tear production, saliva production, taste sensation, and small ear muscle movement can help to determine if only a small branch of the facial nerve is damaged. This is known as topographic localization.

When would an otolaryngologist be consulted to help manage facial paralysis?

An otolaryngologist is consulted to help surgically treat many causes of facial nerve paralysis that will not resolve on their own. These conditions include a trapped nerve that needs to be released to function normally, which can be seen with facial trauma, tumors, or severe otitis media. The otolaryngologist is also skilled in surgically connecting a facial nerve that has been divided by trauma.

In these instances, the facial nerve will continue to die until a surgical procedure is undertaken. This underscores the urgency in which facial nerve paralysis should be evaluated.

Section 20.4

Hearing Loss

This section excerpted from "Communication Considerations for Parents of
Deaf and Hard-of-Hearing Children," National Institute on Deafness and
Other Communication Disorders (www.nidcd.nih.gov), April 25, 2011.

Deafness or hearing impairment affects not only a child who is
deaf or has a hearing loss, but also the child's family, friends, and
teachers. For hundreds of years, people have debated the best ways
to develop communication skills and provide education for deaf and
hard-of-hearing children.

Here are a few points upon which scientific and health professionals, educators, and experienced parents commonly agree:

Newborn Hearing Screening

The earlier that deafness or hearing loss is identified, the better
the chances a child will acquire language, whether spoken or signed. A
hearing screening can be an important indicator of deafness or hearing
loss in a child. For this reason, all infants should be screened while still
in the hospital or within the first month of life. But children who do not
pass their screening need to go for a follow-up examination. The follow-
up examination includes precise audiological testing that confirms the
extent and type of hearing loss. It also allows parents, health professionals, and teachers to determine the best intervention strategy for the
child. The term *intervention* refers to the different steps that families
can take to overcome communication barriers caused by a hearing loss.
When intervention is introduced early, the child can take advantage of
the unique window of opportunity during the first few years of life when
a person acquires language, whether spoken or signed.

Each Child Is Unique

Each child is unique. It is important to understand the full nature
and extent of a child's hearing loss or deafness. It is also important to
understand how each family member and caregiver will communicate

with the child. Get to know the services that are provided in your community for children in preschool and elementary school.

Optimizing Residual Hearing

Optimizing residual hearing may be advantageous. Children may benefit from hearing aids or cochlear implants. This is a decision that you should discuss with your child's health care providers and other professionals who work with deaf children and language development.

Explore Your Options and Work with Professionals

Exploring the options and, if possible, working with professionals in teams can be beneficial. Your child may visit a pediatrician, an otolaryngologist (ear, nose, and throat doctor), an audiologist (hearing specialist), and a speech-language pathologist (specialist in speech and language disorders). Some otolaryngologists and audiologists are specially trained to work with infants and children. Ask each professional to inform other professionals who work with your child about your child's visits. Coordinated care can be a big help to you and your child. Many parents find it useful to include educational and social service professionals on the team.

Interact with Your Child Often

Parents should interact often with a deaf or hard-of-hearing infant. All of the caregivers in your child's life should interact with him or her as much as possible. You can do this by holding, facing, smiling at, and responding to your infant from the very beginning. Children need love, encouragement, and care from their families and caregivers.

Work with Your Child's Teachers

Teachers who are experienced in working with deaf and hard-of-hearing children can help parents understand how to improve long-term outcomes for a child. Talk to your child's teachers. Get to know the educational system your child will be entering and the services it provides for children who are deaf or hard-of-hearing.

Organizations and federal agencies can provide helpful information to families of deaf or hard-of-hearing children. Some organizations offer differing perspectives on the best way to develop the skills and talents of your deaf or hard-of-hearing child.

Section 20.5

Hoarseness

What is hoarseness?

Hoarseness is the name for the breathy, coarse, or harsh-sounding speech produced from a variety of causes. It is important to find the cause of a hoarse voice, so the appropriate treatment plan can be developed.

What are some of the causes of a hoarse voice?

Any illness or process that directly or indirectly affects the vocal cords in the larynx (voice box), that does not allow the vocal cords to close completely, will result in a hoarse voice.

The vocal cords can be affected directly by colds and croup or may be affected indirectly by non-infectious processes, environmental or traumatic causes, and congenital and genetic syndromes.

Hoarseness also may be caused by any process that affects the nerve that moves the vocal cords (the recurrent laryngeal nerve). This results vocal cord paralysis.

What are some of the more common infectious causes of hoarseness?

Viral and bacterial infections can directly affect the throat and vocal cords, resulting in hoarseness. These illnesses are known as laryngitis, laryngotracheitis (croup), and laryngotracheobronchitis (bronchiolitis). These do not usually last more than a week or so, and can usually be identified and treated by your primary care physician. However, it is important to realize that hoarseness can continue for a month or so after the primary infection.

Sinusitis or any infection involving a runny/stuffy nose resulting in drainage of the secretions into the throat (post-nasal drip) may also affect the vocal cords, resulting in hoarseness.

Which non-infectious processes can result in hoarseness?

Allergies are a common non-infectious processes that can result in hoarseness. The secretions produced in common allergies can drip into the throat (post-nasal drip) irritating the throat and vocal cords. Allergies can also cause swelling of the vocal cords resulting in hoarseness. Successful treatment of the allergies will result in resolution of the hoarse voice.

Excessive use or misuse of the voice leading to formation of vocal cord nodules is another relatively common cause of hoarseness.

Gastroesophageal reflux disease (GERD) or reflux of stomach acid into the back of the throat will also cause hoarseness and may be more common than previously thought. Because reflux can be silent in many children, examination of the vocal cords and testing for reflux may be necessary to establish this cause of hoarseness.

Other non-infectious processes are much unusual causes of hoarseness. These can include vocal cord polyps, endocrine (glandular) problems, and tumors of the larynx among others.

What are some of the more common traumatic causes of hoarseness?

Traumatic causes of hoarseness refer to damage of the neck or vocal cords through trauma. Some examples include caustic ingestions (acid, poisons), intubation (breathing tube placement), feeding tube placement, birth trauma, or other trauma (car or bike accidents).

What are some of the congenital and genetic causes of hoarseness?

An infant may be born with a deformity of the larynx (voice box), or a nerve problem causing hoarseness. In many cases, there may be stridor or noisy breathing as well. These causes of hoarseness can include vocal cord paralysis, laryngomalacia, cysts, webs (a membrane blocking the opening), or clefts in the voice box. Some genetic (inherited) syndromes also involve deformities causing hoarseness.

What are some of the indirect causes of hoarseness?

Anything that could damage the nerve (recurrent laryngeal nerve) that moves the vocal cords may result in hoarseness. This may include many rare diseases involving the brain or nerves in the body. Occasionally a child is born with damage to this nerve. Surgery in the chest and around the heart and large blood vessels may also result in damage to the nerve.

Does an ear, nose, and throat specialist (otolaryngologist) always evaluate hoarseness?

An ear, nose and throat specialist focuses on disorders of the head and neck (not including the eyes, brain, or spinal cord). As hoarseness results from a variety of causes, the best person to evaluate hoarseness is an ear, nose, and throat specialist. Treatment may include other specialists depending on the final diagnosis.

When should hoarseness be a concern?

In otherwise healthy children, hoarseness that has been present for four months or longer should be evaluated. In newborn children, children with a history of chest surgery, or those with other congenital problems, hoarseness should be evaluated more promptly. If your child has had a hoarse voice since they began speaking and it has not improved, it should be evaluated.

What does an evaluation consist of?

Not every child is similar, so each patient is evaluated according to their particular history. A thorough history and physical exam is performed. Your doctor may also order a hearing test to rule out hearing loss that sometimes accompanies hoarseness. Finally, an evaluation of the voice box with a special camera is performed. This is called a flexible laryngoscopy. Most often, it can be performed in the office under local (topical) anesthesia placed in the nose.

Section 20.6

Nosebleeds

Although they can be scary, nosebleeds are rarely cause for alarm. Common in kids ages 3 to 10 years, nosebleeds often stop on their own and can be treated safely at home.

What to do:

- Stay calm and reassure your child.

- With your child upright in a chair or in your lap, tilt his or her head slightly forward.

- Gently pinch the soft part of the nose (just below the bony ridge) with a tissue or clean washcloth.

- Keep pressure on the nose for about 10 minutes; if you stop too soon, bleeding may start again.

- Do not have your child lean back. This may cause blood to flow down the back of the throat, which tastes bad and may cause gagging, coughing, or vomiting.

- Have your child relax awhile after a nosebleed. Discourage nose-blowing, picking, or rubbing, and any rough play.

Call the doctor if your child:

- has frequent nosebleeds;

- may have put something in his or her nose;

- tends to bruise easily;

- has heavy bleeding from minor wounds or bleeding from another place, such as the gums;

- recently started taking new medicine.

Seek emergency care or call the doctor if bleeding:

- is heavy, or is accompanied by dizziness or weakness;

- is the result of a fall or blow to the head;

- continues after two attempts of applying pressure for 10 minutes each.

Different Kinds of Nosebleeds

The most common kind of nosebleed is an anterior nosebleed, which comes from the front of the nose. Capillaries, or very small blood vessels, inside the nose may break and bleed, causing this type of nosebleed.

A posterior nosebleed comes from the deepest part of the nose. Blood flows down the back of the throat even if the person is sitting or standing. Kids rarely have posterior nosebleeds, which occur more often in older adults, those with high blood pressure, and people who have had nose or face injuries.

Causes and Remedies

The most common cause of anterior nosebleeds is dry air. A dry climate or heated indoor air irritates and dries out nasal membranes, causing crusts that may itch and then bleed when scratched or picked. Colds also may irritate the lining of the nose, and bleeding can occur after repeated nose-blowing. When you combine a cold with dry winter air, you have the perfect formula for nosebleeds.

Allergies also can cause problems, and a doctor may prescribe medications such as antihistamines or decongestants to control an itchy, runny, or stuffy nose. This can also dry out the nasal membranes and contribute to nosebleeds.

An injury or blow to the nose can cause bleeding and usually is not a serious problem. If your child ever has a facial injury, use the tips outlined to stop a nosebleed. If you can't stop the bleeding after 10 minutes or you are concerned about other facial injuries, take your child to see a medical professional right away.

Nosebleeds are rarely cause for alarm, but frequent nosebleeds might indicate a more serious problem. If your child gets nosebleeds more than once a week, you should contact your doctor. Most cases of frequent nosebleeds are easily treated. Sometimes tiny blood vessels inside the nose become irritated and don't heal. This happens more frequently in kids who have ongoing allergies or frequent colds. A doctor may have a solution if your child has this problem.

If bleeding is not due to a sinus infection, allergies, or irritated blood vessels, the doctor may order other tests to see why your child is getting frequent nosebleeds. Rarely, a bleeding disorder or abnormally formed blood vessels could be a possibility.

Preventing Future Nosebleeds

Since most nosebleeds in kids are caused by nose picking, or irritation due to hot dry air, using a few simple tips may help your kids avoid them in the future.

To help prevent nosebleeds:

- Keep your child's nails short to prevent injuries from nose-picking.

- Keep the inside of your child's nose moist with saline nasal spray or dab antibiotic ointment gently around the opening of the nostrils.

- Humidify bedrooms with a vaporizer (or humidifier) if the air in your home is dry. Look for a cool mist model, as a hot steam humidifier could scald a child. Keep the machine clean to prevent mildew buildup.

- Make sure your kids wear protective athletic equipment when participating in sports that could cause a nose injury.

Even when taking proper precautions, kids can still get a bloody nose occasionally. So the next time your child gets a nosebleed, try not to panic. They're usually harmless and are almost always easy to stop.

Section 20.7

Obstructive Sleep Apnea

This section excerpted from "What Is Sleep Apnea?" National Heart,
Lung, and Blood Institute (www.nhlbi.nih.gov), August 1, 2010.

Sleep apnea is a common disorder in which you have one or more
pauses in breathing or shallow breaths while you sleep. Sleep apnea
usually is a chronic (ongoing) condition that disrupts your sleep. You
often move out of deep sleep and into light sleep when your breathing
pauses or becomes shallow.

This results in poor sleep quality that makes you tired during the
day. Sleep apnea is one of the leading causes of excessive daytime
sleepiness.

Most people who have sleep apnea don't know they have it because
it only occurs during sleep. A family member and/or bed partner may
first notice the signs of sleep apnea.

Causes

When you're awake, throat muscles help keep your airway stiff and
open so air can flow into your lungs. When you sleep, these muscles are
more relaxed. If you have obstructive sleep apnea, your airway can be
blocked or narrowed during sleep. This can cause loud snoring and a
drop in your blood oxygen level.

If the oxygen drops to a dangerous level, it triggers your brain to
disturb your sleep. This helps tighten the upper airway muscles and
open your windpipe. Normal breaths then start again, often with a
loud snort or choking sound.

The frequent drops in oxygen level and reduced sleep quality trigger
the release of stress hormones. These compounds raise your heart rate
and increase your risk of high blood pressure, heart attack, stroke, and
arrhythmias (irregular heartbeats). The hormones also raise the risk
of, or worsen, heart failure.

Untreated sleep apnea also can lead to changes in how your
body uses energy. These changes increase your risk of obesity and
diabetes.

Signs and Symptoms

One of the most common signs of obstructive sleep apnea is loud and chronic (ongoing) snoring. Pauses may occur in the snoring. Choking or gasping may follow the pauses.

The snoring usually is loudest when you sleep on your back; it may be less noisy when you turn on your side. Snoring may not happen every night. Over time, the snoring may happen more often and get louder. Not everyone who snores has sleep apnea.

Another common sign of sleep apnea is fighting sleepiness during the day, at work, or while driving. You may find yourself rapidly falling asleep during the quiet moments of the day when you're not active. Even if you don't have daytime sleepiness, talk with your doctor if you have problems breathing during sleep.

In children, sleep apnea can cause hyperactivity, poor school performance, and angry or hostile behavior. Children who have sleep apnea also may have unusual sleeping positions, bedwetting, and may breathe through their mouths instead of their noses during the day.

Diagnosis

Doctors diagnose sleep apnea based on medical and family histories, a physical exam, and results from sleep studies. Usually, your primary care doctor evaluates your symptoms first. He or she then decides whether you need to see a sleep specialist.

Your doctor will ask you and your family questions about how you sleep and how you function during the day. Your doctor also will want to know how loudly and often you snore or make gasping or choking sounds during sleep. Often you're not aware of such symptoms and must ask a family member or bed partner to report them.

Your doctor will check your mouth, nose, and throat for extra or large tissues. The tonsils may be enlarged in children who have sleep apnea. A physical exam and medical history may be all that's needed to diagnose sleep apnea in children.

A sleep study is the most accurate test for diagnosing sleep apnea. It records what happens with your breathing while you sleep. There are different kinds of sleep studies. If your doctor suspects you have sleep apnea, he or she may recommend a polysomnogram (also called a PSG) or a home-based portable monitor.

Polysomnogram

A PSG is the most common sleep study for diagnosing sleep apnea. This test records the following:

- Brain activity
- Eye movement and other muscle activity
- Breathing, heart rate, and blood pressure
- How much air moves in and out of your lungs while you're sleeping
- The amount of oxygen in your blood

A PSG is painless. You'll go to sleep as usual, except you'll have sensors on your scalp, face, chest, limbs, and finger. The staff at the sleep center will use the sensors to check on you throughout the night. A sleep specialist reviews the results of your PSG to see whether you have sleep apnea and how severe it is.

Home-Based Portable Monitor

Your doctor may recommend a home-based sleep test with a portable monitor. The portable monitor will record some of the same information as a PSG. A sleep specialist may use the results from a home-based sleep test to help diagnose sleep apnea or may use the results to determine whether you need a full PSG study in a sleep center.

Treatment

Lifestyle changes, mouthpieces, breathing devices, and surgery are used to treat sleep apnea. Medicines typically aren't used to treat the condition.

Treatment may improve other medical problems linked to sleep apnea, such as high blood pressure. Treatment also can reduce your risk of heart disease, stroke, and diabetes.

Lifestyle Changes

If you have mild sleep apnea, some changes in daily activities or habits may be all the treatment you need.

- Avoid alcohol and medicines that make you sleepy.
- Lose weight if you're overweight or obese
- Sleep on your side instead of your back to help keep your throat open.
- Keep your nasal passages open at night with nasal sprays or allergy medicines.
- If you smoke, quit.

Mouthpieces

A mouthpiece may help some people who have mild sleep apnea. The mouthpiece will adjust your lower jaw and your tongue to help keep your airways open while you sleep. You may need periodic office visits so your doctor can adjust your mouthpiece to fit better.

Breathing Devices

CPAP (continuous positive airway pressure) is the most common treatment for moderate to severe sleep apnea in adults. A CPAP machine uses a mask that fits over your mouth and nose, or just over your nose. The machine gently blows air into your throat.

The air presses on the wall of your airway. The air pressure is adjusted so that it's just enough to stop the airways from becoming narrowed or blocked during sleep.

CPAP treatment may cause side effects in some people. These side effects include a dry or stuffy nose, irritated skin on your face, dry mouth, and headaches. If your CPAP isn't adjusted properly, you may get stomach bloating and discomfort while wearing the mask.

Surgery

Some people who have sleep apnea may benefit from surgery. Surgery is done to widen breathing passages. It usually involves shrinking, stiffening, or removing excess tissue in the mouth and throat or resetting the lower jaw.

Surgery to remove the tonsils, if they're blocking the airway, may be very helpful for some children. Your child's doctor may suggest waiting some time to see whether these tissues shrink on their own. This is common as small children grow.

Section 20.8

Perforated Eardrum

A ruptured eardrum is an opening or hole in the thin layer of tissue (eardrum) that separates the outer and middle ear.

Causes, Incidence, and Risk Factors

The eardrum vibrates when sound waves strike it. These vibrations then pass through the bones of the middle ear. They stimulate the inner ear, sending nerve impulses to the brain. When the eardrum is damaged, the hearing process is interrupted.

Ear infections may cause a ruptured eardrum, more often in children. The infection causes pus or fluid to build up behind the eardrum. As the pressure increases, the eardrum may break open or rupture.

Damage to the eardrum can also occur from:

- a very loud noise (acoustic trauma);
- difference in pressure between the inside and outside of the eardrum (barotrauma), which may occur when flying, scuba diving, or driving in the mountains;
- foreign objects in the ear;
- injury to the ear (such as a powerful slap or explosion);
- inserting cotton-tipped swabs or small objects into the ear to clean them.

Symptoms

- Drainage from the ear (drainage may be clear, pus, or bloody)
- Ear noise/buzzing
- Earache or ear discomfort
  - May be severe and increasing

- There may be a sudden decrease in ear pain followed by drainage from the ear

- Hearing loss in the affected ear (hearing loss may not be total)

- Weakness of the face, or dizziness (in more severe cases)

Signs and Tests

The doctor will look in your ear with an instrument called an otoscope or a microscope. If the eardrum is ruptured, the doctor will see an opening in it, and may even see the bones of the middle ear.

Sometimes it is hard for the doctor to see the eardrum because of drainage (pus) from the ear.

Audiology testing can measure how much hearing has been lost.

Treatment

The goal of treatment is to relieve pain and prevent or treat infection.

Putting warmth on the ear may help relieve discomfort. Keep the ear clean and dry while it is healing. Place cotton balls in the ear while showering or shampooing to prevent water from entering the ear. Avoid swimming or putting your head underneath the water.

Antibiotics (oral or ear drops) may be used to prevent infection or to treat an infection you already have. Painkillers (analgesics), including over-the-counter medications, may be used to relieve pain.

Sometimes the health care provider may place a patch over the eardrum to speed healing. Surgical repair of the eardrum (tympanoplasty) may be needed if the eardrum does not heal on its own.

Expectations (Prognosis)

The opening in the eardrum usually heals by itself within two months. Any hearing loss is most often short-term.

Complications

- Ear infection (otitis media) (the eardrum prevents bacteria from entering the middle ear)

- Long-term hearing loss

- Spread of infection to the bone behind the ear (mastoiditis)

- Vertigo

Calling Your Health Care Provider

Call your health care provider if you:

- have symptoms of a ruptured eardrum;

- have drainage from the ear, fever, a general ill feeling, or hearing loss that do not improve or that return after being treated;

- have any symptoms that last longer than two months after treatment.

Prevention

Do not insert objects into the ear canal, even to clean it. Foreign objects should only be removed by a health care provider. Have ear infections treated promptly.

Section 20.9

Sinusitis

This section excerpted from "Sinus Infection (Sinusitis)," Centers for Disease Control and Prevention (www.cdc.gov), September 1, 2010.

Sinusitis, or a sinus infection, occurs when the sinuses and nasal passages become inflamed. If you or your child is diagnosed with sinusitis, the infection does not need to be treated with antibiotics unless you or your child has acute bacterial sinusitis, which is caused by bacteria. Acute bacterial sinusitis can last up to 4 weeks and subacute bacterial sinusitis can last 4 to 12 weeks, occurring less than four times per year.

Acute viral sinusitis, caused by a virus, typically lasts for less than 4 weeks and occurs less than three times per year. Acute viral sinusitis usually occurs after having an upper respiratory infection.

Chronic sinusitis typically lasts more than 4 weeks and occurs more than four times per year. If you are diagnosed with chronic sinusitis, you should visit a specialist for evaluation. Chronic sinusitis can be caused by nasal polyps or tumors, allergies, or respiratory tract infections (viral, bacterial, or fungal), among other reasons.

Signs and Symptoms of a Sinus Infection

- Headaches
- Nasal congestion/discharge
- Postnasal drip (mucus drips down the throat from the nose)
- Sore throat
- Fever
- Cough
- Fatigue
- Bad breath

See a health care provider if you or your child has the following:
- Temperature higher than 100.4° F
- Symptoms that last more than 10 days
- Multiple episodes of sinusitis in the past year
- Symptoms that are not relieved with over-the-counter medicines

When Antibiotics Are Needed

Sometimes antibiotics may be needed if the sinus infection is likely to be caused by bacteria. By asking about your symptoms and doing a physical examination, a health care provider can determine if you or your child needs antibiotics.

When Antibiotics Will Not Help

When sinusitis is caused by a virus or irritation in the air (like cigarette smoke), antibiotics will not help it get better. Acute sinusitis will almost always get better on its own. It is better to wait and take antibiotics only when they are needed. Taking antibiotics when they are not needed can be harmful.

If symptoms continue for more than 10 days, schedule a follow-up appointment with a health care provider for reevaluation to avoid any complications.

How to Feel Better

Rest, over-the-counter medicines, and other self-care methods may help you or your child feel better. Remember, always use over-the-counter products as directed. Many over-the-counter products are not recommended for children younger than certain ages.

Preventing a Sinus Infection

- Practice good hand hygiene.

- Keep you and your child up-to-date with recommended immunizations.

- Avoid close contact with people who have colds or other upper respiratory infections.

- Avoid smoking or exposure to secondhand smoke and do not expose children to secondhand smoke.

- Use a clean humidifier to moisten the air at home.

Section 20.10

Stridor

Stridor is an abnormal, high-pitched, musical breathing sound caused by a blockage in the throat or voice box (larynx). It is usually heard when taking in a breath.

Considerations

Children are at higher risk of airway blockage because they have narrower airways than adults. In young children, stridor is a sign of airway blockage and must be treated right away to prevent total airway obstruction.

The airway can be blocked by an object, swelling of the tissues of the throat or upper airway, or spasm of the airway muscles or the vocal cords.

Causes

Common causes of stridor include:

- abscess on the tonsils;
- airway injury;
- allergic reaction;
- croup;
- diagnostic tests such as bronchoscopy or laryngoscopy;
- epiglottitis, inflammation of the cartilage that covers the trachea (windpipe);
- inhaling an object such as a peanut or marble (foreign body aspiration);
- laryngitis;
- neck surgery;

- use of a breathing tube for a long time;

- secretions such as phlegm (sputum);

- smoke inhalation or other inhalation injury;

- swelling of the neck or face;

- swollen tonsils or adenoids (such as with tonsillitis);

- vocal cord cancer.

When to Contact a Medical Professional

Stridor may be a sign of an emergency. Call your health care provider right away if there is unexplained stridor, especially in a child.

What to Expect at Your Office Visit

In an emergency, the health care provider will check the person's temperature, pulse, breathing rate, blood pressure, and may need to do the Heimlich maneuver.

A breathing tube may be needed if the person can't breathe properly.

After the person is stable, the health care worker may ask questions about the patient's medical history and perform a physical exam. This includes listening to the lungs.

Parents or caregivers may be asked the following medical history questions:

- Is the abnormal breathing a high-pitched sound?

- Did the breathing problem start suddenly?

- Could the child have put something in the mouth?

- Has the child been ill recently?

- Is the child's neck or face swollen?

- Has the child been coughing or complaining of a sore throat?

- What other symptoms does the child have? (for example, nasal flaring or bluish color to the skin, lips, or nails)

- Is the child using chest muscles to breathe (intercostal retractions)?

Tests that may be done include:

- arterial blood gas analysis;

- bronchoscopy;

- CT scan, thoracic;

- laryngoscopy (examination of the voice box);

- pulse oximetry to measure blood oxygen level;

- X-ray of the chest or neck.

Section 20.11

Swimmer's Ear (Otitis Externa)

This section excerpted from "Swimmer's Ear (Otitis Externa)," Centers for Disease Control and Prevention (www.cdc.gov), August 31, 2011.

Swimmer's ear is a common problem that can cause pain and discomfort for children and swimmers of all ages. In the United States, swimmer's ear results in an estimated 2.4 million health care visits every year and nearly half a billion dollars in health care costs.

What is swimmer's ear?

Swimmer's ear (also known as otitis externa) is an infection of the outer ear canal. Symptoms of swimmer's ear usually appear within a few days of swimming and include the following:

- Itchiness inside the ear

- Redness and swelling of the ear

- Pain when the infected ear is tugged or when pressure is placed on the ear

- Pus draining from the infected ear

Although all age groups are affected by swimmer's ear, it is more common in children and can be extremely painful.

How is swimmer's ear spread at recreational water venues?

Swimmer's ear can occur when water stays in the ear canal for long periods of time, providing the perfect environment for germs to grow and infect the skin. Germs found in pools and at other recreational water venues are one of the most common causes of swimmer's ear.

Swimmer's ear cannot be spread from one person to another.

If you think you have swimmer's ear, consult your health care provider. Swimmer's ear can be treated with antibiotic ear drops.

Is there a difference between a childhood middle ear infection and swimmer's ear?

Yes. Swimmer's ear is not the same as the common childhood middle ear infection. If you can wiggle the outer ear without pain or discomfort then your ear condition is probably not swimmer's ear.

How do I protect myself and my family?

Take these steps to reduce the risk of swimmer's ear:

- Keep your ears as dry as possible.
  - Use a bathing cap, ear plugs, or custom-fitted swim molds when swimming.
- Dry your ears thoroughly after swimming or showering.
  - Use a towel to dry your ears well.
  - Tilt your head to hold each ear facing down to allow water to escape the ear canal.
  - Pull your earlobe in different directions while your ear is faced down to help water drain out.
  - If you still have water left in your ears, consider using a hair dryer to move air within the ear canal. Put the dryer on the lowest heat and speed/fan setting and hold it several inches from your ear.
- Don't put objects in your ear canal (including cotton-tip swabs, pencils, paperclips, or fingers).
- Don't try to remove ear wax. Ear wax helps protect your ear canal from infection.
  - If you think that your ear canal is blocked by ear wax, consult your health care provider.
- Consult your health care provider about using ear drops after swimming.

- Drops should not be used by people with ear tubes, damaged ear drums, outer ear infections, or ear drainage (pus or liquid coming from the ear).

- Consult your health care provider if you have ear pain, discomfort, or drainage from your ears.

- Ask your pool/hot tub operator if disinfectant and pH levels are checked at least twice per day—hot tubs and pools with proper disinfectant and pH levels are less likely to spread germs.

- Use pool test strips to check the pool or hot tub yourself for adequate disinfectant and pH levels.

Section 20.12

Tonsillitis

"Tonsillitis," June 2010, reprinted with permission from www.kidshealth .org. Copyright © 2010 The Nemours Foundation. This information was provided by KidsHealth, one of the largest resources online for medically reviewed health information written for parents, kids, and teens. For more articles like this one, visit www.KidsHealth.org, or www.TeensHealth.org.

The tonsils are lumps of tissue located on either side of the back of the throat. They are part of the body's immune system, designed to protect us by trapping bacteria and viruses that try to enter the body through the mouth.

But sometimes infections are too much for the tonsils to handle, and these fighters of infection become infected themselves. When that happens, it's called tonsillitis.

Tonsillitis can be caused by certain types of bacteria or viruses. It also can be caused by certain types of bacteria. For example, you've probably heard of strep throat. It's an infection in your throat or tonsils caused by a specific type of bacteria called group A streptococci.

What Are the Signs and Symptoms?

If you have healthy tonsils, you probably don't even notice them— even if you look at the back of your throat in a mirror. The tonsils become a lot easier to see when someone has tonsillitis because they swell up and become red. Here are some of the signs of tonsillitis:

- Sore throat, which can be mild to severe
- Swelling of the tonsils
- Swelling of the lymph nodes (glands) in your neck
- Redness in the tonsils
- White spots or pus on the tonsils
- Changes in your voice
- Fever
- Difficulty swallowing

If you have symptoms of tonsillitis, it's a good idea to visit your doctor.

What Do Doctors Do?

Your doctor will ask about your symptoms and examine your throat and neck. If your doctor thinks you have tonsillitis, he or she may use a soft swab to gently collect a sample from your tonsils and the back of your throat. The sample is then tested to see if strep bacteria are present. The test is quick and easy and it will tell you and your doctor whether you will need medication to get better.

If the test shows that bacteria caused your sore throat, your doctor will usually prescribe an antibiotic to kill the bacteria. Not only will this help you feel better, it will also help prevent complications of untreated strep throat. (When strep throat isn't treated properly with antibiotics, people can develop serious complications, such as kidney disease.)

If your doctor prescribes antibiotics, be sure to follow the directions carefully. You'll need to finish taking all the medicine even if your symptoms go away and you feel better. That will prevent the infection from flaring up again and help protect you against any complications.

If a strep test comes back negative, it's probably a virus causing the tonsillitis. If this is the case, antibiotics won't help. Just like with a cold (also caused by a virus), you'll have to take it easy for several days and let the virus run its course.

If you have frequent episodes of tonsillitis, your doctor or an otolaryngologist (a doctor who specializes in ear, nose, and throat problems) may recommend a tonsillectomy. This is a surgical procedure to remove the tonsils. Tonsillectomy may also be recommended if the infection is not responding to antibiotics.

How Can I Prevent Tonsillitis?

Tonsillitis is contagious. This means you can get it from someone else who has it. Sneezing and coughing can pass the tonsillitis-causing virus or bacteria from one person to the next. But you can protect yourself from catching tonsillitis or passing it to somebody else:

- Wash your hands frequently.

- If someone in your household or a friend has tonsillitis, don't use that person's cups, glasses, silverware, toothbrush, or other utensils. And if you have tonsillitis, keep your stuff separate and don't share it with anyone.

- Don't kiss your boyfriend or girlfriend until you're completely over the tonsillitis.

- Once you've started the antibiotic for strep, throw out your toothbrush and buy a new one. That way you won't reinfect yourself.

What Can I Do to Help Myself Feel Better?

If you have tonsillitis, take it easy. Get plenty of rest and drink lots of fluids. You can take acetaminophen or ibuprofen to relieve any pain or discomfort. (Don't take aspirin or other products that contain aspirin, though, because these may put you at risk of developing Reye syndrome, an illness that can have serious complications.)

Call your doctor right away if your condition gets worse; for example, if you have difficulty breathing or swallowing. Also talk to your doctor if your fever comes back or if you're not feeling better in a couple of days.

Avoid smoking or anything that will irritate your throat. It's best to drink lots of liquids. You may prefer softer foods, like applesauce, flavored gelatin, or ice cream. If you don't feel like eating, try drinking liquids that contain calories, such as fruit juices, milkshakes, and soups and broths.

If you're on antibiotics, it's usually okay to return to school 24 hours after you start taking them if your fever is gone and you feel better. If you're still feeling weak, tired, or achy, it may be best to stay home for another day or two. Rest and relaxation sometimes can be the best medicine.

Chapter 21

Endocrine and Growth Disorders in Children

Chapter Contents

Section 21.1

Adrenal Gland Disorders

"Adrenal Gland Disorders," National Institute of Child Health and
Human Development (www.nichd.nih.gov), July 28, 2010.

What are the adrenal glands?

The adrenal glands are the part of the body responsible for releasing three different classes of hormones. These hormones control many important functions in the body:

- Maintaining metabolic processes, such as managing blood sugar levels and regulating inflammation

- Regulating the balance of salt and water

- Controlling the "fight or flight" response to stress

- Maintaining pregnancy

- Initiating and controlling sexual maturation during childhood and puberty

The adrenal glands are also an important source of sex steroids, such as estrogen and testosterone.

What are adrenal gland disorders?

Adrenal gland disorders occur when the adrenal glands don't work properly. Sometimes, the cause is a problem in another gland that helps to regulate the adrenal gland. In other cases, the adrenal gland itself may have the problem. Some examples include the following:

- **Cushing syndrome:** Cushing syndrome happens when a person's body is exposed to too much of the hormone cortisol. In this syndrome, a person's body makes more cortisol than it needs. For example, adrenal tumors can cause the body to produce too much cortisol. In some cases, children are born with a form of adrenal hyperplasia that leads to Cushing syndrome. Or, in some cases, certain medications can cause the body to make too much cortisol.

- **Congenital adrenal hyperplasia:** Congenital adrenal hyperplasia is a genetic disorder of adrenal gland deficiency. In this disorder, the body doesn't make enough of the hormone cortisol. The bodies of people with congenital adrenal hyperplasia may also have other hormone imbalances, such as not making enough aldosterone, but making too much androgen.

- **Pituitary tumors:** The pituitary gland is located in the brain and helps to regulate the activity of most other glands in the body, including the adrenal glands. In rare cases, benign (non-cancerous) tumors may grow on the pituitary gland, which may restrict the hormones it releases.

  In some cases, tumors on the pituitary can lead to Cushing syndrome—this is called Cushing disease. In other cases, the tumors reduce the adrenal gland's release of hormones needed for the "fight or flight" response to stress. If the body is unable to handle physiological stress—a condition called Addison disease—it can be fatal.

What are the treatments for adrenal gland disorders?

The treatment for adrenal gland disorders depends on the specific disorder or the specific cause of the disorder.

- The treatment for Cushing syndrome depends on the cause. If the excess cortisol is caused by medication, your health care provider can change dosages or try a different medication to correct the problem. If the Cushing syndrome is caused by the body making too much cortisol, treatments may include oral medication, surgery, radiation, or a combination of these treatments.

- Congenital adrenal hyperplasia can't be cured, but it can be treated and controlled. People with congenital adrenal hyperplasia can take medication to help replace the hormones their bodies are not making. Some people with congenital adrenal hyperplasia only need these medications when they are sick, but others may need to take them every day.

- Doctors can successfully treat most pituitary tumors with microsurgery, radiation therapy, surgery, drugs, or a combination of these treatments. Surgery is currently the treatment of choice for tumors that grow rapidly, especially if they threaten or affect vision. The treatment plan for other pituitary tumors differs according to the type and size of the tumor.

Section 21.2

Constitutional Growth Delay

What is constitutional delay of growth?

One of the most common diagnoses made after a growth evaluation
is constitutional delay of growth. These children, often called "late
bloomers," have a characteristic pattern of growth. Constitutional delay of growth (CDG) is considered more of a variant of normal growth,
rather than a "disease process."

Children with constitutional delay of growth are typically born with
a normal birth weight and length, but in the first two years of life, they
show slow growth and thus lose height percentiles. There may be delayed
dental development in childhood. A similar pattern of growth was often
experienced by a parent. For example, the mother might recall her first
menstrual cycle occurring late, such as after age 15, or the father might
recall being short but catching up towards the end of high school.

Constitutional delay of growth is diagnosed more frequently in
boys than girls but can occur in either sex. The growth rate between
ages 3 and 10 should be normal so there should not be a further loss
in percentiles. If there is a concern about the growth rate, further
workup is recommended. However, when peers go through pubertal
growth acceleration, children with constitutional delay of growth will
lose percentiles as their onset into puberty is delayed.

Bone age X-ray of the left hand and wrist is delayed in CDG, but
is also delayed in many other conditions. Thus, a delayed bone age
supports the diagnosis of constitutional delay of growth, but is not
conclusive.

Should I take my child to see a growth specialist?

Your primary care team will help decide whether a consultation is
needed. You should point out whether there was a similar pattern of
growth in any of the family members.

What are questions to ask your primary care physician?

- Is my child short but growing well, such as at least 2¼ inches per year?

- Do you think the growth pattern is consistent with constitutional delay or suggestive of another diagnosis?

- Is the bone age or skeletal age delayed?

- Does it look like my child will catch up to his/her genetic potential?

How is constitutional delay of growth diagnosed?

Your primary care team can diagnose CDG, though sometimes a consultation with an endocrinologist is sought to confirm the diagnosis.

What should I expect at the endocrinologist's office?

The endocrinologist will take a detailed family history of heights and get an appreciation of the timing of growth of other family members. You can help out by asking grandparents about their height and timing of pubertal development.

Hand carry a copy of the growth charts. The more information you provide, the more accurate will be the assessment.

A detailed examination will be performed including a brief assessment of how far along your child is in terms of pubertal development.

There may be no laboratory tests requested, or there might be a bone age X-ray of the left hand and wrist as well as a blood test screening for other tests that can mimic constitutional delay of growth. There is no specific blood test to diagnose constitutional delay of growth.

Section 21.3

Growth Hormone Deficiency

Growth hormone deficiency refers to abnormally short height in childhood due to the lack of growth hormone.

Causes

Growth hormone is produced in the pituitary gland, which is located at the base of the brain.

- Different hormones made in the brain tell the pituitary gland how much growth hormone is needed.

- Growth hormone enters the blood and stimulates the liver to produce a hormone called insulin-like growth factor (IGF-1), which plays a key role in childhood growth.

Abnormally short height in childhood (called short stature) may occur if not enough growth hormone is produced.
Most of the time, no single clear cause of growth hormone deficiency is found.

- Growth hormone deficiency may be present at birth (congenital).

- It may also develop after birth, as the result of a brain injury, tumor, or medical condition.

Children with physical defects of the face and skull, such as cleft lip or cleft palate, are more likely to have decreased growth hormone levels.
Growth hormone deficiency is usually not passed from parent to child.
Although it is uncommon, growth hormone deficiency may also be diagnosed in adults. Possible causes include:

- brain radiation treatments for cancer;

- hormonal problems involving the pituitary gland or hypothalamus;

- severe head injury.

Symptoms

Children with growth hormone deficiency have a slow or flat rate of growth, usually less than two inches per year. The slow growth may not appear until a child is two or three years old.

The child will be much shorter than most or all children of the same age and gender.

Children with growth hormone deficiency still have normal body proportions, as well as normal intelligence. However, their face often appears younger than children of the same age. They may also have a chubby body build.

In older children, puberty may come late or may not come at all.

Exams and Tests

A growth chart is used to compare a child's current height, and how fast he or she is growing, to other children of the same age and gender.

A physical examination including weight, height, and body proportions will show signs of slowed growth rate. The child will not follow the normal growth curves.

Several blood tests are used to help diagnose growth hormone deficiency and its causes:

- GNRH-arginine test

- Growth hormone levels in the blood

- Growth hormone stimulation test

- Insulin tolerance test (ITT, often used to diagnose adults)

- Tests to measure levels of other hormones made by the pituitary gland

Imaging or X-ray tests may include the following:

- Dual energy X-ray absorptiometry (DEXA) scans can also determine bone age.

- Hand X-ray (usually the left hand) can determine bone age. Normally, the size and shape of bones change as a person grows. These changes can be seen on an X-ray and usually follow a pattern as a child grows older.

- Measuring growth hormone and binding protein levels (IGF-I and IGFBP-3) will show whether the growth problem is caused by a problem with the pituitary gland.

- MRI [magnetic resonance imaging] of the head can show the hypothalamus and pituitary glands.

Treatment

A child's short stature will often affect self-esteem. Providing emotional support is an important part of treatment. Children may be teased by classmates and playmates. Family, friends, and teachers should emphasize the child's other skills and strengths.

Treatment involves growth hormone injections given at home. Patients may receive growth hormone several times a week or once a day.

Many children gain four or more inches over the first year, and three or more inches during the next two years. Then the growth rate slowly decreases.

Serious side effects of growth hormone therapy are rare. The most common side effects are:

- fluid retention;

- muscle and joint aches.

Outlook (Prognosis)

The earlier the condition is treated, the better the chance that a child will grow to be a near-normal adult height.

Growth hormone replacement therapy does not work for all children.

Possible Complications

If left untreated, growth hormone deficiency will lead to short stature and delayed puberty.

Growth hormone deficiency may occur with deficiencies of other hormones.

Prevention

Most cases are not preventable.

Review your child's growth chart with your physician after each check-up. If your child's growth rate is dropping or your child's projected adult height is much shorter than an average height of both parents, evaluation by a specialist is recommended.

Section 21.4

Hypothyroidism and Hyperthyroidism (Graves Disease)

This section excerpted from "Hypothyroidism" and "Hyperthyroidism," National Endocrine and Metabolic Diseases Information Service, National Institute of Diabetes and Digestive and Kidney Diseases (endocrine.niddk.nih.gov), 2012.

Hypothyroidism

Hypothyroidism is a disorder that occurs when the thyroid gland does not make enough thyroid hormone to meet the body's needs. Thyroid hormone regulates metabolism—the way the body uses energy—and affects nearly every organ in the body. Without enough thyroid hormone, many of the body's functions slow down.

What is the thyroid?

The thyroid is one of the glands that make up the endocrine system. The glands of the endocrine system produce, store, and release hormones into the bloodstream. The thyroid gland makes two thyroid hormones, triiodothyronine (T3) and thyroxine (T4). Thyroid hormones affect metabolism, brain development, breathing, heart and nervous system functions, body temperature, muscle strength, skin dryness, menstrual cycles, weight, and cholesterol levels.

Thyroid hormone production is regulated by thyroid-stimulating hormone (TSH), which is made by the pituitary gland in the brain. When thyroid hormone levels in the blood are low, the pituitary releases more TSH. When thyroid hormone levels are high, the pituitary responds by dropping TSH production.

What causes hypothyroidism?

Hashimoto disease: Hashimoto disease, also called chronic lymphocytic thyroiditis, is the most common cause of hypothyroidism in the United States.

Thyroiditis: Thyroiditis is an inflammation of the thyroid that causes stored thyroid hormone to leak out of the thyroid gland.

Congenital hypothyroidism: Some babies are born with a thyroid that is not fully developed or does not function properly. If untreated, congenital hypothyroidism can lead to mental retardation and growth failure. Early treatment can prevent these complications, so most newborns in the United States are screened for hypothyroidism.

Surgical removal of the thyroid: When part of the thyroid is removed, the remaining part may produce normal amounts of thyroid hormone, but some people who have this surgery develop hypothyroidism.

Radiation treatment of the thyroid: Radioactive iodine, a common treatment for hyperthyroidism, gradually destroys the cells of the thyroid. Almost everyone who receives radioactive iodine treatment eventually develops hypothyroidism.

Medications: Some drugs can interfere with thyroid hormone production and lead to hypothyroidism.

What are the symptoms of hypothyroidism?

Hypothyroidism has many symptoms that can vary from person to person. Some common symptoms of hypothyroidism are the following:

- Fatigue
- Weight gain
- Puffy face
- Cold intolerance
- Joint and muscle pain
- Constipation
- Dry skin
- Dry, thinning hair
- Decreased sweating
- Heavy or irregular menstrual periods and impaired fertility
- Depression
- Slowed heart rate

How is hypothyroidism diagnosed?

Many symptoms of hypothyroidism are the same as those of other diseases, so hypothyroidism usually cannot be diagnosed based on symptoms alone. With suspected hypothyroidism, health care providers take a medical history and perform a thorough physical examination. Health care providers may then use several blood tests to confirm a diagnosis of hypothyroidism and find its cause:

TSH test: The ultrasensitive TSH test is usually the first test a health care provider performs. This test detects even tiny amounts of TSH in the blood and is the most accurate measure of thyroid activity available.

T4 test: This test measures the actual amount of circulating thyroid hormone in the blood.

Thyroid autoantibody test: This test looks for the presence of thyroid autoantibodies. Most people with Hashimoto disease have these antibodies, but people whose hypothyroidism is caused by other conditions do not.

How is hypothyroidism treated?

Health care providers treat hypothyroidism with synthetic thyroxine, a medication that is identical to the hormone T4 made by the thyroid. Health care providers test TSH levels about six to eight weeks after a patient begins taking thyroid hormone and make any necessary adjustments to the dose. Once a stable dose is reached, blood tests are normally repeated in six months and then once a year.

Hypothyroidism can almost always be completely controlled with synthetic thyroxine, as long as the recommended dose is taken every day as instructed.

Hyperthyroidism

Hyperthyroidism is a disorder that occurs when the thyroid gland makes more thyroid hormone than the body needs.

What causes hyperthyroidism?

Graves disease: Graves disease, also known as toxic diffuse goiter, is the most common cause of hyperthyroidism in the United States. In Graves disease, the immune system makes an antibody called thyroid stimulating immunoglobulin (TSI), which mimics TSH and causes the thyroid to make too much thyroid hormone.

Thyroid nodules: Thyroid nodules, also called adenomas, are lumps in the thyroid. Thyroid nodules are common and usually non-cancerous. However, nodules may become overactive and produce too much hormone.

Thyroiditis: Several types of thyroiditis can cause hyperthyroidism. It causes stored thyroid hormone to leak out of the inflamed gland and raise hormone levels in the blood.

Iodine ingestion: The thyroid gland uses iodine to make thyroid hormone, so the amount of iodine you consume influences the amount of thyroid hormone your thyroid makes.

Overmedicating with thyroid hormone: Some people who take thyroid hormone for hypothyroidism may take too much. If you take synthetic thyroid hormone, see your doctor at least once a year to have your thyroid hormone levels checked and follow your doctor's instructions about the dose you take.

What are the symptoms of hyperthyroidism?

Hyperthyroidism has many symptoms that can vary from person to person. Some common symptoms of hyperthyroidism are the following:

- Nervousness or irritability
- Fatigue or muscle weakness
- Trouble sleeping
- Heat intolerance
- Hand tremors
- Rapid and irregular heartbeat
- Frequent bowel movements or diarrhea
- Weight loss
- Mood swings
- Goiter, which is an enlarged thyroid that may cause your neck to look swollen

How is hyperthyroidism diagnosed?

Your doctor will begin by asking you about your symptoms and performing a thorough physical examination. Your doctor may then use several tests to confirm a diagnosis of hyperthyroidism and to find its cause.

TSH test: The ultrasensitive TSH test will probably be the first test your doctor performs. The TSH test is especially useful in detecting mild hyperthyroidism.

T3 and T4 test: This test will show the levels of T3 and T4 in your blood. If you have hyperthyroidism, the levels of one or both of these hormones in your blood will be higher than normal.

TSI test: This test, also called a thyroid-stimulating antibody test, measures the level of TSI in your blood. Most people with Graves disease have this antibody, but people whose hyperthyroidism is caused by something else do not.

Radioactive iodine uptake test: The radioactive iodine uptake test measures the amount of iodine your thyroid collects from the bloodstream.

Thyroid scan: A thyroid scan shows how and where iodine is distributed in your thyroid. This information helps your doctor diagnose the cause of your hyperthyroidism by providing images of nodules and other possible thyroid irregularities.

How is hyperthyroidism treated?

Treatment depends on the cause of hyperthyroidism and how severe it is. When choosing a treatment, doctors consider a patient's age, possible allergies to or side effects of the medications, other conditions such as pregnancy or heart disease, and the availability of an experienced thyroid surgeon. The three treatment options are medications, radioiodine therapy, and surgery.

Medications: Your doctor may prescribe a drug called a beta blocker to reduce your symptoms until other treatments take effect. Beta blockers act quickly to relieve many of the symptoms of hyperthyroidism, such as tremors, rapid heartbeat, and nervousness.

Antithyroid drugs interfere with thyroid hormone production by blocking the way the thyroid gland uses iodine to make thyroid hormone. Antithyroid drugs are not used to treat thyroiditis.

Once you begin treatment with antithyroid drugs, your thyroid hormone levels may not move into the normal range for several weeks or months. The average treatment time is about one to two years, but treatment can continue for many years. Antithyroid therapy is the easiest way to treat hyperthyroidism but often does not produce permanent results.

Radioiodine therapy: Radioactive iodine-131 is a common and effective treatment for hyperthyroidism. Because your thyroid gland collects iodine to make thyroid hormone, it will collect the radioactive iodine in the same way. The radioactive iodine will gradually destroy the cells that make up the thyroid gland but will not affect other tissues in the body.

Thyroid surgery: The least-used treatment is surgery to remove part or most of the thyroid gland. Doctors sometimes choose surgery to treat pregnant women who cannot tolerate antithyroid drugs, people with very large goiters, or people who have cancerous thyroid nodules.

Section 21.5

Idiopathic Short Stature

Idiopathic short stature (also known as ISS) is a big name for children who are short with no known cause. Idiopathic short stature is a problem that can be present in both girls and boys. Many causes of short stature have been discovered over the past few years, but there are still factors that are not yet understood. ISS falls into to this latter category. Although the reasons for ISS are not yet totally understood, it is known that the administration of growth-promoting treatments may help affected children.

Idiopathic short stature is defined as having a height significantly shorter than the normal population (i.e., shorter than 1.2% of the population of the same age and gender), a poor adult height prediction (generally defined as less than 5'4" for males and less than 4'11" for females), and no detectable cause for the short stature.

Should I take my child to see a growth specialist?

You should first take your child to visit your local pediatrician who will refer your child to a growth specialist (pediatric endocrinologist) if necessary.

You should remember that the window of opportunity for growth ends when the growth plates fuse after puberty; therefore, the earlier you take your child for an assessment the better.

What are questions to ask your pediatrician?

1. Is my child growing at an appropriate rate for his/her age?
2. Is my child within the normal range of expected position on the growth chart?
3. Is my child on track to reach a normal expected height which is appropriate for our family?
4. Is my child at an appropriate stage of puberty for his/her age?

How is ISS diagnosed?

Idiopathic short stature is normally diagnosed by a pediatric endocrinologist after a full investigation of the medical history, a complete physical examination, and the exclusion of any chronic medical condition or other hormonal abnormality.

The workup for a diagnosis of idiopathic short stature, although a simple diagnosis, may require a series of blood and/or other tests to be done to rule out various medical conditions that are known to affect height.

Do growth-promoting therapies work in children with ISS?

Growth hormone was first approved by the Federal Drug Administration for use in patients with idiopathic short stature in 2003 based on the successful results of clinical trials conducted in the USA and in Europe.

When started at an early enough age, growth hormone can significantly increase the final height of a child with idiopathic short stature.

After completion of puberty, no further growth in height is possible. An early diagnosis is, therefore, critical to the success of the treatment.

Section 21.6

Klinefelter Syndrome

"Klinefelter Syndrome," National Institute of Child Health and
Human Development (www.nichd.nih.gov), May 24, 2007. Reviewed by
David A. Cooke, MD, FACP, April 2012.

What is Klinefelter syndrome?

Klinefelter syndrome, also known as the XXY condition, is a term
used to describe males who have an extra X chromosome in most of
their cells. Instead of having the usual XY chromosome pattern that
most males have, these men have an XXY pattern. Even though all
men with Klinefelter syndrome have the extra X chromosome, not
every XXY male has all of those symptoms.

Because not every male with an XXY pattern has all the symptoms
of Klinefelter syndrome, it is common to use the term XXY male to
describe these men, or XXY condition to describe the symptoms.

Scientists believe the XXY condition is one of the most common
chromosome abnormalities in humans. About one of every 500 males
has an extra X chromosome, but many don't have any symptoms.

What are the symptoms of the XXY condition?

Not all males with the condition have the same symptoms or to the
same degree. Symptoms depend on how many XXY cells a man has,
how much testosterone is in his body, and his age when the condition
is diagnosed.

The XXY condition can affect three main areas of development:

- **Physical development:** As babies, many XXY males have
  weak muscles and reduced strength. They may sit up, crawl, and
  walk later than other infants. After about age four, XXY males
  tend to be taller and may have less muscle control and coordination than other boys their age.

  - As XXY males enter puberty, they often don't make as much
    testosterone as other boys. This can lead to a taller, less mus-
    cular body, less facial and body hair, and broader hips than

other boys. As teens, XXY males may have larger breasts, weaker bones, and a lower energy level than other boys.

- By adulthood, XXY males look similar to males without the condition, although they are often taller. They are also more likely than other men to have certain health problems, such as autoimmune disorders, breast cancer, vein diseases, osteoporosis, and tooth decay.

- XXY males can have normal sex lives, but they usually make little or no sperm. Between 95% and 99% of XXY males are infertile because their bodies don't make a lot of sperm.

- **Language development:** As boys, between 25% and 85% of XXY males have some kind of language problem, such as learning to talk late, trouble using language to express thoughts and needs, problems reading, and trouble processing what they hear.

  - As adults, XXY males may have a harder time doing work that involves reading and writing, but most hold jobs and have successful careers.

- **Social development:** As babies, XXY males tend to be quiet and undemanding. As they get older, they are usually quieter, less self-confident, less active, and more helpful and obedient than other boys.

  - As teens, XXY males tend to be quiet and shy. They may struggle in school and sports, meaning they may have more trouble "fitting in" with other kids.

  - However, as adults, XXY males live lives similar to men without the condition; they have friends, families, and normal social relationships.

What are the treatments for the XXY condition?

The XXY chromosome pattern cannot be changed. But, there are a variety of ways to treat the symptoms of the XXY condition.

- **Educational treatments:** As children, many XXY males qualify for special services to help them in school. Teachers can also help by using certain methods in the classroom, such as breaking bigger tasks into small steps.

- **Therapeutic options:** A variety of therapists, such as physical, speech, occupational, behavioral, mental health, and family therapists, can often help reduce or eliminate some of the symptoms of the XXY condition, such as poor muscle tone, speech or language problems, or low self-confidence.

- **Medical treatments:** Testosterone replacement therapy (TRT) can greatly help XXY males get their testosterone levels into normal range. Having a more normal testosterone level can help develop bigger muscles, deepen the voice, and grow facial and body hair. TRT often starts when a boy reaches puberty. Some XXY males can also benefit from fertility treatment to help them father children.

One of the most important factors for all types of treatment is starting it as early in life as possible.

Section 21.7

Precocious Puberty

"Precocious Puberty," National Institute of Child Health and Human Development (www.nichd.nih.gov), January 15, 2007. Reviewed by David A. Cooke, MD, FACP, April 2012.

What is precocious puberty?

Precocious puberty is puberty that begins before age eight years for girls and before age nine years for boys. The word *precocious* means developing unusually early.

What are the signs of precocious puberty?

The signs of precocious puberty are the same as those for regular puberty. The difference is that they start to occur at a younger age than normal.

- For females, signs include development of breasts, pubic hair, and underarm hair; increased growth rate; and menstrual bleeding.

- In boys, signs include growth of the penis and testicles, development of pubic and underarm hair, muscle growth, voice changes, and increased growth rate.

What causes precocious puberty?

Sometimes precocious puberty is the result of a structural problem in the brain that triggers puberty to begin too early. There are many conditions that may lead to precocious puberty, such as the following:

- Congenital adrenal hyperplasia

- McCune-Albright syndrome

- Gonadal (testicles or ovaries) or adrenal gland disorders or tumors

- hCG (human chorionic gonadotrophin)-secreting tumors

- Hypothalamic hamartoma

But in many cases, there is no identifiable cause for the precocious puberty. Puberty just starts earlier than normal. If you think your child is beginning puberty early, talk to your child's health care provider.

What is the treatment for precocious puberty?

Treatment for precocious puberty can help stop puberty until the child is closer to the normal time for sexual development. One reason to consider treating precocious puberty is that rapid growth and bone maturation can prevent a child from reaching his or her full height potential.

Children grow rapidly in height during puberty and reach their final adult height after puberty. Children who go through puberty too early may not reach their full adult height potential because their growth stops too soon.

Another reason to consider treating precocious puberty is that a young child may not be psychologically ready for the physical and hormonal changes that occur in puberty.

If precocious puberty is caused by a specific medical problem, treating the underlying problem can often stop the puberty. In addition, precocious puberty can often be stopped by medical treatment to block the hormones that cause puberty.

Section 21.8

Turner Syndrome

This section excerpted from "Turner Syndrome,"
Genetics Home Reference, U.S. National Library of Medicine
(ghr.nlm.nih.gov), January 2012.

What is Turner syndrome?

Turner syndrome is a chromosomal condition that affects development in females. The most common feature of Turner syndrome is short stature, which becomes evident by about age five. An early loss of ovarian function (ovarian hypofunction or premature ovarian failure) is also very common. The ovaries develop normally at first, but egg cells (oocytes) usually die prematurely and most ovarian tissue degenerates before birth. Many affected girls do not undergo puberty unless they receive hormone therapy, and most are unable to conceive (infertile). A small percentage of females with Turner syndrome retain normal ovarian function through young adulthood.

About 30% of females with Turner syndrome have extra folds of skin on the neck (webbed neck), a low hairline at the back of the neck, puffiness or swelling (lymphedema) of the hands and feet, skeletal abnormalities, or kidney problems. One third to one half of individuals with Turner syndrome are born with a heart defect, such as a narrowing of the large artery leaving the heart (coarctation of the aorta) or abnormalities of the valve that connects the aorta with the heart (the aortic valve). Complications associated with these heart defects can be life-threatening.

Most girls and women with Turner syndrome have normal intelligence. Developmental delays, nonverbal learning disabilities, and behavioral problems are possible, although these characteristics vary among affected individuals.

How common is Turner syndrome?

This condition occurs in about 1 in 2,500 newborn girls worldwide, but it is much more common among pregnancies that do not survive to term (miscarriages and stillbirths).

What are the genetic changes related to Turner syndrome?

Turner syndrome is related to the X chromosome, which is one of the two sex chromosomes. People typically have two sex chromosomes in each cell: females have two X chromosomes, while males have one X chromosome and one Y chromosome. Turner syndrome results when one normal X chromosome is present in a female's cells and the other sex chromosome is missing or structurally altered. The missing genetic material affects development before and after birth.

Some women with Turner syndrome have a chromosomal change in only some of their cells, which is known as mosaicism. Women with Turner syndrome caused by X chromosome mosaicism are said to have mosaic Turner syndrome.

Researchers have not determined which genes on the X chromosome are associated with most of the features of Turner syndrome. They have, however, identified one gene called SHOX that is important for bone development and growth. The loss of one copy of this gene likely causes short stature and skeletal abnormalities in women with Turner syndrome.

Can Turner syndrome be inherited?

Most cases of Turner syndrome are not inherited. When this condition results from monosomy X, the chromosomal abnormality occurs as a random event during the formation of reproductive cells (eggs and sperm) in the affected person's parent. An error in cell division called nondisjunction can result in reproductive cells with an abnormal number of chromosomes. If one of these atypical reproductive cells contributes to the genetic makeup of a child, the child will have a single X chromosome in each cell and will be missing the other sex chromosome.

Mosaic Turner syndrome is also not inherited. In an affected individual, it occurs as a random event during cell division in early fetal development. As a result, some of an affected person's cells have the usual two sex chromosomes, and other cells have only one copy of the X chromosome. Other sex chromosome abnormalities are also possible in females with X chromosome mosaicism.

Rarely, Turner syndrome caused by a partial deletion of the X chromosome can be passed from one generation to the next.

Chapter 22

Gastrointestinal Disorders in Children

Chapter Contents

Section 22.1

Abdominal Pain

Overview

What is functional abdominal pain?

Abdominal pain that cannot be explained by any visible or detectable abnormality, after a thorough physical examination and appropriate further testing if needed, is known as functional abdominal pain. Functional abdominal pain can be intermittent (recurrent abdominal pain or RAP) or continuous. Although the exact cause is not known, nerve signals or chemicals secreted by the gut or brain may cause the gut to be more sensitive to triggers that normally do not cause significant pain (such as stretching or gas bloating). Because of this change in bowel function, this type of abdominal pain is often referred to as "functional abdominal pain."

How common is functional abdominal pain?

Functional abdominal pain is one of the most common complaints of children and adolescents who are seen by gastroenterologists who care for young patients. In fact, almost a quarter of all children seen for stomach or intestinal complaints have functional abdominal pain.

Causes

Is functional abdominal pain related to other types of chronic abdominal pain? complaints?

Functional abdominal pain includes several different types of chronic abdominal pain, including recurrent abdominal pain, functional dyspepsia, and irritable bowel syndrome. Recurrent abdominal pain

(RAP) was originally defined about 50 years ago as three or more bouts of abdominal pain (bellyache) in children 4–16 years old over a three-month period severe enough to interfere with his/her activities. Usually, this pain is located around the umbilicus (belly button), however the pattern or location of abdominal pain is not always predictable. The pain may occur suddenly or slowly increase in severity. The pain may be constant or may increase and decrease in severity.

Some children with functional abdominal pain may experience dyspepsia, or upper abdominal pain associated with nausea, vomiting, and/or a feeling of fullness after just a few bites (early satiety). Others may experience abdominal pain with bowel movements. Pain that is usually relieved by bowel movements, or associated with changes in bowel movement habits (mainly constipation, diarrhea, or constipation alternating with diarrhea), is the classic irritable bowel syndrome (IBS).

What else can cause chronic abdominal pain in children?

Most young children will point to the umbilicus (belly button) when asked to describe the location of abdominal pain. However, pain centered around the belly button could be due to a number of causes that should be considered when evaluating a child with chronic abdominal pain. Some of those causes are not very serious while other causes require close and long-term care. Possible causes that should be considered based on the history, physical examination, and testing are acid reflux, constipation, lactose intolerance, parasitic infections of the small and large intestines, infections of the stomach with a germ called *Helicobacter pylori* (that is associated with ulcers in the first portion of the small bowel), inflammatory bowel diseases (IBD) such as Crohn's disease and ulcerative colitis, celiac disease which is a sensitivity to cereal grains, food allergies, inflammation of the liver (hepatitis), gall bladder problems, an inflamed pancreas, an intestinal obstruction (blockage), appendicitis, and many more rare disorders. It must be emphasized that typically, none of these more severe problems cause abdominal pain in most children with chronic or recurrent bellyaches. Instead, the pain is usually "functional."

Is functional abdominal pain a serious condition?

Parents and children need to be reassured that functional abdominal pain is not life threatening. However, functional abdominal pain may have negative effects on the child's physical and psychological state. The pain may interfere with school attendance, participation in sports, and other extracurricular activities. Infrequently, it may affect appetite and sleep. The changes in the daily routine may affect the child's mood and emotions, and in turn cause depression and anxiety. In some cases, children previously suffering from anxiety, depression, and other psychiatric disorders may show an exaggerated pain response. Sometimes, the parent and the child may not be consciously aware of any stress or emotional disturbances.

Diagnosis

How can serious causes of abdominal pain be separated from non-serious causes such as functional abdominal pain?

Detailed information regarding the location of abdominal pain, the frequency (number of times per week) and duration of a typical episode, and association with other complaints will in most cases provide useful clues about the cause, and will guide further testing. Other important pieces of information, known as "red flags" or "alarm signs," that a physician may inquire about include weight loss, poor growth, fever, joint pains, mouth ulcers, unusual rashes, loss of appetite, blood that appears in the vomiting or stool, and nighttime awakening due to diarrhea and abdominal pain. The doctor will also ask about the effects of foods and beverages upon the pain, and relationship to stools, sleep, physical activities, and emotional stress.

Will there be any tests to diagnose the cause of abdominal pain?

The diagnosis of functional abdominal pain is often based on the report of symptoms and normal physical examination. It is also quite possible that the doctor may obtain some tests. The reason for these tests is to look for signs of any serious disease. These screening tests may initially include blood and stool tests. The results of screening tests often guide the doctor in deciding whether further tests are needed or whether a trial of diet changes, stress management or medication may be started. Testing should be limited if the history is typical for functional abdominal pain and the child's physical examination is normal. In that case, many doctors prefer to treat without testing in order to avoid the discomfort of testing or the slight risk associated with testing. Of course, if the history, the physical examination, or the results of screening tests are abnormal, further testing may be required. This further testing may include a test to confirm lactose intolerance, ultrasound of the abdomen, a CT [computed tomography] of the abdomen, and upper GI [gastrointestinal] series (radiology test), and possibly an endoscopy (scope). The scope allows the doctor to use a special camera on the scope to look at the inner lining of the food pipe, stomach, first and last portion of the small intestine, and the large intestine. At the time of the scope, biopsies (small pinches of the lining) are also obtained and examined under the microscope for signs of certain infections and disorders like IBD and celiac disease. Normal test results in a child without alarm signs or red flags strongly suggest RAP or one of the other types of functional abdominal pain, such as irritable bowel syndrome or functional dyspepsia.

Treatments

What is the management of children with functional abdominal pain?

If a specific cause for abdominal pain is discovered during the evaluation, the physician will discuss specific management of conditions like constipation, lactose intolerance, infections, IBD, celiac disease, and food allergies. If no specific cause is found and functional abdominal pain is suspected, the child needs to be reassured that his or her abdominal pain is accepted as a real disorder and not something that is "just in the head." The goal of managing functional abdominal pain is to provide a satisfactory quality of life through support, education, medicines, and better coping skills. Reassurance about the good outcome of functional abdominal pain and the positive aspects of the child's health are crucial. Addressing the parents' and child's concerns and fears and identifying emotional or psychological stressors are also important. As noted before, some tests may be needed during the evaluation of functional abdominal pain, but it is also important for parents and children to know that doing too many unnecessary tests may be frustrating to the family and child. If functional abdominal pain is strongly suspected as the likely diagnosis, testing should be limited to the most useful, simple, and relatively noninvasive tests.

The child may benefit from certain dietary changes depending on his/her history. These are recommended on a case-by-case basis. The physician may advise avoidance of greasy and spicy foods, caffeine, juices, and carbonated drinks. Eliminating lactose (a natural sugar in milk and other dairy products) from the diet may benefit those who suffer from lactose intolerance in addition to functional abdominal pain. Some children with abdominal pain who also experience "gas" may improve by eating food slowly and by avoiding carbonated drinks and gas-forming foods such as cabbage or beans. In addition, fruit drinks, sugar-free chewing gum, and sugar-free candy sweetened with an alcohol called sorbitol should be avoided. Sorbitol, which tastes sweet, cannot be properly digested, and when taken in large amounts, it can cause cramping, bloating, and even diarrhea.

Some children may be candidates for medications, if functional abdominal pain is significantly limiting the daily routine. These medications include anti-spasmodic medicines for those with crampy pain in relation to bowel movements, laxatives for those with constipation, and acid-suppressing medicines for those with pain and dyspepsia. If the child does not respond to any of these treatments, he or she may benefit from low doses of medicines called tricyclic antidepressants (used at much higher doses to treat depression). At low doses, these medicines can be excellent pain relievers for some children. A fearful, anxious, or depressed child, however, should be fully assessed by a psychiatrist or psychologist. Some psychological treatments that help children cope with functional abdominal pain and other stressors include behavioral therapy, relaxation exercises, and hypnosis. It is very important that the physician, parents, and school encourage the child resume a normal routine.

What are the effects of the functional abdominal pain in the long term?

Fortunately, the diagnosis of functional abdominal pain has a good outcome overall, with almost half of these children getting better on their own or with treatment within a few weeks to months. A supportive and understanding environment at home and school is important to keep the child physically and mentally healthy.

Section 22.2

Appendicitis

This section excerpted from "Appendicitis," National Digestive Diseases Information Clearinghouse, National Institute of Diabetes and Digestive and Kidney Diseases (digestive.niddk.nih.gov), November 2008.

What is appendicitis?

Appendicitis is a painful swelling and infection of the appendix.

What is the appendix?

The appendix is a fingerlike pouch attached to the large intestine and located in the lower right area of the abdomen. Scientists are not sure what the appendix does, if anything, but removing it does not appear to affect a person's health. The inside of the appendix is called the appendiceal lumen. Mucus created by the appendix travels through the appendiceal lumen and empties into the large intestine.

What causes appendicitis?

Obstruction of the appendiceal lumen causes appendicitis. Mucus backs up in the appendiceal lumen, causing bacteria that normally live inside the appendix to multiply. As a result, the appendix swells and becomes infected. Sources of obstruction include the following:

- Feces, parasites, or growths that clog the appendiceal lumen

- Enlarged lymph tissue in the wall of the appendix, caused by infection in the gastrointestinal tract or elsewhere in the body

- Inflammatory bowel disease, including Crohn disease and ulcerative colitis

- Trauma to the abdomen

An inflamed appendix will likely burst if not removed. Bursting spreads infection throughout the abdomen—a potentially dangerous condition called peritonitis.

379

Who gets appendicitis?

Anyone can get appendicitis, but it is more common among people 10 to 30 years old. Appendicitis leads to more emergency abdominal surgeries than any other cause.

What are the symptoms of appendicitis?

Most people with appendicitis have classic symptoms that a doctor can easily identify. The main symptom of appendicitis is abdominal pain. The abdominal pain usually follows these patterns:

- Occurs suddenly, often causing a person to wake up at night
- Occurs before other symptoms
- Begins near the belly button and then moves lower and to the right
- Is new and unlike any pain felt before
- Gets worse in a matter of hours
- Gets worse when moving around, taking deep breaths, coughing, or sneezing

Other symptoms of appendicitis may include the following:

- Loss of appetite
- Nausea
- Vomiting
- Constipation or diarrhea
- Inability to pass gas
- A low-grade fever that follows other symptoms
- Abdominal swelling
- The feeling that passing stool will relieve discomfort

Symptoms vary and can mimic other sources of abdominal pain, including these:

- Intestinal obstruction
- Inflammatory bowel disease
- Pelvic inflammatory disease and other gynecological disorders
- Intestinal adhesions
- Constipation

How is appendicitis diagnosed?

A doctor or other health care provider can diagnose most cases of appendicitis by taking a person's medical history and performing a physical examination. If a person shows classic symptoms, a doctor may suggest surgery right away to remove the appendix before it bursts. Doctors may use laboratory and imaging tests to confirm appendicitis if a person does not have classic symptoms. Tests may also help diagnose appendicitis in people who cannot adequately describe their symptoms, such as children or the mentally impaired.

Details about the abdominal pain are key to diagnosing appendicitis. The doctor will assess pain by touching or applying pressure to specific areas of the abdomen.

Responses that may indicate appendicitis include the following:

- **Guarding:** Guarding occurs when a person subconsciously tenses the abdominal muscles during an examination.

- **Rebound tenderness:** A doctor tests for rebound tenderness by applying hand pressure to a patient's abdomen and then letting go. Pain felt upon the release of the pressure indicates rebound tenderness.

- **Rovsing sign:** A doctor tests for Rovsing sign by applying hand pressure to the lower left side of the abdomen. Pain felt on the lower right side of the abdomen upon the release of pressure on the left side indicates the presence of Rovsing sign.

- **Psoas sign:** The right psoas muscle runs over the pelvis near the appendix. Flexing this muscle will cause abdominal pain if the appendix is inflamed.

- **Obturator sign:** The right obturator muscle also runs near the appendix. A doctor tests for the obturator sign by asking the patient to lie down with the right leg bent at the knee.

Women of childbearing age may be asked to undergo a pelvic exam to rule out gynecological conditions, which sometimes cause abdominal pain similar to appendicitis. The doctor may also examine the rectum, which can be tender from appendicitis.

How is appendicitis treated?

Typically, appendicitis is treated by removing the appendix. If appendicitis is suspected, a doctor will often suggest surgery without conducting extensive diagnostic testing. Prompt surgery decreases the likelihood the appendix will burst.

Surgery to remove the appendix is called appendectomy and can be done two ways. The older method, called laparotomy, removes the appendix through a single incision in the lower right area of the abdomen. The newer method, called laparoscopic surgery, uses several smaller incisions and special surgical tools fed through the incisions to remove the appendix. Laparoscopic surgery leads to fewer complications, such as hospital-related infections, and has a shorter recovery time.

Surgery occasionally reveals a normal appendix. In such cases, many surgeons will remove the healthy appendix to eliminate the future possibility of appendicitis.

Sometimes an abscess forms around a burst appendix—called an appendiceal abscess. An abscess is a pus-filled mass that results from the body's attempt to keep an infection from spreading. An abscess may be addressed during surgery or, more commonly, drained before surgery.

Nonsurgical treatment may be used if surgery is not available, if a person is not well enough to undergo surgery, or if the diagnosis is unclear. Some research suggests that appendicitis can get better without surgery. Nonsurgical treatment includes antibiotics to treat infection and a liquid or soft diet until the infection subsides. A soft diet is low in fiber and easily breaks down in the gastrointestinal tract.

With adequate care, most people recover from appendicitis and do not need to make changes to diet, exercise, or lifestyle. Full recovery from surgery takes about four to six weeks. Limiting physical activity during this time allows tissues to heal.

What should people do if they think they have appendicitis?

Appendicitis is a medical emergency that requires immediate care. People who think they have appendicitis should see a doctor or go to the emergency room right away. Swift diagnosis and treatment reduce the chances the appendix will burst and improve recovery time.

Section 22.3

Celiac Disease

This section excerpted from "Celiac Disease," National Digestive Diseases Information Clearinghouse, National Institute of Diabetes and Digestive and Kidney Diseases (digestive.niddk.nih.gov), September 2008.

What is celiac disease?

Celiac disease is a digestive disease that damages the small intestine and interferes with absorption of nutrients from food. People who have celiac disease cannot tolerate gluten, a protein in wheat, rye, and barley. Gluten is found mainly in foods but may also be found in everyday products such as medicines, vitamins, and lip balms.

When people with celiac disease eat foods or use products containing gluten, their immune system responds by damaging or destroying villi—the tiny, fingerlike protrusions lining the small intestine. Villi normally allow nutrients from food to be absorbed through the walls of the small intestine into the bloodstream. Without healthy villi, a person becomes malnourished, no matter how much food one eats.

Celiac disease is both a disease of malabsorption—meaning nutrients are not absorbed properly—and an abnormal immune reaction to gluten. Celiac disease is genetic, meaning it runs in families. Sometimes the disease is triggered—or becomes active for the first time—after surgery, pregnancy, childbirth, viral infection, or severe emotional stress.

What are the symptoms of celiac disease?

Symptoms of celiac disease vary from person to person. Symptoms may occur in the digestive system or in other parts of the body. Digestive symptoms are more common in infants and young children and may include the following:

- Abdominal bloating and pain

- Chronic diarrhea

- Vomiting

- Constipation

- Pale, foul-smelling, or fatty stool

- Weight loss

Irritability is another common symptom in children. Malabsorption of nutrients during the years when nutrition is critical to a child's normal growth and development can result in other problems such as failure to thrive in infants, delayed growth and short stature, delayed puberty, and dental enamel defects of the permanent teeth.

Adults are less likely to have digestive symptoms and may instead have one or more of the following:

- Unexplained iron-deficiency anemia

- Fatigue

- Bone or joint pain

- Arthritis

- Bone loss or osteoporosis

- Depression or anxiety

- Tingling numbness in the hands and feet

- Seizures

- Missed menstrual periods

- Infertility or recurrent miscarriage

- Canker sores inside the mouth

- An itchy skin rash called dermatitis herpetiformis

People with celiac disease may have no symptoms but can still develop complications of the disease over time. Long-term complications include malnutrition—which can lead to anemia, osteoporosis, and miscarriage, among other problems—liver diseases, and cancers of the intestine.

Why are celiac disease symptoms so varied?

Researchers are studying the reasons celiac disease affects people differently. The length of time a person was breastfed, the age a person started eating gluten-containing foods, and the amount of gluten-containing foods one eats are three factors thought to play a role in when and how celiac disease appears.

Symptoms also vary depending on a person's age and the degree of damage to the small intestine. Many adults have the disease for a decade or more before they are diagnosed.

How common is celiac disease?

More than 2 million people in the United States have the disease, or about 1 in 133 people. Among people who have a first-degree relative—a parent, sibling, or child—diagnosed with celiac disease, as many as 1 in 22 people may have the disease.

How is celiac disease diagnosed?

Recognizing celiac disease can be difficult because some of its symptoms are similar to those of other diseases. Celiac disease can be confused with irritable bowel syndrome, iron-deficiency anemia caused by menstrual blood loss, inflammatory bowel disease, diverticulitis, intestinal infections, and chronic fatigue syndrome. As a result, celiac disease has long been underdiagnosed or misdiagnosed.

Blood tests: People with celiac disease have higher than normal levels of certain autoantibodies—proteins that react against the body's own cells or tissues—in their blood. To diagnose celiac disease, doctors will test blood for high levels of anti-tissue transglutaminase antibodies (tTGA) or anti-endomysium antibodies (EMA).

Before being tested, one should continue to eat a diet that includes foods with gluten, such as breads and pastas. If a person stops eating foods with gluten before being tested, the results may be negative for celiac disease even if the disease is present.

Intestinal biopsy: If blood tests and symptoms suggest celiac disease, a biopsy of the small intestine is performed to confirm the diagnosis.

Dermatitis herpetiformis (DH): DH is an intensely itchy, blistering skin rash that affects 15% to 25% of people with celiac disease. The rash usually occurs on the elbows, knees, and buttocks. Most people with DH have no digestive symptoms of celiac disease. DH is diagnosed through blood tests and a skin biopsy.

Screening: Screening for celiac disease means testing for the presence of autoantibodies in the blood in people without symptoms. Americans are not routinely screened for celiac disease. However, because celiac disease is hereditary, family members of a person with the disease may wish to be tested.

How is celiac disease treated?

The only treatment for celiac disease is a gluten-free diet. Doctors may ask a newly diagnosed person to work with a dietitian on a gluten-free diet plan. Someone with celiac disease can learn from a dietitian how to read ingredient lists and identify foods that contain gluten in order to make informed decisions at the grocery store and when eating out.

For most people, following this diet will stop symptoms, heal existing intestinal damage, and prevent further damage. Improvement begins within days of starting the diet. The small intestine usually heals in three to six months in children but may take several years in adults.

To stay well, people with celiac disease must avoid gluten for the rest of their lives. Eating even a small amount of gluten can damage the small intestine. Depending on a person's age at diagnosis, some problems will not improve, such as short stature and dental enamel defects.

Some people with celiac disease show no improvement on the gluten-free diet. The most common reason for poor response to the diet is that small amounts of gluten are still being consumed. Hidden sources of gluten include additives such as modified food starch, preservatives, and stabilizers made with wheat.

Rarely, the intestinal injury will continue despite a strictly gluten-free diet. People with this condition, known as refractory celiac disease, have severely damaged intestines that cannot heal. Because their intestines are not absorbing enough nutrients, they may need to receive nutrients directly into their bloodstream through a vein, or intravenously.

What is the gluten-free diet?

A gluten-free diet means not eating foods that contain wheat, rye, and barley. Foods and products made from these grains should also be avoided. In other words, a person with celiac disease should not eat most grain, pasta, cereal, and many processed foods.

Despite these restrictions, people with celiac disease can eat a well-balanced diet with a variety of foods. They can use potato, rice, soy, amaranth, quinoa, buckwheat, or bean flour instead of wheat flour. They can buy gluten-free bread, pasta, and other products from stores that carry organic foods or order products from special food companies. Gluten-free products are increasingly available from mainstream stores.

"Plain" meat, fish, rice, fruits, and vegetables do not contain gluten, so people with celiac disease can freely eat these foods.

The gluten-free diet requires a completely new approach to eating. Newly diagnosed people and their families may find support groups helpful as they learn to adjust to a new way of life.

Gluten is also used in some medications. People with celiac disease should ask a pharmacist if prescribed medications contain wheat. Because gluten is sometimes used as an additive in unexpected products—such as lipstick and play dough—reading product labels is important. If the ingredients are not listed on the label, the manufacturer should provide a list upon request. With practice, screening for gluten becomes second nature.

Section 22.4

Crohn Disease

This section excerpted from "Crohn's Disease," National Digestive Diseases Information Clearinghouse, National Institute of Diabetes and Digestive and Kidney Diseases (digestive.niddk .nih.gov), January 18, 2011.

Crohn disease is a disease that causes inflammation, or swelling, and irritation of any part of the digestive tract—also called the GI tract. The part most commonly affected is the end part of the small intestine, called the ileum.

In Crohn disease, inflammation extends deep into the lining of the affected part of the GI tract. Swelling can cause pain and can make the intestine—also called the bowel—empty frequently, resulting in diarrhea. Chronic—or long-lasting—inflammation may produce scar tissue that builds up inside the intestine to create a stricture. A stricture is a narrowed passageway that can slow the movement of food through the intestine, causing pain or cramps.

Crohn disease is an inflammatory bowel disease, the general name for diseases that cause inflammation and irritation in the intestines. Crohn disease can be difficult to diagnose because its symptoms are similar to other intestinal disorders.

Crohn disease affects men and women equally and seems to run in some families. Crohn disease occurs in people of all ages, but it most commonly starts in people between the ages of 13 and 30.

Causes

The cause of Crohn disease is unknown, but researchers believe it is the result of an abnormal reaction by the body's immune system. Normally, the immune system protects people from infection by identifying and destroying bacteria, viruses, or other potentially harmful foreign substances. Researchers believe that in Crohn disease the immune system attacks bacteria, foods, and other substances that are actually harmless or beneficial. During this process, white blood cells accumulate in the lining of the intestines, producing chronic inflammation, which leads to ulcers, or sores, and injury to the intestines.

Symptoms

The most common symptoms of Crohn disease are abdominal pain, often in the lower right area, and diarrhea. Rectal bleeding, weight loss, and fever may also occur. Bleeding may be serious and persistent, leading to anemia—a condition in which red blood cells are fewer or smaller than normal, which means less oxygen is carried to the body's cells. The range and severity of symptoms varies.

Diagnosis

A doctor will perform a thorough physical exam and schedule a series of tests to diagnose Crohn disease.

- **Blood tests** can be used to look for anemia caused by bleeding. Blood tests may also uncover a high white blood cell count, which is a sign of inflammation or infection somewhere in the body.

- **Stool tests** are commonly done to rule out other causes of GI diseases, such as infection.

- **Flexible sigmoidoscopy and colonoscopy** tests are used to help diagnose Crohn disease and determine how much of the GI tract is affected. For either test, the person will lie on a table while the doctor inserts a flexible tube into the anus. A small camera on the tube sends a video image of the intestinal lining to a computer screen. The doctor can see inflammation, bleeding, or ulcers on the colon wall. The doctor may also perform a biopsy by snipping a bit of tissue from the intestinal lining.

- **CT** scans use a combination of X-rays and computer technology to create three-dimensional (3-D) images.

- An **upper or lower GI series** may be done to look at the small or large intestine.

Complications

The most common complication of Crohn disease is an intestinal blockage caused by thickening of the intestinal wall because of swelling and scar tissue. Crohn disease may also cause ulcers that tunnel through the affected area into surrounding tissues. The tunnels, called fistulas, are a common complication—especially in the areas around the anus and rectum—and often become infected. Most fistulas can be treated with medication, but some may require surgery. In addition to fistulas, small tears called fissures may develop in the lining of the mucus membrane of the anus. The health care provider may prescribe a topical cream and may suggest soaking the affected area in warm water.

Some Crohn disease complications occur because the diseased area of intestine does not absorb nutrients effectively, resulting in deficiencies of proteins, calories, and vitamins.

People with Crohn disease often have anemia, which can be caused by the disease itself or by iron deficiency. Anemia may make a person feel tired. Children with Crohn disease may fail to grow normally and may have low height for their age.

Other complications include osteoporosis, restless legs syndrome, arthritis, skin problems, inflammation in the eyes or mouth, kidney stones, gallstones, or diseases related to liver function.

Treatment

Treatment may include medications, surgery, nutrition supplementation, or a combination of these options. The goals of treatment are to control inflammation, correct nutritional deficiencies, and relieve symptoms such as abdominal pain, diarrhea, and rectal bleeding.

Treatment can help control Crohn disease and make recurrences less frequent, but no cure exists. Someone with Crohn disease may need long-lasting medical care and regular doctor visits to monitor the condition. Some people have long periods—sometimes years—of remission when they are free of symptoms, and predicting when a remission may occur or when symptoms will return is not possible. This changing pattern of the disease makes it difficult to be certain a treatment has helped.

Despite possible hospitalizations and the need to take medication for long periods of time, most people with Crohn disease have full lives—balancing families, careers, and activities.

Medications

Anti-inflammation medications: Most people are first treated with medications containing mesalamine, a substance that helps control inflammation.

Cortisone or steroids: These medications, also called corticosteroids, are effective at reducing inflammation. During the earliest stages of Crohn disease, when symptoms are at their worst, corticosteroids are usually prescribed in a large dose.

Immune system suppressors: Medications that suppress the immune system are also used to treat Crohn disease. Immunosuppressive medications work by blocking the immune reaction that contributes to inflammation.

Biological therapies: Biological therapies are medications given by an injection in the vein or an injection in the skin. Biological therapies bind to TNF [tumor necrosis factor] substances to block the body's inflammation response.

Antibiotics: Antibiotics are used to treat bacterial overgrowth in the small intestine caused by stricture, fistulas, or surgery.

Antidiarrheal medications and fluid replacements: Diarrhea and abdominal cramps are often relieved when the inflammation subsides, but additional medication may be needed.

Surgery

About two-thirds of people with Crohn disease will require surgery at some point in their lives. Surgery becomes necessary to relieve symptoms that do not respond to medical therapy or to correct complications such as intestinal blockage, perforation, bleeding, or abscess—a painful, swollen, pus-filled area caused by infection. Surgery to remove part of the intestine can help people with Crohn disease, but it does not eliminate the disease. People with Crohn disease commonly need more than one operation because inflammation tends to return to the area next to where the diseased intestine was removed.

Because Crohn disease often recurs after surgery, people considering surgery should carefully weigh its benefits and risks compared with other treatments.

Nutrition Supplementation

The health care provider may recommend nutritional supplements, especially for children whose growth has been slowed. Special high-calorie liquid formulas are sometimes used. A small number of people may receive nutrition intravenously for a brief time through a small tube inserted into an arm vein.

Eating, Diet, and Nutrition

No special diet has been proven effective for preventing or treating Crohn disease, but it is important that people who have Crohn disease follow a nutritious diet and avoid any foods that seem to worsen symptoms. People with Crohn disease often experience a decrease in appetite, which can affect their ability to receive the daily nutrition needed for good health and healing. In addition, Crohn disease is associated with diarrhea and poor absorption of necessary nutrients. Foods do not cause Crohn disease, but foods such as bulky grains, hot spices, alcohol, and milk products may increase diarrhea and cramping.

Section 22.5

Constipation

This section excerpted from "Constipation in Children," National Digestive Diseases Information Clearinghouse, National Institute of Diabetes and Digestive and Kidney Diseases (digestive.niddk .nih.gov), October 2008.

What is constipation?

Constipation is a condition in which bowel movements occur less frequently than usual or stools tend to be hard, dry, and difficult and painful to pass. It is common in children and is usually without long-term consequences; however, it can diminish a child's quality of life, cause emotional problems, and create family stress. Rarely, constipation is a sign of a more serious health problem.

What causes constipation in children?

Children often develop constipation as a result of stool withholding. They may withhold stool because they are stressed about potty training, are embarrassed to use a public bathroom, do not want to interrupt playtime, or are fearful of having a painful or unpleasant bowel movement.

Delaying a bowel movement causes stool to become hard, dry, and difficult to pass—sometimes resulting in a large mass of stool in the rectum called a fecal impaction. Stool builds up behind the impaction and may unexpectedly leak, soiling a child's underwear. Parents often mistake this soiling as a sign of diarrhea.

Other causes of constipation in children include the following:

- A low-fiber diet
- Certain medications or drugs, such as antacids, opiates, and antidepressants
- Diseases, such as Hirschsprung disease, diabetes, and Down syndrome
- Anatomic abnormalities, such as a birth defect

What are the symptoms of constipation in children?

Symptoms of constipation in children include the following:

- Fewer bowel movements than usual
- Postures that indicate the child is withholding stool, such as standing on tiptoes and then rocking back on the heels of the feet, clenching buttocks muscles, and other unusual dancelike behaviors; parents often mistake such postures as attempts to "push"
- Abdominal pain and cramping
- Painful or difficult bowel movements
- Hard, dry, or large stools
- Stool in the child's underwear

When should a child with constipation see a doctor?

A child should see a doctor if symptoms of constipation last for more than two weeks. A child should see a doctor sooner if the constipation is accompanied by one or more of these symptoms that may indicate a more serious health problem:

- Fever
- Vomiting
- Blood in the stool
- A swollen abdomen
- Weight loss
- Painful cracks in the skin around the anus, called anal fissures
- Intestine coming out of the anus, called rectal prolapse

The doctor will ask questions about the child's history of symptoms and will perform a physical examination. The doctor may perform a rectal exam by inserting a gloved finger into the child's anus to check for anatomical abnormalities and for the presence of a fecal impaction.

How is constipation in children treated?

Constipation is treated by changing diet, taking laxatives, and adopting healthy bowel habits. Treatment depends on the child's age and the severity of the problem. Dietary changes include eating more high-fiber foods, such as whole grains, fruits, and vegetables. Laxatives are frequently used to clear a fecal impaction and sometimes to re-store regular bowel movements. A doctor should be consulted before giving a laxative to a child. Parents should encourage their child to spend time on the toilet after meals and when their child shows signs of withholding stool.

A child should be seen again by a doctor if treatment fails or if the child begins to show symptoms that suggest a more serious health problem.

Section 22.6

Cyclic Vomiting Syndrome

This section excerpted from "Cyclic Vomiting Syndrome," National Digestive Diseases Information Clearinghouse, National Institute of Diabetes and Digestive and Kidney Diseases (digestive.niddk.nih .gov), December 2008.

What is cyclic vomiting syndrome (CVS)?

CVS is characterized by episodes or cycles of severe nausea and vomiting that last for hours, or even days, that alternate with inter-vals with no symptoms. Although originally thought to be a pediatric disease, CVS occurs in all age groups. Medical researchers believe CVS and migraine headaches are related.

Each episode of CVS is similar to previous ones, meaning the epi-sodes tend to start at the same time of day, last the same length of time, and occur with the same symptoms and level of intensity. Although CVS can begin at any age, in children it starts most often between the ages of three and seven.

Episodes can be so severe that a person has to stay in bed for days, unable to go to school or work. The exact number of people with CVS is unknown, but medical researchers believe more people may have the disorder than commonly thought. Because other more common diseases and disorders also cause cycles of vomiting, many people with CVS are initially misdiagnosed until other disorders can be ruled out. CVS can be disruptive and frightening not just to people who have it but to family members as well.

What are the four phases of CVS?

CVS has four phases:

- **Symptom-free interval phase:** This phase is the period between episodes when no symptoms are present.

- **Prodrome phase:** This phase signals that an episode of nausea and vomiting is about to begin. Often marked by nausea—with or without abdominal pain—this phase can last from just a few minutes to several hours. Sometimes, taking medicine early in the phase can stop an episode in progress. However, sometimes there is no warning; a person may simply wake up in the morning and begin vomiting.

- **Vomiting phase:** This phase consists of nausea and vomiting; an inability to eat, drink, or take medicines without vomiting; paleness; drowsiness; and exhaustion.

- **Recovery phase:** This phase begins when the nausea and vomiting stop. Healthy color, appetite, and energy return.

What triggers CVS?

Many people can identify a specific condition or event that triggered an episode, such as an infection. Common triggers in children include emotional stress and excitement. Anxiety and panic attacks are more common triggers in adults. Colds, allergies, sinus problems, and the flu can also set off episodes in some people.

Other reported triggers include eating certain foods such as chocolate or cheese, eating too much, or eating just before going to bed. Hot weather, physical exhaustion, menstruation, and motion sickness can also trigger episodes.

What are the symptoms of CVS?

A person who experiences the following symptoms for at least three months—with first onset at least six months prior—may have CVS:

- Vomiting episodes that start with severe vomiting—several times per hour—and last less than one week

- Three or more separate episodes of vomiting in the past year

- Absence of nausea or vomiting between episodes

A person with CVS may experience abdominal pain, diarrhea, fever, dizziness, and sensitivity to light during vomiting episodes. Continued vomiting may cause severe dehydration that can be life threatening. Symptoms of dehydration include thirst, decreased urination, paleness, exhaustion, and listlessness. A person with any symptoms of dehydration should see a health care provider immediately.

How is CVS diagnosed?

CVS is hard to diagnose because no tests—such as a blood test or X-ray—can establish a diagnosis of CVS. A doctor must look at symptoms and medical history to rule out other common diseases or disorders that can cause nausea and vomiting. Making a diagnosis takes time because the doctor also needs to identify a pattern or cycle to the vomiting.

What is the relationship between CVS and migraine?

The relationship between migraine and CVS is still unclear, but medical researchers believe the two are related.

- Migraine headaches, which cause severe head pain; abdominal migraines, which cause stomach pain; and CVS are all marked by severe symptoms that start and end quickly and are followed by intervals without pain or other symptoms.

- Many of the situations that trigger CVS also trigger migraines, including stress and excitement.

- Research has shown that many children with CVS either have a family history of migraine or develop migraines as they grow older.

Because of the similarities between migraine and CVS, doctors treat some people with severe CVS with drugs that are also used for migraine headaches. The drugs are designed to prevent episodes, reduce frequency, and lessen severity.

How is CVS treated?

Treatment varies, but people with CVS generally improve after learning to control their symptoms. People with CVS are advised to get plenty of rest and sleep and to take medications that prevent a vomiting episode, stop one in progress, speed up recovery, or relieve associated symptoms.

Once a vomiting episode begins, treatment usually requires the person to stay in bed and sleep in a dark, quiet room. Severe nausea and vomiting may require hospitalization and intravenous fluids to prevent dehydration. Sedatives may help if the nausea continues.

Sometimes, during the prodrome phase, it is possible to stop an episode from happening. For example, people with nausea or abdominal pain before an episode can ask their doctor about taking ondansetron (Zofran) or lorazepam (Ativan) for nausea or ibuprofen (Advil, Motrin) for pain. Other medications that may be helpful are ranitidine (Zantac) or omeprazole (Prilosec), which help calm the stomach by lowering the amount of acid it makes.

During the recovery phase, drinking water and replacing lost electrolytes are important. Electrolytes are salts the body needs to function and stay healthy. Symptoms during the recovery phase can vary. Some people find their appetite returns to normal immediately, while others need to begin by drinking clear liquids and then move slowly to solid food.

People whose episodes are frequent and long-lasting may be treated during the symptom-free intervals in an effort to prevent or ease future episodes. Medications that help people with migraine headaches are sometimes used during this phase, but they do not work for everyone. Taking the medicine daily for one to two months may be necessary before one can tell if it helps.

The symptom-free interval phase is a good time to eliminate anything known to trigger an episode. For example, if episodes are brought on by stress or excitement, a symptom-free interval phase is the time to find ways to reduce stress and stay calm. If sinus problems or allergies cause episodes, those conditions should be treated.

What are the complications of CVS?

The severe vomiting that defines CVS is a risk factor for several complications:

- **Dehydration:** Vomiting causes the body to lose water quickly. Dehydration can be severe and should be treated immediately.

- **Electrolyte imbalance:** Vomiting causes the body to lose important salts it needs to keep working properly.

- **Peptic esophagitis:** The esophagus becomes injured from stomach acid moving through it while vomiting.

- **Hematemesis:** The esophagus becomes irritated and bleeds, so blood mixes with vomit.

- **Mallory-Weiss tear:** The lower end of the esophagus may tear open or the stomach may bruise from vomiting or retching.

- **Tooth decay:** The acid in vomit can hurt teeth by corroding tooth enamel.

Section 22.7

Diarrhea

This section excerpted from "Diarrhea," National Digestive Diseases Information Clearinghouse, National Institute of Diabetes and Digestive and Kidney Diseases (digestive.niddk.nih.gov), January 2011.

What is diarrhea?

Diarrhea is loose, watery stools. Having diarrhea means passing loose stools three or more times a day. Acute diarrhea is a common problem that usually lasts one or two days and goes away on its own.

Diarrhea lasting more than two days may be a sign of a more serious problem. Chronic diarrhea—diarrhea that lasts at least four weeks—may be a symptom of a chronic disease. Chronic diarrhea symptoms may be continual or they may come and go.

Diarrhea of any duration may cause dehydration, which means the body lacks enough fluid and electrolytes—chemicals in salts, including sodium, potassium, and chloride—to function properly. Loose stools contain more fluid and electrolytes and weigh more than solid stools.

People of all ages can get diarrhea. In the United States, adults average one bout of acute diarrhea each year, and young children have an average of two episodes of acute diarrhea each year.

What causes diarrhea?

Acute diarrhea is usually caused by a bacterial, viral, or parasitic infection. Chronic diarrhea is usually related to a functional disorder such as irritable bowel syndrome or an intestinal disease such as Crohn disease.

The most common causes of diarrhea include the following:

- **Bacterial infections:** Several types of bacteria consumed through contaminated food or water can cause diarrhea.

- **Viral infections:** Many viruses cause diarrhea. Infection with the rotavirus is the most common cause of acute diarrhea in children. Rotavirus diarrhea usually resolves in three to seven days but can cause problems digesting lactose for up to a month or longer.

- **Parasites:** Parasites can enter the body through food or water and settle in the digestive system.

- **Functional bowel disorders:** Diarrhea can be a symptom of irritable bowel syndrome.

- **Intestinal diseases:** Inflammatory bowel disease, ulcerative colitis, Crohn disease, and celiac disease often lead to diarrhea.

- **Food intolerances and sensitivities:** Some people have difficulty digesting certain ingredients, such as lactose, the sugar found in milk and milk products. Some people may have diarrhea if they eat certain types of sugar substitutes in excessive quantities.

- **Reaction to medicines:** Antibiotics, cancer drugs, and antacids containing magnesium can all cause diarrhea.

Some people develop diarrhea after stomach surgery, which may cause food to move through the digestive system more quickly.

People who visit certain foreign countries are at risk for traveler's diarrhea, which is caused by eating food or drinking water contaminated with bacteria, viruses, or parasites. Traveler's diarrhea can be a problem for people traveling to developing countries in Africa, Asia, Latin America, and the Caribbean.

In many cases, the cause of diarrhea cannot be found. As long as diarrhea goes away on its own within one to two days, finding the cause is not usually necessary.

What other symptoms accompany diarrhea?

Diarrhea may be accompanied by cramping, abdominal pain, nausea, an urgent need to use the bathroom, or loss of bowel control. Some infections that cause diarrhea can also cause a fever and chills or bloody stools.

Diarrhea can cause dehydration. Loss of electrolytes through dehydration affects the amount of water in the body, muscle activity, and other important functions.

Dehydration is particularly dangerous in children, older adults, and people with weakened immune systems. Dehydration must be treated promptly to avoid serious health problems. Severe dehydration may require hospitalization.

Signs of dehydration in adults include the following:

- Thirst

- Less frequent urination than usual
- Dark-colored urine
- Dry skin
- Fatigue
- Dizziness
- Light-headedness

Signs of dehydration in infants and young children include these symptoms:

- Dry mouth and tongue
- No tears when crying
- No wet diapers for three hours or more
- Sunken eyes, cheeks, or soft spot in the skull
- High fever
- Listlessness or irritability

Also, when people are dehydrated, their skin does not flatten back to normal right away after being gently pinched and released.

Although drinking plenty of water is important in preventing dehydration, water does not contain electrolytes. Adults can prevent dehydration by also drinking liquids that contain electrolytes, such as fruit juices, sports drinks, caffeine-free soft drinks, and broths. Children with diarrhea should be given oral rehydration solutions such as Pedialyte to prevent dehydration.

When should children with diarrhea see a health care provider?

Children with any of the following symptoms should see a health care provider:

- Signs of dehydration
- Diarrhea for more than 24 hours
- A fever of 102 degrees or higher
- Stools containing blood or pus
- Stools that are black and tarry

If children have diarrhea, parents or caregivers should not hesitate to call a health care provider for advice. Diarrhea is especially dangerous in newborns and infants, leading to severe dehydration in just a day or two. Children can die from dehydration within a day.

How is the cause of diarrhea diagnosed?

If acute diarrhea lasts two days or less, diagnostic tests are usually not necessary. If diarrhea lasts longer or is accompanied by symptoms such as fever or bloody stools, a doctor may perform tests to determine the cause.

Diagnostic tests to find the cause of diarrhea may include the following:

- Medical history and physical examination

- Stool culture: A sample of stool is analyzed in a laboratory to check for bacteria, parasites, or other signs of disease and infection.

- Blood tests

- Fasting tests: To find out if a food intolerance or allergy is causing the diarrhea, the doctor may ask a person to avoid foods with lactose, carbohydrates, wheat, or other ingredients to see whether the diarrhea responds to a change in diet.

- Sigmoidoscopy or colonoscopy: These tests may be used to look for signs of intestinal diseases that cause chronic diarrhea.

How is diarrhea treated?

In most cases of diarrhea, the only treatment necessary is replacing lost fluids and electrolytes to prevent dehydration.

Over-the-counter medicines such as loperamide (Imodium) and bismuth subsalicylate (Pepto-Bismol and Kaopectate) may help stop diarrhea in adults. However, people with bloody diarrhea—a sign of bacterial or parasitic infection—should not use these medicines. If diarrhea is caused by bacteria or parasites, over-the-counter medicines may prolong the problem, so doctors usually prescribe antibiotics instead.

Medications to treat diarrhea in adults can be dangerous for infants and children and should only be given with a doctor's guidance.

Until diarrhea subsides, avoiding caffeine and foods that are greasy, high in fiber, or sweet may lessen symptoms. These foods can aggravate diarrhea. Some people also have problems digesting lactose during or after a bout of diarrhea. Yogurt, which has less lactose than milk, is often better tolerated. Yogurt with active, live bacterial cultures may even help people recover from diarrhea more quickly.

As symptoms improve, soft, bland foods can be added to the diet. Once the diarrhea stops, the health care provider will likely encourage children to return to a normal and healthy diet if it can be tolerated. Infants with diarrhea should be given breast milk or full-strength formula as usual, along with oral rehydration solutions.

Can diarrhea be prevented?

Two types of diarrhea can be prevented—rotavirus diarrhea and traveler's diarrhea.

Rotavirus diarrhea: Two oral vaccines have been approved by the U.S. Food and Drug Administration to protect children from rotavirus infections. Parents of infants should discuss rotavirus vaccination with a health care provider. For more information, parents can visit the Centers for Disease Control and Prevention rotavirus vaccination webpage at www.cdc.gov/vaccines/vpd-vac/rotavirus.

Traveler's diarrhea: To prevent traveler's diarrhea, people traveling from the United States to developing countries should avoid the following:

- Drinking tap water, using tap water to brush their teeth, or using ice made from tap water
- Drinking unpasteurized milk or milk products
- Eating raw fruits and vegetables, unless they peel the fruits or vegetables themselves
- Eating raw or rare meat and fish
- Eating meat or shellfish that is not hot when served
- Eating food from street vendors

Travelers can drink bottled water, soft drinks, and hot drinks such as coffee or tea.

Section 22.8

Dysphagia
(Difficulty Swallowing)

Dysphagia is a term that means "difficulty swallowing." It is the inability of food or liquids to pass easily from the mouth, into the throat, and down into the esophagus to the stomach during the process of swallowing.

What Causes Dysphagia?

To understand dysphagia, we must first understand how we swallow. Swallowing involves three stages. These three stages are controlled by nerves that connect the digestive tract to the brain.

Oral preparation stage: Food is chewed and moistened by saliva. The tongue pushes food and liquids to the back of the mouth toward the throat. (This phase is voluntary: we have control over chewing and beginning to swallow.)

Pharyngeal stage: Food enters the pharynx (throat). A flap called the epiglottis closes off the passage to the windpipe so food cannot get into the lungs. The muscles in the throat relax. Food and liquid are quickly passed down the pharynx (throat) into the esophagus. The epiglottis opens again so we can breathe. (This phase starts under voluntary control, but then becomes an involuntary phase that we cannot consciously control.)

Esophageal stage: Liquids fall through the esophagus into the stomach by gravity. Muscles in the esophagus push food toward the stomach in wave-like movements known as peristalsis. A muscular band between the end of the esophagus and the upper portion of the esophagus (known as the lower esophageal sphincter) relaxes in response to swallowing, allowing food and liquids to enter the stomach. (The events in this phase are involuntary.)

Swallowing disorders occur when one or more of these stages fails to take place properly. Children's health problems that can affect swallowing include:

- cleft lip or cleft palate;

- dental problems (teeth that do not meet properly, such as with an overbite);

- large tongue;

- diseases that affect the nerves and muscles, such as a stroke, tumor, nerve injury, brain injury, or muscular dystrophy, and can cause paralysis or poor function of the tongue or the muscles in the throat and esophagus;

- large tonsils;

- tumors or masses in the throat;

- problems with the prenatal development of the bones of the skull and the structures in the mouth and throat (known as craniofacial anomalies);

- prenatal malformations of the digestive tract, such as esophageal atresia or tracheoesophageal fistula;

- oral sensitivity that can occur in very ill children who have been on a ventilator for a prolonged period of time;

- irritation of the vocal cords after being on a ventilator for long periods of time (as may occur with premature babies or very ill children);

- paralysis of the vocal cords;

- having a tracheostomy (artificial opening in the throat for breathing);

- irritation or scarring of the esophagus or vocal cords by acid in gastroesophageal reflux disease (GERD);

- compression of the esophagus by other body parts, such as the heart, thyroid gland, blood vessels, or lymph nodes;

- foreign bodies in the esophagus, such as a swallowed coin;

- developmental delays;

- prematurity.

Why Is Dysphagia a Concern?

Dysphagia can result in aspiration, which occurs when food or liquids go into the windpipe and lungs. Aspiration of food and liquids may cause pneumonia and/or other serious lung conditions. Children with dysphagia usually have trouble eating enough, leading to inadequate nutrition and failure to gain weight or grow properly.

Symptoms of Dysphagia

The symptoms that children with dysphagia have may be obvious, or they can be difficult to associate with swallowing trouble. The following are the most common symptoms of dysphagia. However, each individual may experience symptoms differently. Symptoms may include:

- eating slowly;
- trying to swallow a single mouthful of food several times;
- difficulty coordinating sucking and swallowing;
- gagging during feeding;
- drooling;
- a feeling that food or liquids are sticking in the throat or esophagus, or that there is a lump in these areas;
- discomfort in the throat or chest;
- congestion in the chest after eating or drinking;
- coughing or choking when eating or drinking (or very soon afterwards);
- wet or raspy sounding voice during or after eating;
- tiredness or shortness of breath while eating or drinking;
- frequent respiratory infections;
- color change during feeding, such as becoming blue or pale;
- spitting up or vomiting frequently;
- food or liquids coming out of the nose during or after a feeding;
- frequent sneezing after eating;
- weight loss.

Symptoms of dysphagia may resemble other conditions or medical problems. Please consult your child's physician for a diagnosis.

Diagnosing Dysphagia

A physician or health care provider will examine your child and obtain a medical history. You will be asked questions about how your child eats and any problems you notice during feeding. Imaging tests may also be done to evaluate the mouth, throat, and esophagus. These tests can include:

- **Oral-pharyngeal video swallow:** Your child is given small amounts of a liquid containing barium to drink with a bottle, spoon, or cup, or spoon fed a solid food containing barium. Barium shows up well on X-ray. A series of X-rays are taken to evaluate what happens as your child swallows the liquid.

- **Barium swallow/upper GI series:** Your child is given a liquid containing barium (a metallic, chemical, chalky liquid used to coat the inside of organs so that they will show up on an X-ray) to drink, and a series of X-rays are taken. The physician can watch what happens as your child swallows the fluid, and note any problems that may occur in the throat, the esophagus, or the stomach.

- **Endoscopy:** A test that uses a small, flexible tube with a light and a camera lens at the end (endoscope) to examine the inside of part of the digestive tract. Under anesthesia, an endoscopy is performed. Pictures are taken of the inside of the throat, the esophagus, and the stomach to look for abnormalities. Small tissue samples, called biopsies, can also be taken to look for problems.

Other tests that may be performed to evaluate dysphagia include the following:

- **Esophageal manometry:** Under sedation, a small tube containing a pressure gauge is guided through your child's mouth and into the esophagus. The pressure inside the esophagus is then measured to evaluate the esophageal motility.

- **Laryngoscopy:** Under anesthesia, a physician places a tube into your child's throat and looks through it for narrowed areas and other problems.

Treatment for Dysphagia

Specific treatment for dysphagia will be determined by your child's physician based on the following:

- Your child's age, overall health, and medical history
- The extent of the disease
- The type of disease
- Your child's tolerance for specific medications, procedures, or therapies

- Expectations for the course of the disease
- Your opinion or preference

Speech or occupational therapy can be helpful for some children. These therapists can give your child exercises to help make swallowing more effective, or suggest techniques for feeding that may help improve swallowing problems.

Infants and children with dysphagia are often able to swallow thick fluids and soft foods (such as baby foods or pureed foods) better than thin liquids. Some infants who had trouble swallowing formula will do better when they are old enough to eat baby foods. The following suggestions should also be considered when caring for a child with dysphagia:

- Adding a small amount of rice cereal to infant formula or pumped breast milk may help dysphagia. Blending the formula/cereal mixture before adding it to a baby bottle can remove the lumps and make the mixture easier to suck through a nipple, as well as easier to swallow.

- Do not cut holes in nipples, since this can increase the risk for choking and aspiration, as well as interfere with the baby's oral development. Future feeding and speech skills may be affected.

- Baby foods should not be offered to infants from a spoon until they are at least four months old, since they do not have the proper coordination to swallow foods from a spoon until this age.

- Your child's speech or occupational therapist may be able to recommend other commercial products that help thicken liquids and make them easier to swallow.

Babies who have "oral aversion," which can occur after oral surgery or being on a ventilator for a prolonged period of time, may benefit from exercises and activities to desensitize them to having objects in their mouths.

- Provide safe toys and other objects for babies to chew on and mouth. Try things that have varying textures and temperatures.

- Vary the taste, texture, and temperature of soft foods for children over the age of four months.

- Allow your child to play with foods and get messy at mealtime.

When symptoms of gastroesophageal reflux disease (GERD) are also present with dysphagia, treating this condition may produce improvements in your child's ability to swallow. (More on GERD at http://www.childrensmemorial.org/depts/gastroenterology/digestion/gerd.asp.) As the esophagus and throat are less irritated by acid reflux, their function may improve. Treatment of GERD may include:

- remaining upright for at least an hour after eating;
- medications to decrease stomach acid production;
- medications to help food move through the digestive tract faster;
- an operation to help keep food and acid in the stomach (fundoplication).

Children who have scarring or narrowing of the esophagus (esophageal stricture) may be able to be dilated, or widened, under anesthesia. This procedure may have to be repeated periodically.

The Long-Term Outlook for a Child with Dysphagia

Some children with dysphagia will have long-term problems. Children who have other health problems, especially those that affect the nerves and muscles (such as muscular dystrophy and brain injury), may not be able to experience much improvement with their swallowing difficulties. Other children may learn to eat and drink successfully.

Consult your child's physician regarding the prognosis for your child.

Section 22.9

Encopresis (Overflow Soiling)

What is constipation?

When your child's bowel movements are very hard, difficult or painful to pass, and/or occur less often than every three days, it is called constipation. This may happen if your child doesn't eat enough fiber, doesn't get enough exercise, or doesn't drink enough liquids (especially water). It can also happen if your child ignores the urge to poop because they are embarrassed to use the public bathroom, or don't want to stop playing. Constipation can make pooping painful, so that your child may hold their poop in to avoid a painful bowel movement. Functional constipation means that the constipation is not due to an underlying disease process.

What is soiling?

Soiling, overflow incontinence, or fecal incontinence is when liquid or formed poop leaks into the child's underwear. The child has no control over this leakage. It usually happens when a big, hard blockage of poop from constipation is blocking the rectum. This is called an impaction. When a child has an impaction, poop can leak around the blockage into the underwear.

What is encopresis?

Encopresis is overflow soiling that happens because of constipation. In children with encopresis, formed, soft, or liquid poop leaks from the anus around a mass of poop that is stuck in the lower bowel. The bowel can get so stretched that your child can no longer feel the urge to poop, and the anal sphincter (the muscle around the anus that

409

holds the poop in) can get very weak. Sometimes the poop takes up so much room that your child's bladder doesn't have enough space. This can cause bedwetting.

How common are constipation and encopresis?

About 16%–37% of school-aged kids have to deal with constipation. Constipation with overflow (encopresis) soiling affects at least 4% of preschool kids and 1–2% of school-aged kids. In school-aged kids, encopresis is most likely to affect boys.

How do I know when to see the doctor?

If you feel there may be a problem with your child's bowel function, don't delay. Talk to your pediatrician. Current studies show that children do better with early diagnosis and treatment.

You should call your child's doctor if:

- you are worried about constipation in your child;

- any constipation symptoms last longer than one week;

- you see blood on the stool (poop), or worry about small skin tears at the anus;

- your child has hemorrhoids;

- normal pushing is not enough to get the poop out;

- your child's bowel movements are painful;

- liquid or soft poop leaks out between bowel movements;

- your child is constipated and vomiting;

- your child has a swollen belly;

- you are concerned about your child's growth and weight gain.

How does the doctor tell if my child has encopresis?

The doctor will need to talk to you and your child. The doctor may need to do a finger exam of your child's rectal vault to feel whether it is full of impacted poop, and may need your child to get an abdominal X-ray and/or barium enema. Keep a "bowel movement monitoring sheet" (available at http://www.med.umich.edu/1libr/guides/BMchart.pdf) of your child's pooping patterns, and bring it to your doctor appointment. This will help the doctor and you figure out what is going on.

What kind of treatment will my child need?

Only a doctor should start treatment for your child. Never give laxatives, suppositories, enemas, or other bowel medication to a child without your child's doctor's instructions to do so.

Treatment may include:

- starting with a "clean-out" to clear the impaction from the rectal vault (your doctor may prescribe a high dose of mineral oil, enemas, or a combination of things);

- changing your child's diet to include more fluids (especially water) and fiber-rich foods;

- making sure your child gets lots of exercise;

- behavioral training, which includes having your child sit on the toilet several times a day, and using rewards for sitting and for pooping (keep the tone positive; never try to embarrass or punish your child);

- giving your child medicines by mouth to help soften the stools;

- following up with your doctor on a regular schedule to make sure the impaction does not happen again.

Remember: it is very important to use both the medicines and the behavior training. You are the key to helping your child solve this problem. Consistency is important. Get your child's school to work with you on the program.

How do I work with my child's school?

Talk with your child's teacher, principal, and school nurse, to make sure they know what is going on. They will need to be involved with making sure that your child gets enough fluids during the school day, and can get to the toilet often and on time. School personnel may also need to help with your child's clean-up if they soil themselves. Teachers have an important role to play in making sure your child can take care of the problem privately and avoid being teased by the other kids.

Section 22.10

Gastroenteritis

This section excerpted from "Viral Gastroenteritis," Centers for Disease Control and Prevention (www.cdc.gov), February 25, 2011.

What is viral gastroenteritis?

Gastroenteritis means inflammation of the stomach and small and large intestines. Viral gastroenteritis is an infection caused by a variety of viruses that results in vomiting or diarrhea. It is often called the "stomach flu," although it is not caused by the influenza viruses.

What causes viral gastroenteritis?

Many different viruses can cause gastroenteritis, including rotaviruses; noroviruses; adenoviruses, types 40 and 41; sapoviruses; and astroviruses. Viral gastroenteritis is not caused by bacteria or parasites, or by medications or other medical conditions, although the symptoms may be similar.

What are the symptoms of viral gastroenteritis?

The main symptoms of viral gastroenteritis are watery diarrhea and vomiting. The affected person may also have headache, fever, and abdominal cramps ("stomach ache"). In general, the symptoms begin 1 to 2 days following infection with a virus that causes gastroenteritis and may last for 1 to 10 days, depending on which virus causes the illness.

Is viral gastroenteritis a serious illness?

For most people, it is not. People who get viral gastroenteritis almost always recover completely without any long-term problems. Gastroenteritis is a serious illness, however, for persons who are unable to drink enough fluids to replace what they lose through vomiting or diarrhea. Infants, young children, and persons who are unable to care for themselves, such as the disabled or elderly, are at risk for dehydration from loss of fluids. Immune-compromised persons are at risk for dehydration because they may get a more serious illness, with greater vomiting or diarrhea. They may need to be hospitalized for treatment to correct or prevent dehydration.

Is the illness contagious? How are these viruses spread?

Yes, viral gastroenteritis is contagious. The viruses that cause gastroenteritis are spread through close contact with infected persons. Individuals may also become infected by eating or drinking contaminated foods or beverages.

How does food get contaminated by gastroenteritis viruses?

Food may be contaminated by food preparers or handlers who have viral gastroenteritis, especially if they do not wash their hands regularly after using the bathroom. Shellfish may be contaminated by sewage, and persons who eat raw or undercooked shellfish harvested from contaminated waters may get diarrhea. Drinking water can also be contaminated by sewage and be a source of spread of these viruses.

Where and when does viral gastroenteritis occur?

Viral gastroenteritis affects people in all parts of the world. Each virus has its own seasonal activity. For example, in the United States, rotavirus and astrovirus infections occur during the cooler months of the year (October to April), whereas adenovirus infections occur throughout the year. Norovirus infections occur year round but tend to increase in cooler months. Norovirus outbreaks can occur in institutional settings, such as schools, child care facilities, and nursing homes.

Who gets viral gastroenteritis?

Anyone can get it. Viral gastroenteritis occurs in people of all ages and backgrounds. However, some viruses tend to cause diarrheal disease primarily among people in specific age groups. Rotavirus infections are the most common cause of diarrhea in infants and young children under five years old. Adenoviruses and astroviruses cause diarrhea mostly in young children, but older children and adults can also be affected. Noroviruses infect persons of all ages.

How is viral gastroenteritis diagnosed?

Generally, viral gastroenteritis is diagnosed by a physician on the basis of the symptoms and medical examination of the patient. Rotavirus infection can be diagnosed by laboratory testing of a stool specimen.

How is viral gastroenteritis treated?

The most important goal of treating viral gastroenteritis in children and adults is to prevent severe loss of fluids (dehydration). This treatment should begin at home. Your physician may give you specific instructions about what kinds of fluid to give. Centers for Disease Control and Prevention (CDC) recommends that families with infants and young children keep a supply of oral rehydration solution (ORS) at home at all times and use the solution when diarrhea first occurs in the child. ORS is available at pharmacies without a prescription. Medications, including antibiotics (which have no effect on viruses) and other treatments, should be avoided unless specifically recommended by a physician.

Can viral gastroenteritis be prevented?

Persons can reduce their chance of getting infected by frequent handwashing, prompt disinfection of contaminated surfaces with household chlorine bleach-based cleaners, and prompt washing of soiled articles of clothing. If food or water is thought to be contaminated, it should be avoided.

Currently there are two licensed rotavirus vaccines available that protect against severe diarrhea from rotavirus infection in infants and young children. These vaccines are given to children in their first year of life with other childhood vaccines.

Section 22.11

Gastroesophageal Reflux

This section excerpted from "Gastroesophageal Reflux in Children and Adolescents," National Digestive Diseases Information Clearinghouse, National Institute of Diabetes and Digestive and Kidney Diseases (digestive.niddk.nih .gov), August 2006. Revised by David A. Cooke, MD, FACP, April 2012.

What is gastroesophageal reflux (GER)?

Gastroesophageal reflux occurs when stomach contents reflux, or back up, into the esophagus during or after a meal. The esophagus is the tube that connects the mouth to the stomach. A ring of muscle at the bottom of the esophagus opens and closes to allow food to enter the stomach. This ring of muscle is called the lower esophageal sphincter (LES). Reflux can occur when the LES opens, allowing stomach contents and acid to come back up into the esophagus.

GER often begins in infancy, but only a small number of infants continue to have GER as older children.

What are the symptoms of GER?

Almost all children and adults have a little bit of reflux, often without being aware of it. When refluxed material rapidly returns to the stomach, it does not harm the esophagus. However, in some children, the stomach contents remain in the esophagus and damage the esophageal lining. In other children, the stomach contents go up to the mouth and are swallowed again. When the refluxed material passes into the back of the mouth or enters the airways, the child may become hoarse, have a raspy voice, or a chronic cough. Other symptoms include the following:

- Recurrent pneumonia

- Wheezing

- Difficult or painful swallowing

- Vomiting

- Sore throat

- Weight loss

- Heartburn (in older children)

How is GER diagnosed?

You may want to visit an internist or a gastroenterologist. The doctor can talk with you about your child's symptoms, examine your child, and recommend tests to determine if reflux is the cause of the symptoms. These tests check the esophagus, stomach, and small intestine for problems. Sometimes a doctor will start treatment without running tests if the symptoms strongly indicate GER.

The most common tests used to diagnose GER are the following:

- **Upper GI series X-ray:** X-rays are taken to check for damage to the esophagus, stomach, or intestines. A doctor cannot make a diagnosis of GER based on X-rays alone, but X-rays help rule out other problems that cause the same symptoms as GER.

- **Endoscopy:** A sedative is given before this procedure to make the child sleepy. A small, flexible tube with a very tiny camera on the end is then inserted through the mouth and esophagus and into the stomach. The camera gives the doctor a view of the lining of the esophagus, stomach, and small intestine.

- **Esophageal pH probe:** A thin, light wire with an acid sensor at its tip is inserted through the nose into the lower part of the esophagus. This probe detects and records the amount of stomach acid coming back up into the esophagus and indicates whether acid is in the esophagus when the child has symptoms such as crying, coughing, or arching her back. Wireless pH probes, which are more comfortable, are becoming increasingly available.

Speak with your child's health care provider if any of the following occur:

- Increased amounts of vomiting or persistent projectile (forceful) vomiting

- Vomiting fluid that is green or yellow or looks like coffee grounds or blood

- Difficulty breathing after vomiting or spitting up

- Pain related to eating

- Food refusal that causes weight loss or poor weight gain

- Difficult or painful swallowing

What is the treatment for GER?

Treatment for reflux depends on the child's symptoms and age. The doctor or nurse may first suggest a trial of medication to decrease the amount of acid made in the stomach when a child or teenager is uncomfortable, has difficulty sleeping or eating, or fails to grow.

H2-blockers, which are also called H2-receptor agonists, are one class of medication often tried first. These drugs help keep acid from backing up into the esophagus. They are often used to treat children with GER because they come in liquid form.

A second class of medications often used to reduce stomach acid is proton-pump inhibitors (PPIs), which block the production of stomach acid. PPIs have few side effects, but those that have been reported are constipation, nausea, and headaches.

A third class of medications used to treat GER is prokinetic agents. These agents promote forward movement of food and gastric fluids through the intestinal tract to reduce reflux. However, they are not used frequently, as they tend to be less effective than acid-reducing medications. Additionally, serious side effects have been reported in adults and children taking some prokinetic agents, and most of these drugs have been removed from the market. People taking prokinetic agents should tell their doctor if they are taking other medications because there could be an adverse drug reaction.

Besides using medication, you may be able to reduce symptoms other ways.

• Have your child eat more frequent smaller meals.

• Have your child avoid eating two to three hours before bed.

• Raise the head of your child's bed six to eight inches by putting blocks of wood under the bedposts. Just using extra pillows will not help.

• Have your child avoid carbonated drinks, chocolate, caffeine, and foods that are high in fat or contain a lot of acid (citrus fruits) or spices.

If the child continues to have symptoms despite initial treatment, tests may be ordered to help find better treatments. Surgery for GER in children is rare. However, surgery may be the best option for children who have severe symptoms that do not respond to medication.

If surgery is needed, a fundoplication will be performed. During a fundoplication the upper part of the stomach is wrapped around the LES. This procedure adds pressure to the lower end of the esophagus and reduces acid reflux. There are also several procedures performed via an endoscope that can also treat reflux.

Section 22.12

Irritable Bowel Syndrome

This section excerpted from "Irritable Bowel Syndrome in Children," National Digestive Diseases Information Clearinghouse, National Institute of Diabetes and Digestive and Kidney Diseases (digestive.niddk.nih.gov), November 2008.

What is irritable bowel syndrome?

IBS is a functional gastrointestinal disorder marked by abdominal pain or discomfort, bloating, and irregular bowel habits, such as diarrhea or constipation. Functional gastrointestinal disorders are defined by their symptoms. IBS can cause a great deal of discomfort and distress, but it is not life threatening, does not damage the bowel, and does not progress to other diseases. IBS should not be confused with inflammatory bowel disease, a group of diseases including ulcerative colitis and Crohn disease.

What is the bowel?

The bowel is the section of the gastrointestinal tract that begins after the stomach, ends at the anus, and has two main sections: the small intestine and the large intestine—also called the colon.

What causes IBS?

The cause of IBS is unknown. Research suggests people with IBS are more sensitive to gas or stool in the colon. People with IBS can also have abnormalities in how their intestines contract, called motility, which refers to the rate stool moves through the intestines. Whereas a faster rate of movement may cause diarrhea, a slower rate may result in constipation.

Researchers have proposed many explanations for the increased bowel sensitivity and abnormal bowel motility associated with IBS:

- Reactions to certain foods
- Overgrowth of bacteria in the colon
- Psychological stress, including anxiety and depression
- Problems in the way the brain and the gastrointestinal tract communicate with each other, called the brain-gut connection

Who gets IBS?

IBS is common in people of all ages, including children. About 14% of high school students and 6% of middle school students report IBS-like symptoms.

IBS affects boys and girls equally, although in adults it is more common in women than in men.

What are the symptoms of IBS?

The frequency and severity of IBS symptoms vary widely and may include the following:

- Abdominal pain or discomfort
- Intestinal bloating
- Irregular bowel habits, including diarrhea, constipation, or both
- A change in the appearance of stool, including stools that are loose, hard, thin, or pelletlike
- Mucus in the stool
- The need to strain to have a bowel movement
- A sense of urgency when having a bowel movement
- The sensation of not completely emptying the bowels

How is IBS diagnosed?

For a child to be diagnosed with IBS, abdominal pain or discomfort must be present at least one day per week for a period of two months or longer. Two or more of the following must also occur at least 25% of the time:

- The pain or discomfort is relieved by having a bowel movement.
- The pain or discomfort is associated with an increase or decrease in the number of bowel movements.
- The pain or discomfort is associated with a change in the appearance of stool.

No test can show if a person has IBS; however, a doctor may run tests to rule out diseases with symptoms similar to IBS. Signs and symptoms that suggest a problem other than IBS include these:

- Persistent pain in the upper right or lower right area of the abdomen

- Difficulty swallowing

- Persistent vomiting

- Gastrointestinal bleeding

- Waking up during the night with diarrhea or because of abdominal pain

- A family history of IBD, celiac disease, or peptic ulcer disease

- Arthritis

- Inflamed, pus-filled masses around the rectum, also called perirectal disease

- Involuntary weight loss

- A sudden stop in height growth

- Delayed puberty

- Unexplained fever

How is IBS treated?

No cure for IBS exists; however, treatment can reduce symptoms. Treatment is guided by the symptoms present, their severity, and the child's response to treatment. Treatment includes dietary changes, medication, and stress management.

Dietary changes: Reducing or eliminating certain foods may improve symptoms. Common trigger foods include fatty foods, dairy products, carbonated beverages, and caffeine. Keeping a diary of symptoms, bowel habits, and diet may help identify foods that trigger IBS symptoms.

Eating high-fiber foods, such as fruits, vegetables, and whole grain breads and cereals, may also help. Fiber helps relieve constipation and promotes regular bowel movements.

Eating several small meals throughout the day instead of a few large ones may reduce symptoms.

Medications: Medications are used to control constipation and diarrhea.

- Fiber supplements, such as Metamucil or Citrucel, help control constipation.

- Laxatives, such as PEG 3350 (MiraLAX, GlycoLax), mineral oil, or bisacodyl (Dulcolax), relieve moderate to severe constipation.

- Loperamide (Imodium) and bismuth subsalicylate (Pepto-Bismol) help relieve diarrhea.

- Antispasmodics, such as dicyclomine (Bentyl), relax smooth muscle contractions in the bowel and can, theoretically, lessen pain related to IBS but should be used with caution due to potentially serious side effects.

- Antidepressants, including selective serotonin reuptake inhibitors (SSRIs) and tricyclic antidepressants (TCAs), are used to treat IBS, although their effectiveness in children is not well documented.

Before taking any of these medications, children and their parents should seek the advice of a health care provider to help weigh the potential benefits against the risk of possible side effects.

Stress management: Understanding that IBS is not a life-threatening disease can help reduce a child's anxiety, which may in turn lessen IBS symptoms. Certain types of counseling, including cognitive behavior therapy and hypnotherapy, have been shown to help manage IBS symptoms. Parents can help reduce a child's stress by discussing potential IBS-related issues with school personnel—for example, the need for ready access to a private restroom.

What is the outlook for a child with IBS?

IBS symptoms typically fluctuate. Symptoms may go away for a long period of time only to return for no obvious reason. The majority of people with IBS continue to report symptoms five years after initial diagnosis.

Section 22.13

Lactose Intolerance

This section excerpted from "What I Need to Know about Lactose Intolerance," National Digestive Diseases Information Clearinghouse, National Institute of Diabetes and Digestive and Kidney Diseases (digestive.niddk .nih.gov), June 2010.

What is lactose intolerance?

Lactose intolerance means you have trouble digesting lactose. Lactose is the sugar found in milk and foods made with milk. The small intestine needs lactase enzyme to break down lactose. With lactose intolerance, you may not feel well when you eat or drink something with lactose because you don't have enough lactase enzyme.

Who gets lactose intolerance?

Many people have problems digesting lactose. Some people become lactose intolerant as children. In others, the problem starts when they are teenagers or adults. Lactose intolerance is rare in babies. Premature babies may be lactose intolerant for a short time after they are born.

Lactose intolerance is common in certain areas of the world. Certain groups are more likely to be lactose intolerant:

- Asian Americans

- African Americans

- American Indians

- Hispanics/Latinos

- People with southern European heritage

People of northern European descent are least likely to be lactose intolerant.

If your small intestine has been damaged, it may produce less lactase enzyme, causing you to become lactose intolerant. The small intestine can be hurt by the following:

- Diseases such as celiac disease or Crohn disease
- Infections
- Surgery
- Injuries

What are the symptoms of lactose intolerance?

If you have lactose intolerance, you may not feel well after you eat or drink milk and milk products. You may also have these symptoms:

- Cramps or pain in your abdomen
- Bloating or swelling in your abdomen
- Gas
- Diarrhea
- Nausea

Some illnesses can cause these same symptoms. If you have these symptoms after you eat or drink milk and milk products, see your doctor.

How is lactose intolerance diagnosed?

To find out if you have lactose intolerance, your doctor will ask about your symptoms. The doctor may ask you to stop eating or drinking milk and milk products to see if your symptoms improve. Your doctor might perform other tests to confirm your diagnosis:

- **Breath tests:** You will drink a sweet drink with lactose in it. Then your breath is tested to see if you were able to digest the lactose.
- **Stool test:** Your stool can be tested to see if you digest lactose.

What should I do if I think my child is lactose intolerant?

Talk with your doctor before making any changes in your child's diet. While lactose intolerance is more common in adults, children may be lactose intolerant.

How is lactose intolerance managed?

You can change your diet to manage your symptoms. Most people with lactose intolerance do not have to give up milk or milk products.

You may be able to tolerate milk and milk products if you do the following:

- Drink small amounts of milk—four ounces or less—at a time.

- Drink small amounts of milk with meals.

- Gradually add small amounts of milk and milk products to your diet and see how you feel.

- Eat milk products that are easier for people with lactose intolerance to digest, such as yogurt and hard cheeses like cheddar and Swiss.

You can also use over-the-counter products that may help you digest milk and milk products:

- You can take a tablet that contains the lactase enzyme when you eat foods that contain lactose.

- You can add liquid lactase drops to liquid milk products.

You can also find lactose-free and lactose-reduced milk and milk products at the grocery store. These products have the same nutrients and benefits as regular milk.

How will I know if a food has lactose?

Lactose is found in milk and all foods made with milk, such as ice cream, cream, butter, cheese, cottage cheese, and yogurt.

Rarely, people with lactose intolerance are bothered by small amounts of lactose. Some boxed, canned, frozen, packaged, and prepared foods contain small amounts of lactose. Look for certain words on food labels. These words mean the food has lactose in it:

- Milk
- Whey
- Milk by-products
- Nonfat dry milk powder

- Lactose
- Curds
- Dry milk solids

How will I get the calcium I need?

Milk and milk products are the most common sources of calcium. Calcium is a mineral the body needs for strong bones and teeth. If you are lactose intolerant, make sure you get enough calcium each day. Other foods contain calcium, such as the following:

- Canned salmon or sardines with bones

- Broccoli and other leafy green vegetables

- Oranges

- Almonds, Brazil nuts, and dried beans

- Soy milk and tofu

- Products with added calcium, such as orange juice

To absorb calcium, your body needs vitamin D. Be sure to eat foods that contain vitamin D, such as eggs, liver, and certain kinds of fish like salmon and tuna. Also, getting enough sun helps your body make vitamin D.

Vitamin D is added to some milk and milk products. If you're able to drink small amounts of milk or eat yogurt, choose varieties that have vitamin D added.

It's hard to get enough calcium and vitamin D even if you eat and drink milk and milk products. Ask your doctor if you should also take a supplement to get enough calcium, vitamin D, or other nutrients.

Section 22.14

Motion Sickness

This section excerpted from "2012 Yellow Book: Travelers' Health:
Motion Sickness," Centers for Disease Control and Prevention
(www.cdc.gov), July 1, 2011.

Risk for Travelers

All people, given sufficient stimulus, will develop motion sickness,
although some groups are at higher risk:

- Children aged 2–12 years are especially susceptible, but infants
  and toddlers seem relatively immune.

- Women, especially when pregnant, menstruating, or on hormones, are more likely to have motion sickness.

- People who get migraine headaches are prone to motion sickness
  during a migraine and prone to getting a migraine while they
  are experiencing motion sickness.

- People who expect to be sick are likely to experience symptoms.

Treatment

Some providers feel that continued exposure to motions that induce
motion sickness will diminish symptoms; however, most people will
be reluctant to endure the symptoms and will want medication. Antihistamines are the most commonly used and available medications,
although nonsedating ones appear to be the least effective. Sedation
is the primary side effect of all the efficacious drugs.

Medications in Children

For children aged 2–12 years, dimenhydrinate (Dramamine), 1–1.5
mg/kg per dose, or diphenhydramine, 0.5–1 mg/kg per dose up to 25
mg, can be given one hour before travel and every six hours during the trip. Because some children have paradoxical agitation with
these medicines, a test dose should be given at home before departure.

Scopolamine may cause dangerous adverse effects in children and should not be used; prochlorperazine and metoclopramide should be used with caution in children. Antihistamines are not approved by the Food and Drug Administration to treat motion sickness in children. Caregivers should be reminded to always ask a physician, pharmacist, or other clinician if they have any questions about how to use or dose antihistamines in children before they administer the medication. Oversedation of young children with antihistamines can lead to life-threatening side effects.

Preventive Measures for Travelers

Nonpharmacologic interventions to treat or manage motion sickness include the following:

- Being aware of situations that tend to trigger symptoms

- Optimizing positioning—driving a vehicle instead of riding in it, sitting in the front seat of a car or bus, sitting over the wing of an aircraft, or being in the central cabin on a ship

- Eating before the onset of symptoms, which may hasten gastric emptying, but in some people may aggravate motion sickness

- Drinking caffeinated beverages along with medications

- Reducing sensory input by, for example, lying prone, looking at the horizon, or shutting eyes

- Adding distractions—aromatherapy using mint, lavender, or ginger (oral) helps some; flavored lozenges may help, as well (they may function as placebos or, in the case of oral ginger, may hasten gastric emptying)

- Using acupressure or magnets is advocated by some to prevent or treat nausea (not specifically for motion sickness), although scientific data are lacking

Chapter 23

Kidney and Urologic Disorders in Children

Chapter Contents

Section 23.1

Bedwetting and Urinary Incontinence

This section excerpted from "Urinary Incontinence in Children,"
National Kidney and Urologic Diseases Information Clearinghouse
(kidney.niddk.nih.gov), September 2, 2010.

Parents or guardians of children who experience bedwetting at night or accidents during the day should treat this problem with understanding and patience. This loss of urinary control is called urinary incontinence or just incontinence. Although it affects many young people, it usually disappears naturally over time, which suggests that incontinence, for some people, may be a normal part of growing up. It is important to understand that many children experience occasional incontinence and that treatment is available for most children who have difficulty controlling their bladders.

How does the urinary system work?

Urination, or voiding, is a complex activity. The bladder is a balloon-like organ that lies in the lowest part of the abdomen. The bladder stores urine, then releases it through the urethra, the canal that carries urine to the outside of the body. Controlling this activity involves nerves, muscles, the spinal cord, and the brain.

A baby's bladder fills to a set point, then automatically contracts and empties. As the child gets older, the nervous system matures. The child's brain begins to get messages from the filling bladder and begins to send messages to the bladder to keep it from automatically emptying until the child decides it is the time and place to void.

What causes nighttime incontinence?

After age five, wetting at night—often called bedwetting or sleep-wetting—is more common than daytime wetting. Experts do not know what causes nighttime incontinence. Young people who experience nighttime wetting are usually physically and emotionally normal. Most cases probably result from a mix of factors including slower physical development, an overproduction of urine at night, a lack of ability to recognize bladder filling when asleep, and, infrequently, anxiety. For many, there is a strong family history of bedwetting, suggesting an inherited factor.

Slower physical development: Between the ages of 5 and 10, bedwetting may be the result of a small bladder capacity, long sleeping periods, and underdevelopment of the body's alarms that signal a full or emptying bladder. This form of incontinence will fade away as the bladder grows and the natural alarms become operational.

Excessive output of urine during sleep: Normally, the body produces a hormone that can slow the production of urine. This hormone is called antidiuretic hormone, or ADH. If the body doesn't produce enough ADH at night, the production of urine may not be slowed down, leading to bladder overfilling.

Anxiety: Experts suggest that anxiety-causing events occurring in the lives of children ages two to four might lead to incontinence before the child achieves total bladder control. Anxiety experienced after age four might lead to wetting after the child has been dry for a period of six months or more.

Genetics: Certain inherited genes appear to contribute to incontinence. If both parents were bedwetters, a child has an 80% chance of also being a bedwetter.

Obstructive sleep apnea: Nighttime incontinence may be one sign of another condition called obstructive sleep apnea, in which the child's breathing is interrupted during sleep, often because of inflamed or enlarged tonsils or adenoids. In some cases, successful treatment of this breathing disorder may also resolve the associated nighttime incontinence.

Structural problems: Finally, a small number of cases of incontinence are caused by physical problems in the urinary system in children. Rarely, a blocked bladder or urethra may cause the bladder to overfill and leak. Nerve damage associated with the birth defect spina bifida can cause incontinence. In these cases, the incontinence can appear as a constant dribbling of urine.

What causes daytime incontinence?

Daytime incontinence that is not associated with urinary infection or anatomic abnormalities is less common than nighttime incontinence and tends to disappear much earlier than the nighttime versions. One possible cause of daytime incontinence is an overactive bladder. Many children with daytime incontinence have abnormal elimination habits, the most common being infrequent voiding and constipation.

Overactive bladder: Muscles surrounding the urethra have the job of keeping the passage closed, preventing urine from passing out of the body. If the bladder contracts strongly and without warning, the muscles surrounding the urethra may not be able to keep urine from passing. This often happens as a consequence of urinary tract infection (UTI) and is more common in girls.

Infrequent voiding: Infrequent voiding refers to a child's voluntarily holding urine for prolonged intervals. For example, a child may not want to use the toilets at school or may not want to interrupt enjoyable activities, so he or she ignores the body's signal of a full bladder. In these cases, the bladder can overfill and leak urine.

Other causes: Some of the same factors that contribute to nighttime incontinence may act together with infrequent voiding to produce daytime incontinence. These factors include the following:

- Small bladder capacity
- Structural problems
- Anxiety-causing events
- Pressure from a hard bowel movement (constipation)
- Drinks or foods that contain caffeine

What treats or cures incontinence?

Growth and development: Most urinary incontinence fades away naturally. Here are examples of what can happen over time:

- Bladder capacity increases.
- Natural body alarms become activated.
- An overactive bladder settles down.
- Production of ADH becomes normal.
- The child learns to respond to the body's signal that it is time to void.
- Stressful events or periods pass.

Many children overcome incontinence naturally as they grow older. The number of cases of incontinence goes down by 15% for each year after the age of five.

Medications: Nighttime incontinence may be treated by increasing ADH levels. The hormone can be boosted by a synthetic version known as desmopressin, or DDAVP.

Another medication, called imipramine, acts on both the brain and the urinary bladder. Researchers estimate that these medications may help as many as 70% of patients achieve short-term success. Many patients, however, relapse once the medication is withdrawn.

If a young person experiences incontinence resulting from an overactive bladder, a doctor might prescribe a medicine that helps to calm the bladder muscle. This medicine controls muscle spasms and belongs to a class of medications called anticholinergics.

Bladder training and related strategies: Bladder training consists of exercises for strengthening and coordinating muscles of the bladder and urethra and may help the control of urination. These techniques teach the child to anticipate the need to urinate and prevent urination when away from a toilet. Techniques that may help nighttime incontinence include the following:

- Determining bladder capacity
- Drinking less fluid before sleeping
- Developing routines for waking up

Techniques that may help daytime incontinence include the following:

- Urinating on a schedule—timed voiding—such as every two hours
- Avoiding caffeine or other foods or drinks that you suspect may contribute to your child's incontinence
- Following suggestions for healthy urination, such as relaxing muscles and taking your time

Moisture alarms: At night, moisture alarms can awaken a person when he or she begins to urinate. These devices include a water-sensitive pad worn in pajamas, a wire connecting to a battery-driven control, and an alarm that sounds when moisture is first detected. For the alarm to be effective, the child must awaken as soon as the alarm goes off, go to the bathroom, and change the bedding. Using alarms may require having another person sleep in the same room to awaken the bedwetter.

Section 23.2

Childhood Nephrotic Syndrome

This section excerpted from "Childhood Nephrotic Syndrome,"
National Kidney and Urologic Diseases Information Clearinghouse
(kidney.niddk.nih.gov), September 2, 2010.

Nephrotic syndrome is a set of signs or symptoms that may point to kidney problems. The kidneys are two bean-shaped organs found in the lower back. Each is about the size of a fist. They clean the blood by filtering out excess water and salt and waste products from food. Healthy kidneys keep protein in the blood, which helps the blood soak up water from tissues. But kidneys with damaged filters may leak protein into the urine. As a result, not enough protein is left in the blood to soak up the water. The water then moves from the blood into body tissues and causes swelling.

Both children and adults can have nephrotic syndrome. The causes of and treatments for nephrotic syndrome in children are sometimes different from the causes and treatments in adults. Childhood nephrotic syndrome can occur at any age but is most common between the ages of 1½ and 5 years. It seems to affect boys more often than girls.

A child with nephrotic syndrome has these signs:

- High levels of protein in the urine, a condition called proteinuria

- Low levels of protein in the blood

- Swelling resulting from buildup of salt and water

- Less frequent urination

- Weight gain from excess water

Nephrotic syndrome is not itself a disease. But it can be the first sign of a disease that damages the kidney's tiny blood-filtering units, called glomeruli, where urine is made.

Diagnosis

To diagnose childhood nephrotic syndrome, the doctor may ask for a urine sample to check for protein. The doctor may take a blood sample to see how well the kidneys are removing wastes.

In some cases, the doctor may want to examine a small piece of kidney tissue with a microscope to see if something specific is causing the syndrome. The procedure of collecting a small tissue sample from the kidney is called a biopsy, and it is usually performed with a long needle passed through the skin. The child will be awake during the procedure and receive calming drugs and a local painkiller at the site of the needle entry.

Conditions Associated with Childhood Nephrotic Syndrome

Minimal Change Disease

The condition most commonly associated with childhood nephrotic syndrome is minimal change disease. Doctors do not know what causes it. Children with this form of the nephrotic syndrome have normal or nearly normal appearing kidney biopsies. The doctor will probably prescribe prednisone, which belongs to a class of drugs called corticosteroids. Prednisone stops the movement of protein from the blood into the urine, but it does have side effects that the doctor will explain. Following the doctor's directions exactly is essential to protect the child's health. The doctor may also prescribe another type of drug called a diuretic, which reduces the swelling by helping the child urinate more frequently.

When protein is no longer present in the urine, the doctor will begin to reduce the dosage of prednisone. This process takes several weeks. Some children never get sick again, but most experience a relapse, developing swelling and protein in the urine again, usually following a viral illness. However, as long as the child continues to respond to prednisone and the urine becomes protein free, the child has an excellent long-term outlook without kidney damage.

Children who relapse frequently, or who seem to be dependent on prednisone or have side effects from it, may be given a second type of drug called a cytotoxic agent. The agents most frequently used are cyclophosphamide and chlorambucil.

In recent years, doctors have explored the use of mycophenolate mofetil (MMF) instead of cytotoxic agents for children who relapse frequently. MMF is an immunosuppressant used to treat autoimmune diseases and to keep the body from rejecting a transplanted organ. MMF has milder side effects than cytotoxic agents, but taking immunosuppressants can raise the risk of infection and other diseases. The good news is that most children outgrow minimal change disease by their late teens with no permanent damage to their kidneys.

435

Focal Segmental Glomerulosclerosis (FSGS) and Membranoproliferative Glomerulonephritis (MPGN)

In about 20% of children with nephrotic syndrome, a kidney biopsy reveals scarring or deposits in the glomeruli. The two most common diseases that damage these tiny blood-filtering units are FSGS and MPGN.

Because prednisone is less effective in treating these diseases than it is in treating minimal change disease, the doctor may use additional therapies, including cytotoxic agents. Recent experience with another class of drugs called ACE (angiotensin-converting enzyme) inhibitors, usually used to treat high blood pressure, indicates these drugs can help decrease the amount of protein leaking into the urine and keep the kidneys from being damaged in children with FSGS or MPGN.

Congenital Nephropathy

Rarely, a child may be born with congenital nephropathy, a condition that causes nephrotic syndrome. The most common form of this condition is congenital nephropathy of the Finnish type (CNF), inherited as an autosomal recessive trait—meaning the gene for CNF must be inherited from both parents.

Another condition that causes nephrotic syndrome in the first months of life is diffuse mesangial sclerosis (DMS). The pattern of inheritance for DMS is not as clearly understood as the pattern for CNF, although the condition does appear to be genetic.

Since medicines have little effect on congenital nephropathy, transplantation is usually required by the second or third year of life, when the child has grown enough to receive a kidney. Congenital nephropathy can disturb thyroid activity, so the child may need the substitute hormone thyroxine to promote growth and help bones mature. Some children with congenital nephropathy have excessive blood clotting, or thrombosis, which must be treated with a blood thinner like warfarin.

Section 23.3

Hemolytic Uremic Syndrome

This section excerpted from "Hemolytic Uremic Syndrome in Children,"
National Kidney and Urologic Diseases Information Clearinghouse
(kidney.niddk.nih.gov), September 2, 2010.

What is hemolytic uremic syndrome (HUS)?

HUS, a disease that destroys red blood cells, is the most common
cause of sudden, short-term acute kidney failure in children. Although
HUS can cause serious complications and can even be life threatening,
most children who develop HUS recover without permanent damage
to their health.

What causes HUS?

HUS develops when *Escherichia coli* (*E. coli*) bacteria lodged in
the digestive tract make toxins that enter the bloodstream and start
to destroy red blood cells. Most cases of HUS occur after an infection
of the digestive tract by the *E. coli* bacterium, which is found in foods
like meat, dairy products, and juice when they are contaminated. Some
people have contracted HUS after swimming in pools or lakes contaminated with feces.

Infection of the digestive tract is called gastroenteritis and may
cause a child to vomit and have stomach cramps and bloody diarrhea.
Most children who have gastroenteritis recover fully in two or three
days and do not develop HUS.

What are the signs and symptoms of HUS and kidney failure?

With HUS, the child remains pale, tired, and irritable. Other signs
include small, unexplained bruises or bleeding from the nose or mouth
that may occur because the toxins also destroy the platelets, cells that
normally help the blood to clot. Signs and symptoms of HUS may not become apparent until a week after the digestive problems have occurred.

More than half of children with HUS develop acute kidney failure.
With kidney failure, the child's urine output decreases. The urine may

also appear red. The body's inability to rid itself of excess fluid and wastes may in turn cause high blood pressure or swelling of the face, hands, feet, or entire body.

Parents or guardians should call the child's doctor immediately if the child has unexplained bruises, unusual bleeding, swollen limbs or generalized swelling, extreme fatigue, or decreased urine output. A child who goes 12 hours without urinating should be taken to a doctor or an emergency room.

How is HUS diagnosed?

A doctor may suspect that a child has HUS after examining the child and learning the history of symptoms. The diagnosis is confirmed by microscopic examination of a blood sample to see if the red blood cells are misshapen.

How is HUS treated?

Treatments, which consist of maintaining normal salt and water levels in the body, are aimed at easing the immediate symptoms and preventing further problems. A child may need a transfusion of red blood cells delivered through an intravenous, or IV, tube. In severe cases, several sessions of dialysis, a blood-cleansing treatment, may be required to temporarily take over the kidneys' job of filtering wastes and extra fluid from the blood.

Some children may sustain significant kidney damage that slowly develops into permanent kidney failure and will then require long-term dialysis or a kidney transplant. Some studies suggest that limiting protein in the child's diet and treating high blood pressure with a medicine from a class of drugs called ACE inhibitors helps delay or prevent the onset of permanent kidney failure. Most children recover completely with no long-term consequences.

How can HUS be prevented?

Washing and cooking foods adequately, especially meats, and avoiding unclean swimming areas are the best ways to protect a child from this disease.

Section 23.4

Urinary Tract Infections

This section excerpted from "Urinary Tract Infections in Children,"
National Kidney and Urologic Diseases Information Clearinghouse
(kidney.niddk.nih.gov), November 16, 2011.

What is a urinary tract infection (UTI)?

A UTI is an infection in the urinary tract. Bacteria are the most
common cause of UTIs. Normally, bacteria that enter the urinary tract
are rapidly removed by the body before they cause symptoms. However,
sometimes bacteria overcome the body's natural defenses and cause
infection.

What is the urinary tract?

The urinary tract is the body's drainage system for removing wastes
and extra water. The urinary tract includes two kidneys, two ureters,
a bladder, and a urethra. Every minute, a person's kidneys filter about
three ounces of blood, removing wastes and extra water. The urine
travels from the kidneys down two narrow tubes called the ureters.
The bladder fills with urine until it is full enough to signal the need
to urinate.

When the bladder empties, a muscle called the sphincter relaxes
and urine flows out of the body through a tube called the urethra at
the bottom of the bladder

What causes UTIs?

Most UTIs are caused by bacteria that live in the bowel. The bacterium *E. coli* causes the vast majority of UTIs. The urinary tract has
several systems to prevent infection. The points where the ureters
attach to the bladder act like one-way valves to prevent urine from
backing up, or refluxing, toward the kidneys, and urination washes
microbes out of the body. Immune defenses also prevent infection. But
despite these safeguards, infections still occur. Certain bacteria have a
strong ability to attach themselves to the lining of the urinary tract.

Children who often delay urination are more likely to develop UTIs. Regular urination helps keep the urinary tract sterile by flushing away bacteria. Holding in urine allows bacteria to grow. Producing too little urine because of inadequate fluid intake can also increase the risk of developing a UTI. Chronic constipation—a condition in which a child has fewer than two bowel movements a week—can add to the risk of developing a UTI. When the bowel is full of hard stool, it presses against the bladder and bladder neck, blocking the flow of urine and allowing bacteria to grow.

Some children develop UTIs because they are prone to such infections, just as other children are prone to getting coughs, colds, or ear infections.

Who is at risk for a UTI?

Throughout childhood, the risk of having a UTI is 2% for boys and 8% for girls. Having an anomaly of the urinary tract, such as urine reflux from the bladder back into the ureters, increases the risk of a UTI. Boys who are younger than six months old who are not circumcised are at greater risk for a UTI than circumcised boys the same age.

Are UTIs serious?

Most UTIs are not serious, but some infections can lead to serious problems, such as kidney infections. Chronic kidney infections—infections that recur or last a long time—can cause permanent damage, including kidney scars, poor kidney growth, poor kidney function, high blood pressure, and other problems. Some acute kidney infections—infections that develop suddenly—can be life threatening, especially if the bacteria enter the bloodstream, a condition called septicemia.

In some children, a UTI may be a sign of an abnormality in the urinary tract that leads to repeated problems. Young children are at the greatest risk for kidney damage from UTIs and defects in the urinary tract. Children with UTIs should receive careful evaluation with prompt treatment. Because UTIs are less common in boys after the first four weeks of life, boys with a UTI should be assumed to have an abnormality of the urinary tract until proven otherwise.

What are the signs and symptoms of a UTI?

Symptoms of a UTI range from slight burning with urination or unusual-smelling urine to severe pain and high fever. A child with a UTI may also have no symptoms. A UTI causes irritation of the lining of the bladder, urethra, ureters, and kidneys, just as the inside of the nose or the throat becomes irritated with a cold. In infants or children who are only a few years old, the signs of a UTI may not be clear because children that young cannot express exactly how they feel. Children may have a high fever, be irritable, or not eat.

On the other hand, children may have only a low-grade fever; experience nausea, vomiting, and diarrhea; or just not seem healthy. Children who have a high fever and appear sick for more than a day without signs of a runny nose or other obvious cause for discomfort should be checked for a UTI.

Older children with UTIs may complain of pain in the middle and lower abdomen. They may urinate often. Crying or complaining that it hurts to urinate and producing only a few drops of urine at a time are other signs of a UTI. Children may leak urine into clothing or bedsheets. The urine may look cloudy or bloody. If a kidney is infected, children may complain of pain in the back or side below the ribs.

How are UTIs diagnosed?

Only a health care provider can determine whether a child has a UTI. A urine sample will be collected and examined. The way urine is collected depends on the child's age.

Some of the urine will be examined with a microscope. If an infection is present, bacteria and sometimes pus will be found in the urine. A urine culture should also be performed on some of the urine. The health care provider may also order a sensitivity test, which tests the bacteria for sensitivity to different antibiotics to see which medication is best for treating the infection.

How are UTIs treated?

Most UTIs are caused by bacteria, which are treated with bacteria-fighting medications called antibiotics or antimicrobials. The choice of medication and length of treatment depend on the child's history and the type of bacteria causing the infection.

After a few doses of the antibiotic, a child may appear much better, but often several days may pass before all symptoms are gone. In any case, the medication should be taken for as long as the health care provider recommends. Medications should not be stopped because the symptoms have gone away. Infections may return, and bacteria can resist future treatment if the medication is stopped too soon.

Once the infection has cleared, more tests may be recommended to check for abnormalities in the urinary tract. Repeated infections in an abnormal urinary tract may cause kidney damage.

What abnormalities lead to chronic urinary problems?

Many children who get a UTI have normal kidneys and bladders. But if a child has an abnormality, it should be detected as early as possible to protect the kidneys against damage. Abnormalities that could occur include the following:

- **Vesicoureteral reflux (VUR):** Vesicoureteral reflux is the abnormal flow of urine from the bladder to the upper urinary tract. In VUR, urine may reflux into one or both ureters and, in some cases, to one or both kidneys.

- **Urinary obstruction:** Blockages to urinary flow can occur in many places in the urinary tract.

- **Dysfunctional voiding:** Some children develop a habit of delaying a trip to the bathroom and holding their urine because they don't want to leave their play. These children may be unable to empty the bladder completely. Some children may strain during urination. Dysfunctional voiding can lead to VUR, accidental urinary leakage, and UTIs.

How are abnormalities in the urinary tract treated?

Some abnormalities in the urinary tract correct themselves as the child grows, but some may require surgical correction. While milder forms of VUR may resolve on their own, one common procedure to correct VUR is the reimplantation of the ureters. During this procedure, the surgeon repositions the connection between the ureters and the bladder so that urine will not reflux into the ureters and kidneys.

In recent years, health care providers have treated some cases of VUR by injecting substances into the bladder wall, just below the opening where the ureter joins the bladder. This injection creates a kind of narrowing or valve that keeps urine from refluxing into the ureters.

How can UTIs be prevented?

If a child has a normal urinary tract, parents can help the child avoid UTIs by encouraging regular trips to the bathroom. The parents should make sure the child gets enough to drink if infrequent urination is a problem. The child should be taught proper cleaning techniques after using the bathroom to keep bacteria from entering the urinary tract.

Chapter 24

Liver Disorders in Children

Chapter Contents

Section 24.1

Alpha-1 Antitrypsin Deficiency

What is Alpha-1 Antitrypsin Deficiency (Alpha-1)?

Alpha-1 Antitrypsin Deficiency (Alpha-1) is an inherited disease that can cause liver problems in infants, children, or adults and may cause lung problems in adults, particularly if they smoke cigarettes.

In people with Alpha-1, large amounts of the abnormal alpha-1 antitrypsin (A1AT) protein are made in the liver and nearly 85% of this protein gets stuck in the liver. If the liver is not able to break down the abnormal protein, the liver gets damaged and scarred over time. Currently, there is no way to prevent the A1AT protein from getting stuck in the liver of a person with Alpha-1. Since not all people with Alpha-1 get liver disease, there must be some other things that contribute to the liver disease, but these are not currently known. The lack of A1AT in the blood allows the lungs to get damaged by cigarette smoke and air pollution, which usually shows up in adults with Alpha-1.

What are symptoms of liver disease in Alpha-1?

Symptoms of Alpha-1 in infants can include jaundice (eyes and skin turning yellow), swelling of the liver, or poor growth. Most jaundiced infants do not have Alpha-1 or other liver problems, but have another harmless cause of jaundice. Blood tests can tell if the jaundice is due to a liver problem or the common harmless type. Diarrhea and poor weight gain may also happen in infants with Alpha-1 liver disease. Sometimes an infant or child is found to have a large liver or spleen when they are examined by their doctor, or it may be found by a parent when the child is bathed. This can be caused by scarring in the liver caused by Alpha-1 and a number of other liver problems. Scarring in the liver can also lead to swelling of the abdomen by fluid (ascites), intestinal bleeding, or feeling weak and tired. These are the types of symptoms that may occur later in childhood or in adults with Alpha-1 liver disease. Most children and adults with Alpha-1 have no symptoms of liver disease at all.

How do you get Alpha-1?

Alpha-1 is a genetic condition that is passed on from parents to their children through genes. Genes are codes that are found on chromosomes, the genetic material in each cell in our bodies. Each person receives two genes for each trait in their body: one gene from their mother and one from their father. The usual (normal) alpha-1 gene is called M. People with Alpha-1 have received two alpha-1 genes that are different from the usual gene. One changed gene came from their mother and one from their father. There are many types of changed alpha-1 genes, but the most common are called S or Z. People with Alpha-1 who could get liver disease have either two Z genes (called ZZ) or one S and one Z gene (called SZ). People with Alpha-1 who are ZZ or SZ will pass on one of these changed genes to each of their children. The alpha-1 genes tell the liver how to make the protein alpha-1 antitrypsin, which the liver sends into the blood so it can protect the lungs and other parts of the body.

If someone has two changed alpha-1 genes, then the liver makes a form of the protein A1AT that becomes trapped in the liver rather than being released into the blood. The build-up of the A1AT protein in the liver can cause the liver to build up scar tissue (see the following). Also, when the A1AT protein builds up in the liver, the blood doesn't get as much of the protein as it needs to help other parts of the body. This makes the lungs more sensitive to damage from cigarette smoke and other air pollutants that are breathed in.

An Alpha-1 carrier is a person who has one normal M alpha-1 gene and one changed alpha-1 gene (usually Z or S). Most Alpha-1 carriers are called either MS or MZ. Being an Alpha-1 carrier is very common. Over 20 million people in the U.S. are carriers. Alpha-1 carriers have less A1AT protein in their blood than other people, but they hardly ever have liver or lung problems. The parents of children with Alpha-1 are usually both carriers and are completely healthy.

What happens to the liver in Alpha-1?

The liver is one of the largest organs in your body. It is found in the upper right part of your abdomen. It is very important to your health because it cleans your blood and helps fight infections. The liver stores vitamins, sugars, fats, and other nutrients from the foods you eat. The liver makes many substances for your body. It also breaks down alcohol, drugs, and other toxic substances that can hurt your body. The liver also removes a yellow substance from the body, called bilirubin, that builds up in the blood in many liver diseases. The term "liver disease" means a number of conditions that stop the liver from working as well as it should.

Of all babies who are born with two changed alpha-1 genes (ZZ or SZ), about 1 in 20 of them will get liver disease that may be serious in the first year of life. These infants usually have jaundice (yellow color of the skin and the eyes), swelling of the liver, and do not gain weight well. They may develop serious scarring of the liver. Of all infants born with ZZ or SZ, about 1 in 4 will have blood tests showing that the liver is being injured; however, the infants will feel and look fine. In most children with abnormal blood tests, the liver disease improves by itself by the time these children reach their teens, and they remain healthy. Adults with Alpha-1 can also get liver disease, usually involving scarring of the liver (cirrhosis). This is especially true for those over 50 years of age. People with Alpha-1 have up to a 30%-40% chance of developing a liver problem during their lifetime. These problems include cirrhosis (scarring of the liver) and liver cancer.

If the liver does get damaged, there are treatments to prevent or slow down problems that can be caused by liver damage. Healthy living is also important. This includes avoiding alcoholic drinks, maintaining a healthy weight, getting vaccinated against infections that can damage the liver, and eating a healthy diet. If the liver damage becomes severe or life-threatening, then liver transplantation is an option.

Alpha-1 carriers almost never develop liver problems related to Alpha-1. When they do, this is probably caused by something else that damaged the liver, like viruses, drinking too much alcohol, or being overweight.

How is Alpha-1 liver disease found and diagnosed?

Alpha-1 liver disease is found by a physical exam by a doctor and by blood tests. The physical exam may show a large, firm-feeling liver or spleen. The blood tests include measuring how much of the A1AT protein is in the blood and how well the liver works. In addition, ultrasound of the liver may be ordered. Ultrasound is a painless procedure using sound waves (sonar) through the skin to make a picture of the liver. The diagnosis of Alpha-1 is made by a blood test called the A1AT "phenotype" test. This test tells the type (M, Z, or S) of A1AT protein in a person's body. Doctors can also test a person's genes for A1AT from a blood sample or a mouth swab (rubbing a Q-tip on the inside of a person's mouth). A liver biopsy is usually not needed to diagnose Alpha-1. A liver biopsy is a procedure performed by a doctor, after a patient has received medicines to numb the skin and take away pain, in which a needle is pushed into the liver through the skin and a small piece of liver is removed in the needle. But liver biopsies are sometimes used to see how bad the liver disease is and to look for other reasons for liver damage.

How is liver disease treated in people with Alpha-1?

When doctors treat someone with Alpha-1 liver disease, they focus on keeping patients as healthy as they can be and preventing health problems. Treatments are available for intestinal bleeding, ascites (fluid in the abdomen), nutrition, and other problems from scarring of the liver.

There is no cure for Alpha-1, but there are ways to prevent or reduce health problems related to Alpha-1. People with Alpha-1 should do the following important things:

- Get hepatitis A and B vaccinations.

- Get regular physical exams by a doctor.

- Get regular medical tests as suggested by their doctors, such as blood tests and liver ultrasound exams or other X-ray tests (for example, liver CT [CAT, or computed axial tomography] scans).

- Stay away from tobacco smoke and heavy air pollution.

- Don't drink alcohol.

- Eat a balanced diet and maintain a healthy weight.

- Speak to your doctor before using any herbal, vitamin, or other therapies.

Severe liver damage and scarring is called "cirrhosis." In some people with cirrhosis caused by Alpha-1, the liver does not work well enough to keep them healthy and a liver transplant may be necessary. A liver transplant is surgery to remove a sick liver and replace it with a healthy one from another person.

Some adults with lung damage are treated with "intravenous A1AT replacement." This means they are given A1AT protein through a needle into a vein. This treatment is not helpful in reducing or preventing damage to the liver.

What is the outlook for someone with Alpha-1?

There is wide variation in how sick people get from Alpha-1. Some patients have serious problems if the liver is affected, while others have little or no liver disease. Some infants may have rather quick scarring of the liver that leads to the need for a liver transplantation in the first few years of life. However, this is rare and most children affected with Alpha-1 liver disease do well and reach adulthood without major liver problems. Lung problems from Alpha-1 do not occur in childhood, but it is very important for children with Alpha-1 to avoid all exposure to cigarette smoke or heavy air pollution to protect their lungs. It is best to talk with your doctor to figure out how your Alpha-1 might turn out and what can be done to protect the lungs and liver.

How can I learn more about liver disease in people with Alpha-1?

- Ask your health care provider.

- Access information available online.

- Contact local, national, or federal organizations and agencies dedicated to liver disease and/or Alpha-1.

Section 24.2

Hepatitis in Children

Hepatitis is the inflammation of the liver and can result in liver cell damage and destruction.

What Causes Hepatitis?

Hepatitis in children has many different origins or causes. A child may contract hepatitis from exposure to a viral source. The following is a list of some of the viruses associated with hepatitis:

- **Hepatitis viruses:** Six main types of the hepatitis virus have been identified, including hepatitis A, B, C, D, E, and G.

- **Cytomegalovirus (CMV):** A virus that is a part of the herpes virus family that can be transmitted from person to person.

- **Epstein-Barr virus (EBV):** The virus most commonly associated with infectious mononucleosis.

- **Herpes simplex virus (HSV):** Herpes can involve the face and skin above the waist, or the genitalia.

- **Varicella zoster virus (VZV):** Also known as chickenpox, a complication of VZV is hepatitis.

- **Enteroviruses:** A group of viruses commonly seen in children such as coxsackieviruses, hand-foot-mouth disease, and echoviruses.

- **Rubella:** Caused by the Rubivirus, rubella is a mild disease that causes a rash.

- **Adenovirus:** A group of viruses that commonly cause colds, tonsillitis, and ear infections in children. They can also cause diarrhea.

- **Parvovirus:** A virus referred to as fifth disease, which is characterized by a facial rash that is described as having a "slapped-cheek" appearance.

The following is a list of some of the diseases that may cause chronic hepatitis in children:

- **Autoimmune liver disease:** The body's immune system develops antibodies that attack the liver causing an inflammatory process that leads to hepatitis.

- **Chronic viral hepatitis:** Usually caused by hepatitis B, C, or D.

Types of hepatitis viruses: There are six main types of the hepatitis virus that have been identified, including hepatitis A, B, C, D, E, and G.

Hepatitis A

This type of hepatitis is usually spread by fecal-oral contact, or fecal-infected food and water, and may also be spread by blood-borne infection (which is rare). The following is a list of modes of transmission for hepatitis A:

- Consuming food made by someone who touched infected feces

- Drinking water that is contaminated by infected feces—a problem in developing countries with poor sewage removal

- Touching infected person's feces, which may occur with poor handwashing

- Outbreaks in child care centers especially when there are children in diapers

- Residents of American Indian reservations or Native Alaskan villages where hepatitis A may be more common

- International travel to areas where hepatitis A is common

- Sexual contact with an infected person

- Use of intravenous (IV) drugs

- Blood transfusions (very rare)

- Vertical transmission (very rare)

A vaccine for hepatitis A has been developed and is now available. Because the vaccine is not given routinely, please consult your physician if you have questions about its use. The vaccine is recommended for the following children:

- Children living in areas of the country where the infection rate of hepatitis A is above the national average—according to the

American Academy of Pediatrics, these states include: Arizona, Alaska, Oregon, New Mexico, Utah, Washington, Oklahoma, South Dakota, Idaho, Nevada, and California

- Children who live in other areas where there has been a community outbreak

- Children who have a blood clotting disorder, such as hemophilia

- Children who attend child care centers that have had outbreaks of hepatitis A

- Children with chronic liver disease

The vaccine is not recommended for children under two years of age.

Hepatitis B

Hepatitis B has a wide range of clinical presentations. It can be mild, without symptoms, or it may cause chronic hepatitis. In some cases, when infants and young children acquire hepatitis B, they are at high risk for chronic liver disease and liver failure.

Transmission of hepatitis B virus occurs through blood and body fluid exposure such as blood, semen, vaginal secretions, or saliva. Infants may also develop the disease if they are born to a mother who has the virus. Infected children often spread the virus to other children if there is frequent contact (i.e., household contact) or a child has many scrapes or cuts.

The following describes persons who are at risk for developing hepatitis B:

- Children born to mothers who have hepatitis B

- Children who are born to mothers who have immigrated from a country where hepatitis B is widespread such as southeast Asia and China

- Children who live in long-term care facilities or who are disabled

- Children who live in households where another member is infected with the virus

- Children who have a blood clotting disorder such as hemophilia and require blood products

- Children who require dialysis for kidney failure

- Adolescents who may participate in high-risk activities such as IV drug use and/or unprotected heterosexual or homosexual contact

A vaccine for hepatitis B does exist and is now widely used for routine childhood immunization. Children currently receive the first vaccine between birth and 2 months, the second vaccine at 1 to 4 months, and the third vaccine at 6 to 18 months. The vaccine is generally required for all children born on or after January 1, 1992, before they enter school. The vaccine is available for older children who may have not been immunized before 1992 and is recommended before age 11 or 12.

Hepatitis C

The symptoms of hepatitis C are usually mild and gradual. Children often show no symptoms at all. Transmission of hepatitis C occurs primarily from contact with infected blood, but can also occur from sexual contact or from an infected mother to her baby.

Although hepatitis C has milder symptoms initially, it leads to chronic liver disease in a majority of people who are infected. According to the Centers for Disease Control and Prevention (CDC), hepatitis C is the leading indication for liver transplantation in adults. With some cases of hepatitis C, no mode of transmission can be identified.

The following describes persons who may be at risk for contracting hepatitis C:

- Children born to mothers who are infected with the virus

- Persons who have a blood clotting disorder such as hemophilia and received clotting factors before 1987

- Children who require dialysis for kidney failure

- Individuals who received a blood transfusion before 1992

- Adolescents who participate in high-risk activities such as IV drug use and/or unprotected heterosexual or homosexual contact

There is no vaccine for hepatitis C. Persons who are at risk should be checked regularly for hepatitis C. Persons who have hepatitis C should be monitored closely for signs of chronic hepatitis and liver failure.

Hepatitis D

This form of hepatitis can only occur in the presence of hepatitis B. If an individual has hepatitis B and does not show symptoms or shows very mild symptoms, infection with D can put that person at risk for liver failure that progresses rapidly.

Hepatitis D can occur at the same time as the initial infection with B, or it may show up much later. Transmission of hepatitis D occurs the same way as hepatitis B, except the transmission from mother to baby is less common.

Hepatitis D is rare in children born in the U.S. due to the common use of hepatitis B vaccine in infancy.

Hepatitis E

This form of hepatitis is similar to hepatitis A. Transmission occurs through fecal-oral contamination. It is less common in children than hepatitis A. Hepatitis E is most common in poorly developed countries and rarely seen in the United States. There is no vaccine for hepatitis E at this time.

Hepatitis G

This is the newest strain of hepatitis and very little is known about it. Transmission is believed to occur through blood and is most commonly seen in IV drug users, individuals with clotting disorders such as hemophilia, and individuals who require hemodialysis for renal failure. Often hepatitis G shows no clinical symptoms and has not been found to be a cause of acute or chronic hepatitis.

How Often Does Hepatitis Occur?

According to the CDC, in the U.S., each year:

- one-third of Americans will be exposed to hepatitis A;
- there are 60,000 hepatitis B infections;
- 26,000 hepatitis C infections will occur.

Why Is Hepatitis a Concern?

Hepatitis is a concern because it often originates from a virus and is communicable (can be spread from your child to others). In some cases, liver failure or death can occur. However, not everyone who is infected will experience symptoms.

What Are the Symptoms of Hepatitis?

The following are the most common symptoms for hepatitis. However, each child may experience symptoms differently and some children may experience no symptoms at all.

Symptoms of acute (abrupt onset) hepatitis may include the following:

- Flu-like symptoms

- Fever

- Nausea and/or vomiting

- Decreased appetite

- Not feeling well all over

- Abdominal pain or discomfort

- Diarrhea

- Joint pain

- Sore muscles

- Itchy red hives on skin

Later symptoms include dark colored urine and jaundice (yellowing of the skin and eyes). The symptoms of hepatitis may resemble other conditions or medical problems. Always consult your child's physician for a diagnosis.

How Is Hepatitis Diagnosed?

In addition to a complete medical history and examination by your physician, diagnostic procedures and other tests to determine the extent of the disease may include the following:

- Blood testing for the following:

  - Liver function studies

  - Antibody studies (to check for hepatitis)

  - Cellular blood counts

  - Bleeding times

  - Electrolytes

  - Other chemicals in the body

- Ultrasound: A diagnostic imaging technique which uses high-frequency sound waves and a computer to create images of blood vessels, tissues, and organs. Ultrasounds are used to view internal organs of the abdomen such as the liver, spleen, and kidneys and to assess blood flow through various vessels.

- Liver biopsy: A small sample of liver tissue is obtained with a special biopsy needle and examined for abnormalities.

Treatment for Hepatitis

Specific treatment for hepatitis will be determined by your child's physician based on:

- your child's age, overall health, and medical history;
- extent of the disease;
- your child's tolerance for specific medications, procedures, or therapies;
- expectations for the course of the disease;
- your opinion or preference.

Treatment for hepatitis varies depending on the underlying cause of the disease. The goal of treatment is to stop damage to the liver and alleviate symptoms.

Treatment may include one, or more, of the following:

- Supportive care (healthy diet and rest)
- Medications (to help control itching)
- Maintaining adequate growth and development
- Avoiding alcohol and drugs
- Preventing the spread of the disease (if the cause is viral hepatitis)
- Interferon drug therapy—a medication referred to as a "biologic response modifier" that can affect the immune system and has virus-fighting activities
- Frequent blood testing (to determine disease progression)
- Hospitalization (may be required in more severe cases)
- Liver transplantation (may be recommended for end-stage liver failure)

Preventing the Spread of Viral Hepatitis

Proper hygiene is the key to preventing the spread of many diseases, including hepatitis. Other preventative measures include:

- **Vaccinations:** Vaccinations are available for hepatitis A and B.

- **Blood transfusion:** Blood transfusions are routinely screened for hepatitis B and C to reduce the risk of infection.

- **Antibody preparation:** If a person has been exposed to hepatitis A or B, an antibody preparation (immunoglobulin) can be administered to help protect them from contracting the disease.

Chapter 25

Musculoskeletal Disorders in Children

Chapter Contents

Section 25.1

Knock Knees

Knock knees is a condition in which the knees touch, but the ankles do not touch. The legs angle inward.

Causes

Infants start out with bowlegs because of their folded position in the uterus. The infant's bowlegs begin to straighten once the child starts to walk (at about 12 to 18 months). By age three, the child becomes knock-kneed. When the child stands, the knees touch but the ankles are apart.

By puberty, the legs straighten out and most children can stand with the knees and ankles touching (without forcing the position).

Knock knees can also develop as a result of a medical problem or disease, such as:

- injury of the shinbone (only one leg will be knock-kneed);
- osteomyelitis (bone infection);
- overweight or obesity;
- rickets (a disease caused by a lack of vitamin D).

Exams and Tests

If a doctor's examination and review of the child's medical history indicate a specific cause for the knock knees other than normal development, your health care provider will order the appropriate studies.

Treatment

Knock knees are usually not treated.

If the problem is still present after age seven, the child may use a night brace, which is attached to a shoe or orthopedic shoe.

Surgery may be considered for knock knees that persist beyond late childhood and in which the separation between the ankles is severe.

Outlook (Prognosis)

Children normally outgrow knock knees without treatment, unless it is caused by a disease. For cases needing surgery, the procedure provides good cosmetic results.

Possible Complications

- Difficulty walking (very rare)

- Self-esteem changes related to cosmetic appearance of knock knees

- If left untreated, knock knees can lead to early arthritis of the knee

Section 25.2

Flat Feet

"Pediatric Flatfoot," © 2009 The Cleveland Clinic Foundation, 9500 Euclid Avenue, Cleveland, OH 44195. All rights reserved. Reprinted with permission. Additional information is available from the Cleveland Clinic Health Information Center, 216-444-3771, toll-free 800-223-2273 extension 43771, or at http://my.clevelandclinic.org/health.

What is pediatric flatfoot?

Flatfoot is a condition that can affect both adults and children. In children, it is called "pediatric flatfoot." When a child has pediatric flatfoot, the arch of the foot shrinks or disappears when he or she stands. The arch reappears when the child sits or stands on tiptoe. This is called flexible pediatric flatfoot.

Most children who have pediatric flatfoot are born with the condition, though it may not appear for a few years. Children will usually outgrow pediatric flatfoot on their own by the age of five.

A second, more rare kind of pediatric flatfoot is called rigid flatfoot. With this condition, the arches do not reappear when the child sits or stands on tiptoe.

What are the symptoms of pediatric flatfoot?

Most children with pediatric flatfoot have no symptoms. A parent or caregiver usually notices the condition.

Symptoms children may experience include:

- pain, tenderness, and/or cramping in the feet or legs, especially along the bottom of the feet;

- heels that tilt outward;

- a change in walking;

- pain or discomfort while walking.

Parents may also notice their child withdrawing from sports and other physical activities that may cause pain in their feet and legs.

If your child experiences any of these symptoms, you should consult with your pediatrician.

Children affected by rigid flatfoot may experience more severe symptoms. Those affected with tarsal coalition, an abnormal joining of two bones in the feet, may begin to experience symptoms at pre-adolescence.

Children with a condition called congenital vertical talus, which causes a rigid rocker bottom appearance, may begin to experience symptoms at walking age.

How is pediatric flatfoot diagnosed?

Your pediatrician can usually diagnose pediatric flatfoot. He or she may also refer you to a foot and ankle surgical specialist. The condition is usually diagnosed by viewing the foot with the naked eye. The physician will have your child sit, stand, and walk to examine how the feet look in each situation. The physician may also examine your child's shoes to look for patterns of wear.

In more severe cases, an X-ray may be taken to determine the extent of the deformity. Your physician may also examine the child's knees and hips to determine if the foot condition is related to any problems in the leg.

How is pediatric flatfoot treated?

In most cases, children outgrow pediatric flatfoot without treatment. Unless the child is experiencing pain, your physician may recommend a wait-and-watch approach. You will be asked to bring your child for periodic reevaluations.

If the child is experiencing pain, the physician may recommend hard or soft shoe inserts to support the arch. He or she may also create a custom orthotic device to fit into your child's shoe to help support the arch and relieve the pain. In older children and adolescents, stretching exercises and physical therapy may provide relief.

In rare cases, surgery may be needed to treat pediatric flatfoot. This is more common with rigid flatfoot and in children who continue to experience pain despite nonsurgical approaches. Several different types of surgery can be done, depending on the child's age, type of flatfoot, and the degree of his or her deformity.

Section 25.3

Growing Pains

"Growing Pains," August 2009, reprinted with permission from www.kids health.org. Copyright © 2009 The Nemours Foundation. This information was provided by KidsHealth, one of the largest resources online for medically reviewed health information written for parents, kids, and teens. For more articles like this one, visit www.KidsHealth.org, or www.TeensHealth.org.

Your eight-year-old son wakes up crying in the night complaining that his legs are throbbing. You rub them and soothe him as much as you can, but you're uncertain about whether to give him any medication or take him to the doctor.

Sound familiar? Your child is probably experiencing growing pains, a normal occurrence in about 25% to 40% of children. They generally strike during two periods: in early childhood among 3- to 5-year-olds and, later, in 8- to 12-year-olds.

What Causes Them?

No firm evidence shows that the growth of bones causes pain. The most likely causes are the aches and discomforts resulting from the jumping, climbing, and running that active kids do during the day. The pains can occur after a child has had a particularly athletic day.

Signs and Symptoms

Growing pains always concentrate in the muscles, rather than the joints. Most kids report pains in the front of their thighs, in the calves, or behind the knees. Whereas joints affected by more serious diseases are swollen, red, tender, or warm, the joints of kids experiencing growing pains appear normal.

Although growing pains often strike in late afternoon or early evening before bed, pain can sometimes wake a sleeping child. The intensity of the pain varies from child to child, and most kids don't experience the pains every day.

Diagnosing Growing Pains

One symptom that doctors find most helpful in making a diagnosis of growing pains is how the child responds to touch while in pain. Kids who have pain from a serious medical disease don't like to be handled because movement tends to increase the pain. But those with growing pains respond differently—they feel better when they're held, massaged, and cuddled.

Growing pains are what doctors call a diagnosis of exclusion. This means that other conditions should be ruled out before a diagnosis of growing pains is made. A thorough history and physical examination by your doctor can usually accomplish this. In rare instances, blood and X-ray studies may be required before a final diagnosis of growing pains is made.

Helping Your Child

Some things that may help alleviate the pain include:

- massaging the area;
- stretching;
- placing a heating pad on the area;
- giving ibuprofen or acetaminophen. (Never give aspirin to a child under 12 due to its association with Reye syndrome, a rare but potentially fatal disease.)

When to Call the Doctor

Alert your doctor if any of the following symptoms occur with your child's pain:

- Persistent pain, pain in the morning, or swelling or redness in one particular area or joint
- Pain associated with a particular injury
- Fever
- Limping
- Unusual rashes
- Loss of appetite
- Weakness
- Tiredness
- Uncharacteristic behavior

These signs are not due to growing pains and should be evaluated by the doctor.

Although growing pains often point to no serious illness, they can be upsetting to a child—or a parent. Because a child seems completely cured of the aches in the morning, parents sometimes suspect that the child faked the pains. However, this usually is not the case. Support and reassurance that growing pains will pass as kids grow up can help them relax.

Section 25.4

Intoeing

"Intoeing," reproduced with permission from *Your Orthopaedic Connection.* © American Academy of Orthopaedic Surgeons (www.aaos.org), Rosemont, IL, 2011.

Intoeing means that when a child walks or runs, the feet turn inward instead of pointing straight ahead. It is commonly referred to as being "pigeon-toed."

Intoeing is often first noticed by parents when a baby begins walking, but children at various ages may display intoeing for different reasons.

Occasionally, severe intoeing may cause young children to stumble or trip as they catch their toes on the other heel. Intoeing usually does not cause pain, nor does it lead to arthritis.

In the vast majority of children younger than eight years old, intoeing will almost always correct itself without the use of casts, braces, surgery, or any special treatment. A child whose intoeing is associated with pain, swelling, or a limp should be evaluated by an orthopaedic surgeon.

Cause

The cause of intoeing depends on where the change in alignment is centered. There are three common conditions causing intoeing:

- Curved foot (metatarsus adductus)

- Twisted shin (tibia torsion)

- Twisted thighbone (femoral anteversion)

Each of these conditions may run in families. They also can simply occur on their own or in association with other orthopaedic problems. Prevention is not usually possible because they occur from developmental or genetic problems that cannot be controlled for.

Metatarsus Adductus

Metatarsus adductus is when a child's feet bend inward from the middle part of the foot to the toes. Some cases may be mild and flexible, and others may be more obvious and rigid. Severe cases of metatarsus adductus may partially resemble a clubfoot deformity.

Metatarsus adductus improves by itself most of the time, usually over the first four to six months of life. Babies aged six to nine months with severe deformity or feet that are very rigid may be treated with casts or special shoes with a high rate of success. Surgery to straighten the foot is seldom required.

Tibial Torsion

Tibial torsion occurs if the child's lower leg (tibia) twists inward. This can occur before birth, as the legs rotate to fit in the confined space of the womb. After birth, an infant's legs should gradually rotate to align properly. If the lower leg remains turned in, the result is tibial torsion.

When the child begins walking, the feet turn inward because the tibia in the lower leg, just above the foot, points the foot inward. As the tibia grows taller, it usually untwists.

Tibial torsion almost always improves without treatment, and usually before school age. Splints, special shoes, and exercise programs do not help. Surgery to reset the bone may be done in a child who is at least 8 to10 years old and has a severe twist that causes significant walking problems.

Femoral Anteversion

Femoral anteversion (also known as excessive femoral torsion) occurs when a child's thighbone (femur) turns inward. It is often most obvious at about five or six years of age. The upper end of the thighbone, near the hip, has an increased twist, which allows the hip to turn inward more than it turns outward. This causes both the knees and the feet to point inward during walking. Children with this condition often sit in the "W" position, with their knees bent and their feet flared out behind them.

Femoral anteversion spontaneously corrects in almost all children as they grow older. Studies have found that special shoes, braces, and exercises do not help. Surgery is usually not considered unless the child is older than 9 or 10 years and has a severe deformity that causes tripping and an unsightly gait. Like surgery for tibial torsion, during the procedure for femoral anteversion, the femur is cut and rotated back into proper alignment.

Section 25.5

Juvenile Idiopathic (Rheumatoid) Arthritis

This section excerpted from "Questions and Answers about Juvenile Arthritis (Juvenile Idiopathic Arthritis, Juvenile Rheumatoid Arthritis, and Other Forms of Arthritis Affecting Children)," National Institute of Arthritis and Musculoskeletal and Skin Diseases (www.niams.nih.gov), September 2011.

What is juvenile arthritis?

"Arthritis" means joint inflammation. This term refers to a group of diseases that cause pain, swelling, stiffness, and loss of motion in the joints. Juvenile arthritis (JA) is a term often used to describe arthritis in children. Children can develop almost all types of arthritis that affect adults, but the most common type that affects children is juvenile idiopathic arthritis. Both juvenile idiopathic arthritis (JIA) and juvenile rheumatoid arthritis (JRA) are classification systems for chronic arthritis in children.

JIA is currently the most widely accepted term to describe various types of chronic arthritis in children. In general, the symptoms of JIA include joint pain, swelling, tenderness, warmth, and stiffness that last for more than six continuous weeks. It is divided into seven separate subtypes, each with characteristic symptoms.

What causes juvenile arthritis?

Most forms of juvenile arthritis are autoimmune disorders, which means that the body's immune system—which normally helps to fight off bacteria or viruses—mistakenly attacks some of its own healthy cells and tissues. The result is inflammation, marked by redness, heat, pain, and swelling. Inflammation can cause joint damage. Doctors do not know why the immune system attacks healthy tissues in children who develop JA. Scientists suspect that it is a two-step process. First, something in a child's genetic makeup gives him or her a tendency to develop JA; then an environmental factor, such as a virus, triggers the development of the disease.

Not all cases of JA are autoimmune, however. Recent research has demonstrated that some people, such as many with systemic arthritis, have what is more accurately called an autoinflammatory condition. Although the two terms sound somewhat similar, the disease processes behind autoimmune and autoinflammatory disorders are different.

What are its symptoms and signs?

The most common symptom of all types of juvenile arthritis is persistent joint swelling, pain, and stiffness that is typically worse in the morning or after a nap. The pain may limit movement of the affected joint, although many children, especially younger ones, will not complain of pain. JA commonly affects the knees and the joints in the hands and feet. One of the earliest signs of JA may be limping in the morning because of an affected knee. Besides joint symptoms, children with systemic JA have a high fever and a skin rash. The rash and fever may appear and disappear very quickly. Systemic arthritis also may cause the lymph nodes located in the neck and other parts of the body to swell. In some cases (fewer than half), internal organs including the heart and (very rarely) the lungs may be involved.

Eye inflammation is a potentially severe complication that commonly occurs in children with oligoarthritis but can also be seen in other types of JA. All children with JA need to have regular eye exams, including a special exam called a slit lamp exam.

Typically, there are periods when the symptoms of JA are better or disappear (remissions) and times when symptoms "flare," or get worse. JA is different in each child; some may have just one or two flares and never have symptoms again, while others experience many flares or even have symptoms that never go away.

Some children with JA have growth problems. Depending on the severity of the disease and the joints involved, bone growth at the affected joints may be too fast or too slow, causing one leg or arm to be longer than the other. Overall growth also may be slowed.

How is it diagnosed?

Doctors usually suspect JA, along with several other possible conditions, when they see children with persistent joint pain or swelling, unexplained skin rashes, and fever associated with swelling of lymph nodes or inflammation of internal organs.

No single test can be used to diagnose JA. A doctor diagnoses JA by carefully examining the patient and considering his or her medical history and the results of tests that help confirm JA or rule out other conditions.

Symptoms: When diagnosing JA, a doctor must consider not only the symptoms a child has but also the length of time these symptoms have been present. Joint swelling or other objective changes in the joint with arthritis must be present continuously for at least six weeks for the doctor to establish a diagnosis of JA. Because this factor is so important, it may be useful to keep a record of the symptoms and changes in the joints, noting when they first appeared and when they are worse or better.

Family history: It is very rare for more than one member of a family to have JA. But children with a family member who has JA are at a small increased risk of developing it. Research shows that JA is also more likely in families with a history of any autoimmune disease.

Laboratory tests: Laboratory tests, usually blood tests, cannot alone provide the doctor with a clear diagnosis. But these tests can be used to help rule out other conditions and classify the type of JA that a patient has.

X-rays: X-rays are needed if the doctor suspects injury to the bone or unusual bone development. Early in the disease, some X-rays can show changes in soft tissue. In general, X-rays are more useful later in the disease, when bones may be affected.

Other tests: Because there are many causes of joint pain and swelling, the doctor must rule out other conditions before diagnosing JA. These include physical injury, bacterial or viral infection, Lyme disease, inflammatory bowel disease, lupus, dermatomyositis, and some forms of cancer. The doctor may use additional laboratory tests to help rule out these and other possible conditions.

How is it treated?

The main goals of treatment are to preserve a high level of physical and social functioning and maintain a good quality of life. To achieve these goals, doctors recommend treatments to reduce swelling, maintain full movement in the affected joints, relieve pain, and prevent, identify, and treat complications. Most children with JA need a combination of medication and nonmedication treatments to reach these goals.

Treatments with medication: Nonsteroidal anti-inflammatory drugs (NSAIDs) are often the first type of medication used. All NSAIDs work similarly: by blocking substances called prostaglandins that contribute to inflammation and pain. If NSAIDs do not relieve symptoms of JA, the doctor is likely to prescribe disease-modifying anti-rheumatic drugs (DMARDs). DMARDs slow the progression of JA, but because they may take weeks or months to relieve symptoms, they often are taken with an NSAID. Although many different types of DMARDs are available, doctors are most likely to use one particular DMARD, methotrexate, for children with JA.

Researchers have learned that methotrexate is safe and effective for some children with JA whose symptoms are not relieved by other medications. Because only small doses of methotrexate are needed to relieve arthritis symptoms, potentially dangerous side effects rarely occur.

In children with very severe JA, stronger medicines may be needed to stop serious symptoms such as inflammation of the sac around the heart (pericarditis). Corticosteroids such as prednisone may be added to the treatment plan to control severe symptoms. Corticosteroids can interfere with a child's normal growth and can cause other side effects, such as a round face, weakened bones, and increased susceptibility to infections. Once the medication controls severe symptoms, the doctor will reduce the dose gradually and eventually stop it completely. Because it can be dangerous to stop taking corticosteroids suddenly, it is important that the patient carefully follow the doctor's instructions about how to take or reduce the dose. For inflammation in one or just a few joints, injecting a corticosteroid compound into the affected joint or joints can often bring quick relief without the systemic side effects of oral or intravenous medication.

Children with JA who have received little relief from other drugs may be given one of a newer class of drug treatments called biologic response modifiers, or biologic agents.

Treatments without medication: Physical therapy—a regular, general exercise program—is an important part of a child's treatment plan. It can help to maintain muscle tone and preserve and recover the range of motion of the joints. A physiatrist (rehabilitation specialist) or a physical therapist can design an appropriate exercise program for a person with JA. The specialist also may recommend using splints and other devices to help maintain normal bone and joint growth.

Many adults seek alternative ways of treating arthritis, such as special diets, supplements, acupuncture, massage, or even magnetic jewelry or mattress pads. Research shows that increasing numbers of children are using alternative and complementary therapies as well.

Although there is little research to support many alternative treatments, some people seem to benefit from them. If a child's doctor feels the approach has value and is not harmful, it can be incorporated into the treatment plan. However, it is important not to neglect regular health care or treatment of serious symptoms.

Do these children have to limit activities?

Although pain sometimes limits physical activity, exercise is important for reducing the symptoms of juvenile arthritis and maintaining function and range of motion of the joints. Most children with JA can take part fully in physical activities and selected sports when their symptoms are under control. During a disease flare, however, the doctor may advise limiting certain activities, depending on the joints involved. Once the flare is over, the child can start regular activities again.

Swimming is particularly useful because it uses many joints and muscles without putting weight on the joints. A doctor or physical therapist can recommend exercises and activities.

Section 25.6

Juvenile Myositis and Dermatomyositis

Juvenile Myositis (JM), including Juvenile Dermatomyositis (JDM) and Juvenile Polymyositis (JPM), is an autoimmune disease in which the body's immune system attacks its own cells and tissues.

Weak muscles and skin rash are the primary symptoms of JDM, while muscle weakness without a rash is the primary symptom of JPM.

Even within these designations, JM affects every child differently. Some children experience a mild form of the disease, while others follow a more severe and potentially more debilitating course. Some of the more onerous secondary symptoms are calcinosis, vasculitic ulcers and contractures.

Incidence of JM

JM is a rare disease and its exact incidence is unknown. Estimates from various studies suggest that between one and five children per million will develop this disease each year. Approximately 1,000 new cases of JM are diagnosed in the United States every year.

JM begins in childhood or the teen years. The average age of onset for JDM is between six to seven years old; 25% are age four or less. JPM usually develops several years later.

JM affects girls twice as much as boys. Once a child is diagnosed with JM, it is always considered to be the juvenile form, even if the patient continues with the disease into adulthood.

Genesis of the Disease

The immune system is a group of cells that normally protects the body from infection and other environmental factors. In an autoimmune disease like JM, however, the cells get active and they cannot stop. The immune system ends up attacking previously healthy tissues, harming the body instead of protecting it. In JM, the immune system mistakenly targets muscles, skin, and other tissues.

The process that occurs when the immune system attacks healthy tissue is called inflammation. In JDM sufferers, the inflammation primarily occurs in the blood vessels that lie under the skin and in the muscles. With JPM, the attack is focused more directly against the muscle cells.

This inflammation causes the weak muscles and—in the case of JDM—skin rashes. If blood vessels or muscle cells in other parts of the body are inflamed, other systems of the body can be affected, such as the digestive tract, heart, and lungs.

What Causes JM?

Researchers believe the coming together of several factors—both environmental and genetic—cause JM. Children who develop this disease often have a family history of other autoimmune diseases, such as thyroid disorder, type I diabetes, rheumatoid arthritis, lupus, or Crohn's disease. If a child is genetically predisposed to JM, experts suspect a microbe, such as a virus or bacteria, might trigger a runaway immune response that will cause the body to attack itself. Other environmental factors, such as a heavy dose of sun exposure, may also play a role.

What Are the Primary Symptoms of JM?

Weak Muscles

The muscles that are affected the most are near the trunk of the body: the stomach, thigh, neck, and upper arm muscles. Other muscles, however, can become weak as well. Sometimes there is inflammation in the swallowing tube or esophagus, which makes it difficult for the child to swallow. Other times, there is inflammation in the intestinal tract, which causes bowel difficulties and stomach pain.

A child with JM has great difficulty climbing stairs and just getting up from a sitting position. Walking and running become very challenging and exhausting. Some children will literally roll out of bed, because sitting up and lifting the head becomes too difficult.

In addition to weakness, some children with JM experience pain in their muscles.

Skin Rash

The skin rash in JDM usually occurs on the eyelids, knuckles, elbows, knees, and ankles. The rash may appear before, after, or at the same time as the muscle weakness. Sometimes the rash is so faint that it is not noticeable.

The rash appearing on the eyelids is red and purplish in color and is referred to as a heliotrope rash (named after a flower of the same color). Another rash that frequently occurs on the cheeks takes on a red color and looks very similar to a sunburn.

On the knuckles, elbows, and knees, the rash takes the form of patches of red and scaly skin (called Gottron's papules). The fingernails and the nail beds may take on a pinkish color as well.

Fatigue

With JM, the child becomes tired easily and can only walk short distances. The child needs to rest often and lacks the energy for normal activities. It becomes difficult for the child to keep up with friends.

Fever

Sometimes, the child with JM runs low-grade fevers, especially at night.

What Are Other Possible Symptoms?

The following symptoms of JM are less common, but important to understand:

Calcinosis

Researchers believe approximately 20% to one-third of the children with JM will develop calcinosis. Calcinosis is the development of small lumps or linear deposits of calcium under the skin or in the muscle. They may feel like rocks under the skin and can range in size from a small pebble to a large softball. They can also form in a sheet-like appearance.

In many cases, these calcium deposits can grow over time or remain unchanged for years. In some cases, the calcinosis lumps are absorbed back into the body. Other times, the lumps break through the skin where they may leak creamy white calcium. These protrusions can become infected and painful, and sometimes need to be surgically removed. Calcinosis lumps are most likely to break through on the joints, such as the elbows and knees, but they can emerge anywhere on the body, often in pressure points.

Calcinosis can be present at the time of diagnosis, or many years later. It can be associated with a delayed diagnosis or the lack of aggressive treatment.

Vasculitic Ulcers

Vasculitic ulcers are holes in the skin or gastrointestinal tract caused by inflammation of the blood vessels.

When they occur in the skin, they look like open sores and can extend deep into the tissues. The ulcers can be very painful and generally are associated with a more severe course of JM.

When the ulcers occur in the gastrointestinal tract, they can harm the digestive organs and result in very serious illness.

The warning signs of this condition are severe stomach pain, dark black stools, or blood in the stools.

Contractures

Contractures are shortened muscles that cause a joint to stay in a bent position or have limited movement. Contractures can occur due to inflammation, muscle weakness, or calcinosis crossing over a joint.

Lipodystrophy

Lipodystrophy is a loss of body fat. In areas affected by lipodystrophy, the fat cells become damaged, and if widespread and extensive, this can result in problems with storing fat and sugar, resulting in high cholesterol and diabetes.

What Tests Are Used to Diagnose JM?

A doctor will first perform a complete physical exam, specifically looking for rashes and muscle weakness. If JM is suspected, blood tests are the next step in making a diagnosis. Muscle enzymes are measured, including creatine kinase (CK), aldolase, lactate dehydrogenase (LDH), aspartate aminotransferase (AST), and alanine aminotransferase (ALT). If these lab tests are elevated, enzymes are leaking from inflamed or damaged muscles into the bloodstream. Antinuclear antibodies (ANA) are also measured to see if the child's body is producing antibodies against its own cells. Several myositis-specific autoantibodies have also been identified, and these can be tested as well. Other blood tests are sometimes available to check out immune activation and/or blood vessel damage.

The next step in diagnosing JM is usually an MRI [magnetic resonance imaging], which can detect muscle inflammation and damage. If the MRI shows evidence of diseased muscles, a muscle biopsy may be performed to finalize the diagnosis. When the characteristic rashes are not present, it is important that a muscle biopsy be performed to exclude other causes of muscle weakness. A small amount of muscle is removed for examination under a microscope to determine if and how much the muscles and blood vessels have been affected by the disease.

If the patient has the rash and muscle weakness of JM, the lab tests are consistent with JM, and the MRI shows muscle inflammation, some doctors will not perform a muscle biopsy.

What Is the Treatment for JM?

Although medications can help alleviate the symptoms of JM, the disease has no known cure. The primary medications used to treat the symptoms of JM are corticosteroids, immunosuppressants, and chemotherapy. These medications themselves can cause severe side effects, making JM challenging to treat. Many researchers believe that early and aggressive treatment is usually the best predictor of a better outcome of this disease.

High dose oral prednisone or other corticosteroids often coupled with intravenous corticosteroids (Solu-Medrol) are usually the first line of treatment for JM. Since the side effects of corticosteroids can be very troublesome, methotrexate (a chemotherapy drug administered at much lower doses than used for cancer patients) is usually introduced early to allow for tapering of the corticosteroids.

Second-line treatments include cyclosporine and intravenous immunoglobulin (IVIG). Plaquenil is often used to control the rash.

For patients who do not respond to the first and second line of treatments, or in patients severely affected by the disease, rituximab, Cytoxan, and CellCept can be added. Protection from UVB is essential with sunscreens. Vitamin D with adequate calcium intake keeps bones strong.

These medications all have their own side effects, but the most common ones for Prednisone are:

- increased appetite and weight gain;
- rounded face;
- mood changes;
- high blood pressure;
- stretch marks;
- fragile bones and bone damage;
- cataracts;
- slow growth.

In addition to medications, physical therapy is generally prescribed to increase strength and flexibility in muscles and joints.

What Is the Prognosis?

There is no cure for JM, but with advances in early diagnosis and aggressive treatment, the outcome has continued to improve. Some children experience a mild form of the disease and may go into remission. Others follow a more severe and potentially debilitating course that can be life-long. Some JM patients will have a loss of range of motion. Some will battle an array of serious complications, resulting in the inability to walk, ongoing pain, disfigurement, and even death. Whether the course of the disease is mild or severe, JM is life-changing for all of these children and their families.

Section 25.7

Procedures to Correct Leg Length Discrepancy

"Leg Lengthening and Shortening," © 2012 A.D.A.M, Inc.
Reprinted with permission.

Leg lengthening and shortening are types of surgery to treat some children who have legs of unequal lengths.
These procedures may:

- lengthen an abnormally short leg;

- shorten an abnormally long leg;

- limit growth of a normal leg to allow a short leg to grow to a matching length.

Description

Bone Lengthening

This series of treatments involves several surgical procedures, a long recovery period, and a number of risks—but it can add up to six inches of length to a leg.
While the child is under general anesthesia:

- The bone to be lengthened is cut.

- Metal pins or screws are inserted through the skin and into the bone. Pins are placed above and below the cut in the bone, and the surgical cut in the skin is stitched closed.

- A metal device (usually some sort of external frame) is attached to the pins in the bone. It will be used later to very slowly (over months) pull the cut bone apart. This creates a space between the ends of the cut bone that will fill in with new bone.

Later, when the leg has reached the desired length and has healed (usually after several months), another surgical procedure will be done to remove the pins.

Bone Resection or Removal

This is a complicated surgery that can produce a very precise degree of correction.

While the child is under general anesthesia:

- The bone to be shortened is cut and a section of bone is removed.

- The ends of the cut bone will be joined and a metal plate with screws or a nail down the center of the bone is placed across the bone incision to hold it in place during healing.

Bone Growth Restriction

Bone growth takes place at the growth plates (physes) at each end of long bones.

While the child is under general anesthesia, the surgeons make a surgical cut over the growth plate at the end of the bone in the longer leg.

- The growth plate may be destroyed by scraping or drilling it (epiphysiodesis or physeal arrest) to stop further growth at that growth plate.

- Another method is to insert staples on each side of the bony growth plate. These can be removed when both legs are close to the same length.

Why the Procedure is Performed

Leg lengthening is considered for large differences in leg length (more than five centimeters or two inches). Leg lengthening is more likely to be recommended:

- for children whose bones are still growing;

- for patients who were short to begin with.

Leg shortening or restricting is considered for smaller differences. Shortening a longer leg may be recommended for children whose bones are no longer growing.

Bone growth restriction is recommended for children whose bones are still growing. It is used to restrict the growth of a longer bone, while the shorter bone continues to grow to match its length. Proper timing of this treatment is important to ensure good results.

Medical illnesses that lead to severely unequal leg lengths include the following:

- Poliomyelitis and cerebral palsy
- Small, weak (atrophied) muscles or short, tight (spastic) muscles, which may cause deformities and prevent normal leg growth
- Hip diseases such as Legg-Perthes disease
- Previous injuries or bone fractures that may stimulate excessive bone growth
- Birth defects (congenital deformities) of bones, joints, muscles, tendons, or ligaments

Risks

Risks for any anesthesia include:

- reactions to medications;
- problems breathing.

Risks for any surgery include:

- bleeding;
- infection.

Additional risks include:

- bone growth restriction (epiphysiodesis), which may cause short height;
- bone infection (osteomyelitis);
- injury to blood vessels;
- poor bone healing;
- nerve damage.

After the Procedure

After bone growth restriction:

- It is common for children to spend up to a week in the hospital. Sometimes a cast is placed on the leg for 3 to 4 weeks.
- Healing is complete in 8 to 12 weeks, at which time the child can restart full activities.

After bone shortening:

- It is common for children to spend 2 to 3 weeks in the hospital. Sometimes a cast is placed on the leg for 3 to 4 weeks.

- Muscle weakness is common, and muscle strengthening exercises are started soon after surgery.

- Crutches are used for 6 to 8 weeks.

- Some children take 6 to 12 weeks to regain normal knee control and function.

- A metal rod placed inside the bone is removed at one year.

After bone lengthening:

- The child will spend a week or longer in the hospital.

- Frequent visits to the doctor are needed to adjust the lengthening device. How long the lengthening device is used depends on the amount of lengthening needed. Physical therapy is needed to maintain normal range of motion.

- Special care of the pins or screws holding the device is needed to prevent infection.

- How long it takes the bone to heal depends on the amount of lengthening. Each centimeter of lengthening takes 36 days of healing.

Because the blood vessels, muscles, and skin are involved, careful and frequent checking of the skin color, temperature, and sensation of the foot and toes is important. This will help identify any damage to blood vessels, muscles, or nerves as early as possible.

Outlook (Prognosis)

Bone growth restriction (epiphysiodesis) is usually successful when it is performed at the correct time in the growth period. However, it may cause short stature.

Bone shortening may achieve more exact correction than bone restriction, but it requires a much longer recovery period.

Bone lengthening is completely successful only 40% of the time and has a much higher rate of complications.

Section 25.8

Marfan Syndrome

This section excerpted from "Questions and Answers about Marfan Syndrome," National Institute of Arthritis and Musculoskeletal and Skin Diseases (www.niams.nih.gov), October 2011.

What is Marfan syndrome?

Marfan syndrome is a heritable condition that affects the connective tissue. The primary purpose of connective tissue is to hold the body together and provide a framework for growth and development. In Marfan syndrome, the connective tissue is defective and does not act as it should. Because connective tissue is found throughout the body, Marfan syndrome can affect many body systems, including the skeleton, eyes, heart and blood vessels, nervous system, skin, and lungs.

What are the symptoms of Marfan syndrome?

Marfan syndrome affects different people in different ways. Some people have only mild symptoms, while others are more severely affected. In most cases, the symptoms progress as the person ages. The body systems most often affected by Marfan syndrome are the following:

Skeleton: People with Marfan syndrome are typically very tall, slender, and loose-jointed. Because Marfan syndrome affects the long bones of the skeleton, a person's arms, legs, fingers, and toes may be disproportionately long in relation to the rest of the body.

Eyes: More than half of all people with Marfan syndrome experience dislocation of one or both lenses of the eye. The lens may be slightly higher or lower than normal, and may be shifted off to one side. The dislocation may be minimal, or it may be pronounced and obvious. One serious complication that may occur with this disorder is retinal detachment.

Heart and blood vessels (cardiovascular system): Most people with Marfan syndrome have problems associated with the heart and blood vessels. Because of faulty connective tissue, the wall of the aorta (the large artery that carries blood from the heart to the rest of the body) may be weakened and stretch, a process called aortic dilatation. Aortic dilatation increases the risk that the aorta will tear (aortic dissection) or rupture, causing serious heart problems or sometimes sudden death.

Nervous system: The brain and spinal cord are surrounded by fluid contained by a membrane called the dura, which is composed of connective tissue. As someone with Marfan syndrome gets older, the dura often weakens and stretches, then begins to weigh on the vertebrae in the lower spine and wear away the bone surrounding the spinal cord. This is called dural ectasia. These changes may cause only mild discomfort, or they may lead to radiated pain in the abdomen or to pain, numbness, or weakness in the legs.

Skin: Many people with Marfan syndrome develop stretch marks on their skin, even without any weight change. These stretch marks can occur at any age and pose no health risk. However, people with Marfan syndrome are also at increased risk for developing an abdominal or inguinal hernia, in which a bulge develops that contains part of the intestines.

Lungs: Although connective tissue problems make the tiny air sacs within the lungs less elastic, people with Marfan syndrome generally do not experience noticeable problems with their lungs. If, however, these tiny air sacs become stretched or swollen, the risk of lung collapse may increase.

What causes Marfan syndrome?

Marfan syndrome is caused by a defect, or mutation, in the gene that determines the structure of fibrillin-1, a protein that is an important part of connective tissue. A person with Marfan syndrome is born with the disorder, even though it may not be diagnosed until later in life.

The defective gene that causes Marfan syndrome can be inherited: the child of a person who has Marfan syndrome has a 50% chance of inheriting the disease. Sometimes a new gene defect occurs during the formation of sperm or egg cells, making it possible for two parents without the disease to have a child with the disease. But this is rare. Two unaffected parents have only a 1 in 10,000 chance of having a child with Marfan syndrome. Possibly 25% of cases are due to a spontaneous mutation at the time of conception.

How is Marfan syndrome diagnosed?

There is no specific laboratory test, such as a blood test or skin biopsy, to diagnose Marfan syndrome. The doctor and/or geneticist relies on observation and a complete medical history, including the following:

- Information about any family members who may have the disorder or who had an early, unexplained, heart-related death

- A thorough physical examination, including an evaluation of the skeletal frame for the ratio of arm/leg size to trunk size

- An eye examination, including a slit lamp evaluation

- Heart tests such as an echocardiogram (a test that uses ultrasound waves to examine the heart and aorta)

The doctor may diagnose Marfan syndrome if the patient has a family history of the disease, and if there are specific problems in at least two of the body systems known to be affected. For a patient with no family history of the disease, at least three body systems must be affected before a diagnosis is made. Moreover, two of the systems must show clear signs that are relatively specific for Marfan syndrome.

What treatment options are available?

There is no cure for Marfan syndrome. However, a range of treatment options can minimize and sometimes prevent complications. The appropriate specialists will develop an individualized treatment program; the approach the doctors use depends on which systems have been affected.

Skeletal: Annual evaluations are important to detect any changes in the spine or sternum. This is particularly important in times of rapid growth, such as adolescence. A serious malformation not only can be disfiguring, but also can prevent the heart and lungs from functioning properly.

Eyes: Early, regular eye examinations are essential for identifying and correcting any vision problems associated with Marfan syndrome.

Heart and blood vessels: Regular checkups and echocardiograms help the doctor evaluate the size of the aorta and the way the heart is working. The earlier a potential problem is identified and treated, the lower the risk of life-threatening complications.

Surgery should be performed before the aorta reaches a size that puts it at high risk for tear or rupture. Because blood clots can form around artificial heart valves, people who have a valve replaced must take the blood-thinning drug warfarin for the rest of their lives.

Because warfarin carries a risk of some serious side effects, including excessive bleeding, and because it is dangerous to unborn babies, doctors are increasingly opting for a newer aortic root replacement procedure that enables people to keep their own valves. The procedure involves removing and replacing the enlarged part of the aorta with a Dacron tube and resuspending the natural valve into the tube so that the tube supports the valve.

Nervous system: If dural ectasia (swelling of the covering of the spinal cord) develops, medication may help minimize any associated pain.

Lungs: It is especially important that people with Marfan syndrome not smoke, as they are already at increased risk for lung damage. Any problems with breathing during sleep should be assessed.

What are some of the emotional and psychological effects of Marfan syndrome?

Being diagnosed and learning to live with a genetic disorder can cause social, emotional, and financial stress. It often requires a great deal of adjustment in outlook and lifestyle.

The parents and siblings of a child diagnosed with Marfan syndrome may feel sadness, anger, and guilt. It is important for parents to know that nothing that they did caused the fibrillin-1 gene to mutate. Parents may be concerned about the genetic implications for siblings or have questions about the risk to future children.

Some children with Marfan syndrome are advised to restrict their activities. This may require a lifestyle adjustment that is hard for a child to understand or accept.

For both children and adults, appropriate medical care, accurate information, and social support make it easier to live with the disease. Genetic counseling may also be helpful for understanding the disease and its potential impact on future generations.

While Marfan syndrome is a lifelong disorder, the outlook has improved in recent years. As early as the 1970s, the life expectancy of a person with Marfan syndrome was two-thirds that of a person without the disease; however, with improvements in recognition and treatment, people with Marfan syndrome now have a life expectancy similar to that of the average person.

Section 25.9

Muscular Dystrophy

This section excerpted from "Muscular Dystrophy: Hope through Research," National Institute of Neurological Disorders and Stroke (www.ninds.nih.gov), September 9, 2011.

What is muscular dystrophy?

Muscular dystrophy (MD) refers to a group of more than 30 genetic diseases that cause progressive weakness and degeneration of skeletal muscles used during voluntary movement. These disorders vary in age of onset, severity, and pattern of affected muscles. All forms of MD grow worse as muscles progressively degenerate and weaken. Many patients eventually lose the ability to walk.

Some types of MD also affect the heart, gastrointestinal system, endocrine glands, spine, eyes, brain, and other organs. Respiratory and cardiac diseases may occur, and some patients may develop a swallowing disorder. MD is not contagious and cannot be brought on by injury or activity.

What causes MD?

All of the muscular dystrophies are inherited and involve a mutation in one of the thousands of genes that program proteins critical to muscle integrity. The body's cells don't work properly when a protein is altered or produced in insufficient quantity (or sometimes missing completely). Many cases of MD occur from spontaneous mutations that are not found in the genes of either parent, and this defect can be passed to the next generation.

How does MD affect muscles?

Muscles are made up of thousands of muscle fibers. Each fiber is actually a number of individual cells that have joined together during development and are encased by an outer membrane. Muscle fibers that make up individual muscles are bound together by connective tissue.

Although MD can affect several body tissues and organs, it most prominently affects the integrity of muscle fibers. The disease causes muscle degeneration, progressive weakness, fiber death, fiber branching and splitting, phagocytosis (in which muscle fiber material is broken down and destroyed by scavenger cells), and, in some cases, chronic or permanent shortening of tendons and muscles. Also, overall muscle strength and tendon reflexes are usually lessened or lost due to replacement of muscle by connective tissue and fat.

Are there other MD-like conditions?

There are many other heritable diseases that affect the muscles, the nerves, or the neuromuscular junction. These diseases may produce symptoms that are very similar to those found in some forms of MD, but they are caused by different genetic defects. The sharing of symptoms among multiple neuromuscular diseases, and the prevalence of sporadic cases in families not previously affected by MD, often makes it difficult for MD patients to obtain a quick diagnosis.

How do the muscular dystrophies differ?

There are nine major groups of the muscular dystrophies. The disorders are classified by the extent and distribution of muscle weakness, age of onset, rate of progression, severity of symptoms, and family history (including any pattern of inheritance). Although some forms of MD become apparent in infancy or childhood, others may not appear until middle age or later. Overall, incidence rates and severity vary, but each of the dystrophies causes progressive skeletal muscle deterioration, and some types affect cardiac muscle.

There are four forms of MD that begin in childhood:

- **Duchenne MD** is the most common childhood form of MD, as well as the most common of the muscular dystrophies overall, accounting for approximately 50% of all cases. Duchenne MD primarily affects boys, although girls and women who carry the defective gene may show some symptoms. Duchenne MD usually becomes apparent when an affected child begins to walk. Progressive weakness and muscle wasting (a decrease in muscle strength and size) caused by degenerating muscle fibers begins in the upper legs and pelvis before spreading into the upper arms. Other symptoms include loss of some reflexes, a waddling gait, frequent falls and clumsiness (especially when running), difficulty when rising from a sitting or lying position or when climbing stairs, changes to overall posture, impaired breathing, lung weakness, and cardiomyopathy (heart muscle weakness that interferes with pumping ability). As the disease progresses, the muscles in the diaphragm that assist in breathing and coughing may weaken. Patients may experience breathing difficulties, respiratory infections, and swallowing problems. Some children are mildly mentally impaired. Between ages 3 and 6, children may show brief periods of physical improvement followed by progressive muscle degeneration. Children with Duchenne MD are typically wheelchair-bound by age 12 and usually die in their late teens or early twenties from progressive weakness of the heart muscle, respiratory complications, or infection.

- **Becker MD** is less severe than but closely related to Duchenne MD. The disorder usually appears around age 11 but may occur as late as age 25, and patients generally live into middle age or later. The rate of progressive, symmetric (on both sides of the body) muscle atrophy and weakness varies greatly among affected individuals. Many patients are able to walk until they are in their mid-thirties or later, while others are unable to walk past their teens. Some affected individuals never need to use a wheelchair.

- **Congenital MD** refers to a group of autosomal recessive muscular dystrophies that are either present at birth or become evident before age two. Congenital MD affects boys and girls. Weakness may be first noted when children fail to meet landmarks in motor function and muscle control. Muscle degeneration may be mild or severe and is restricted primarily to skeletal muscle. The majority of patients are unable to sit or stand without support, and some affected children may never learn to walk.

- **Emery-Dreifuss MD** primarily affects boys. Onset is usually apparent by age 10, but symptoms can appear as late as the mid-twenties. This disease causes slow but progressive wasting of the upper arm and lower leg muscles and symmetric weakness. Contractures in the spine, ankles, knees, elbows, and back of the neck usually precede significant muscle weakness, which is less severe than in Duchenne MD. Contractures may cause elbows to become locked in a flexed position. The entire spine may become rigid as the disease progresses. Nearly all Emery-Dreifuss MD patients have some form of heart problem by age 30, often requiring a pacemaker or other assistive device. Female carriers of the disorder often have cardiac complications without muscle weakness. Patients often die in mid-adulthood from progressive pulmonary or cardiac failure.

Youth/adolescent-onset muscular dystrophies are classified two ways:

- **Facioscapulohumeral MD (FSHD)** initially affects muscles of the face, shoulders, and upper arms with progressive weakness. Most individuals have a normal life span, but some individuals become severely disabled. Disease progression is typically very slow, with intermittent spurts of rapid muscle deterioration. Onset is usually in the teenage years but may occur as late as age 40. Muscles around the eyes and mouth are often affected first, followed by weakness around the lower shoulders and chest. A particular pattern of muscle wasting causes the shoulders to appear to be slanted and the shoulder blades to appear winged.

- **Limb-girdle MD** refers to more than a dozen inherited conditions marked by progressive loss of muscle bulk and symmetrical weakening of voluntary muscles, primarily those in the shoulders and around the hips. The recessive limb-girdle muscular dystrophies occur more frequently than the dominant forms and usually begin in childhood or the teenage years. The dominant limb-girdle muscular dystrophies usually begin in adulthood. In general, the earlier the clinical signs appear, the more rapid the rate of disease progression. Some forms of the disease progress rapidly, resulting in serious muscle damage and loss of the ability to walk, while others advance very slowly over many years and cause minimal disability, allowing a normal life expectancy.

There are three forms of MD that usually begin in adulthood.

- **Distal MD**, also called distal myopathy, describes a group of at least six specific muscle diseases that primarily affect distal muscles (those farthest away from the shoulders and hips) in the forearms, hands, lower legs, and feet. Distal dystrophies are typically less severe, progress more slowly, and involve fewer muscles than other forms of MD, although they can spread to other muscles.

- **Myotonic MD**, also known as Steinert disease and dystrophia myotonica, may be the most common adult form of MD. Myotonia, or an inability to relax muscles following a sudden contraction, is found only in this form of MD. People with myotonic MD can live a long life, with variable but slowly progressive disability.

- **Oculopharyngeal MD (OPMD)** generally begins in a person's forties or fifties and affects both men and women. Patients first report drooping eyelids, followed by weakness in the facial muscles and pharyngeal muscles in the throat, causing difficulty swallowing. The tongue may atrophy and changes to the voice may occur. Muscle weakness and wasting in the neck and shoulder region is common. Limb muscles may also be affected.

How are the muscular dystrophies diagnosed?

Both the patient's medical history and a complete family history should be thoroughly reviewed to determine if the muscle disease is secondary to a disease affecting other tissues or organs or is an inherited condition. It is also important to rule out any muscle weakness resulting from prior surgery, exposure to toxins, current medications that may affect the patient's functional status, and any acquired muscle diseases. Thorough clinical and neurological exams can rule out disorders of the central and/or peripheral nervous systems, identify any patterns of muscle weakness and atrophy, test reflex responses and coordination, and look for contractions.

Various laboratory tests may be used to confirm the diagnosis of MD.

- Blood and urine tests can detect defective genes and help identify specific neuromuscular disorders.

- Electron microscopy can identify changes in subcellular components of muscle fibers. Electron microscopy can also identify changes that characterize cell death, mutations in muscle cell mitochondria, and an increase in connective tissue seen in muscle diseases such as MD.

- Exercise tests can detect elevated rates of certain chemicals following exercise and are used to determine the nature of the MD or other muscle disorder.

- Genetic testing looks for genes known to either cause or be associated with inherited muscle disease.

- Genetic counseling can help parents who have a family history of MD determine if they are carrying one of the mutated genes that cause the disorder.

- Magnetic resonance imaging (MRI) is used to examine muscle quality, any atrophy or abnormalities in size, and fatty replacement of muscle tissue, as well as to monitor disease progression.

- Muscle biopsies are used to monitor the course of disease and treatment effectiveness.

How are the muscular dystrophies treated?

There is no specific treatment that can stop or reverse the progression of any form of MD. Treatment is aimed at keeping the patient independent for as long as possible and preventing complications that result from weakness, reduced mobility, and cardiac and respiratory difficulties. Treatment may involve a combination of approaches, including physical therapy, drug therapy, and surgery.

Assisted ventilation is often needed to treat respiratory muscle weakness that accompanies many forms of MD, especially in the later stages.

Drug therapy may be prescribed to delay muscle degeneration. Corticosteroids can slow the rate of muscle deterioration in Duchenne MD and help children retain strength and prolong independent walking by as much as several years. However, these medicines have side effects such as weight gain and bone fragility that can be especially troubling in children. Immunosuppressive drugs can delay some damage to dying muscle cells. Certain drugs may provide short-term relief from myotonia (muscle spasms and weakness). Anticonvulsants are used to control seizures and some muscle activity. Respiratory infections may be treated with antibiotics.

Physical therapy can help prevent deformities, improve movement, and keep muscles as flexible and strong as possible. Options include passive stretching, postural correction, and exercise.

Dietary changes have not been shown to slow the progression of MD. Proper nutrition is essential, however, for overall health. Limited mobility or inactivity resulting from muscle weakness can contribute to obesity, dehydration, and constipation. A high-fiber, high-protein, low-calorie diet combined with recommended fluid intake may help.

Corrective surgery is often performed to ease complications from MD.

What is the prognosis?

The prognosis varies according to the type of MD and the speed of progression. Some types are mild and progress very slowly, allowing normal life expectancy, while others are more severe and result in functional disability and loss of ambulation. Life expectancy may depend on the degree of muscle weakness and any respiratory and/or cardiac complications.

Section 25.10

Osgood-Schlatter Disease

Good news: Osgood-Schlatter disease (OSD) is far less frightful than its name. Though it's one of the most common causes of knee pain in adolescents, it's really not a disease, but an overuse injury. OSD can be quite painful, but usually resolves itself within 12 to 24 months.

About Osgood-Schlatter Disease

Osgood-Schlatter disease is an inflammation of the bone, cartilage, and/or tendon at the top of the shinbone (tibia), where the tendon from the kneecap (patella) attaches. Most often only one knee is affected.

OSD usually strikes active adolescents around the beginning of their growth spurts, the approximately two-year period during which they grow most rapidly. Growth spurts can begin any time between the ages of 8 and 13 for girls, or 10 and 15 for boys. OSD has been more common in boys, but as more girls participate in sports, this is changing.

Osgood-Schlatter Disease

Teens increase their risk for OSD if they play sports involving running, twisting, and jumping, such as basketball, football, volleyball, soccer, tennis, figure skating, and gymnastics. Doctors disagree about the mechanics that cause the injury but agree that overuse and physical stress are involved.

Growth spurts make kids vulnerable because their bones, muscles, and tendons are growing quickly and not always at the same time. With exercise, differences in size and strength between the muscle groups place unusual stress on the growth plate at the top of the shinbone. (A growth plate is a layer of cartilage near the end of a bone where most of the bone's growth occurs. It is weaker and more vulnerable to injury than the rest of the bone.)

Most parents call the doctor after their child complains of intermittent pain over several months. The pain may be anywhere from mild and felt only during activity to severe and constant.

Other symptoms may include:

- pain that worsens with exercise;

- relief from pain with rest;

- swelling or tenderness under the knee and over the shinbone;

- limping after exercise;

- tightness of the muscles surrounding the knee (the hamstring and quadriceps muscles).

Symptoms that aren't typical of OSD include pain at rest, thigh pain, or very severe pain that awakens kids from sleep or makes them cry. If your child has any of these symptoms, talk to your doctor.

How Is It Treated?

OSD usually goes away by age 18 or when a teenager's bones mature. Until then, only the symptoms need treatment. Rest is the key to pain relief. Parents find it a cruel irony that the most active kids are most likely to get OSD—and also the ones least likely to rest the affected area.

In mild cases, doctors advise that kids limit the activities that cause pain. They might be able to continue their sports as long as the pain remains mild. When symptoms flare up, a short break from sports might be necessary.

After your child gets back in the game, shock-absorbent insoles can decrease stress on the knee. Applying moist heat for 15 minutes before or icing for 20 minutes after activity can minimize swelling. Wrestling gel pads and basketball knee pads (available at sporting goods stores) can protect a tender shin from bumps and bruises. A good stretching program, focusing primarily on the hamstring and quadriceps muscles, before and after activity is important. Your doctor might also suggest over-the-counter pain medicines, such as ibuprofen, or prescription anti-inflammatory medicines.

More severe cases require more rest, usually a total break from sports and physical activities. Active kids may find this very difficult, but the knee cannot heal without rest. Some teens wind up with a cast or brace to enforce the doctor's orders. After a prolonged time off, kids will need to ease back into activity carefully, usually with physical therapy to learn stretching and strengthening exercises.

Long-term consequences of OSD are usually minor. Some kids may have a permanent, painless bump below the knee. In rare cases, they may develop a painful, bony growth below the kneecap that must be surgically removed. About 60% of adults who had OSD as kids experience some pain with kneeling.

Sports Safety

Sports and exercise offer many benefits, but also the risk of injury. According to the National Youth Sports Safety Foundation, sports activities are the second most frequent cause of injury for both male and female adolescents.

Although OSD cannot be prevented, its impact can be minimized by following sports safety guidelines:

- Parents and coaches must teach young athletes to protect their bodies as their skills develop.

- Trained coaches should supervise sports programs.

- Kids should warm up and stretch for 15 to 30 minutes before and after activities.

- Injured kids should never be encouraged to "play through the pain."

- Always remember that sports exist for the emotional and physical good of the kids, not the team or interested adults.

Section 25.11

Legg-Calvé-Perthes Disease

Legg-Calve-Perthes disease is when the ball of the thighbone in the hip doesn't get enough blood, causing the bone to die.

Causes

Legg-Calve-Perthes disease usually occurs in boys 4–10 years old. There are many theories about the cause of this disease, but little is actually known.

Without enough blood to the area, the bone dies. The ball of the hip will collapse and become flat. Usually only one hip is affected, although it can occur on both sides.

The blood supply returns over several months, bringing in new bone cells. The new cells gradually replace the dead bone over two to three years.

Symptoms

The first symptom is often limping, which is usually painless. Sometimes there may be mild pain that comes and goes.

Other symptoms may include:

- hip stiffness that restricts movement in the hip;

- knee pain;

- limited range of motion;

- persistent thigh or groin pain;

- shortening of the leg, or legs of unequal length;

- wasting of muscles in the upper thigh.

Exams and Tests

During a physical examination, the health care provider will look for a loss in hip motion and a typical limp. A hip X-ray or pelvis X-ray may show signs of Legg-Calve-Perthes disease. An MRI scan may be needed.

Treatment

The goal of treatment is to keep the ball of the thighbone inside the socket. Your health care provider may call this "containment." The key to doing this is to make sure the hip has good range of motion. In some cases, bracing is used to help with containment.

Physical therapy and anti-inflammatory medicine (such as ibuprofen) can relieve stiffness in the hip joint. If your hip is painful or the limp gets worse, limiting the amount of weight placed on the leg or restricting activities such as running may help. Nighttime traction devices may also be used.

Health care providers no longer recommend several months of bedrest, although a short period of bed rest may help those with severe pain.

Surgery may be needed if other treatments fail. Surgery ranges from lengthening a groin muscle to major hip surgery to reshape the pelvis, called an osteotomy. The type of surgery depends on the severity of the problem and the shape of the ball of the hip joint.

It is important to have regular follow-up with your doctor and an orthopedic specialist.

Outlook (Prognosis)

The outlook depends on the child's age and the severity of the disease. In general, the younger the child is when the disease starts, the better the outcome.

Children younger than six years old who receive treatment are more likely to end up with a normal hip joint. Children older than age six are more likely to end up with a deformed hip joint, despite treatment, and may later develop arthritis.

Section 25.12

Scoliosis

This section excerpted from "Questions and Answers about Scoliosis in Children and Adolescents," National Institute of Arthritis and Musculo-skeletal and Skin Disorders (www.niams.nih.gov), July 2008.

What is scoliosis?

Scoliosis is a musculoskeletal disorder in which there is a sideways curvature of the spine, or backbone. The bones that make up the spine are called vertebrae. Some people who have scoliosis require treatment. Other people, who have milder curves, may need to visit their doctor for periodic observation only.

Who gets scoliosis?

People of all ages can have scoliosis, but this section focuses on children and adolescents. Of every 1,000 children, 3 to 5 develop spinal curves that are considered large enough to need treatment. Adolescent idiopathic scoliosis (scoliosis of unknown cause) is the most common type and occurs after the age of 10. Girls are more likely than boys to have this type of scoliosis. Because scoliosis can run in families, a child who has a parent, brother, or sister with idiopathic scoliosis should be checked regularly for scoliosis by the family doctor.

Idiopathic scoliosis can also occur in children younger than 10 years of age but is very rare. Early onset or infantile idiopathic scoliosis occurs in children younger than 3 years old. Juvenile idiopathic scoliosis occurs in children between the ages of 3 and 10.

What causes scoliosis?

In 80% to 85% of people, the cause of scoliosis is unknown; this is called idiopathic scoliosis. Before concluding that a person has idiopathic scoliosis, the doctor looks for other possible causes, such as injury or infection. Causes of curves are classified as either nonstructural or structural.

Nonstructural (functional) scoliosis: A structurally normal spine that appears curved. This is a temporary, changing curve. It is caused by an underlying condition such as a difference in leg length, muscle spasms, or inflammatory conditions such as appendicitis. Doctors treat this type of scoliosis by correcting the underlying problem.

Structural scoliosis: A fixed curve that doctors treat case by case. Sometimes structural scoliosis is one part of a syndrome or disease, such as Marfan syndrome, an inherited connective tissue disorder. In other cases, it occurs by itself. Structural scoliosis can be caused by neuromuscular diseases (such as cerebral palsy, poliomyelitis, or muscular dystrophy), birth defects (such as hemivertebra, in which one side of a vertebra fails to form normally before birth), injury, certain infections, tumors (such as those caused by neurofibromatosis, a birth defect sometimes associated with benign tumors on the spinal column), metabolic diseases, connective tissue disorders, rheumatic diseases, or unknown factors (idiopathic scoliosis).

How is scoliosis diagnosed?

Doctors take the following steps to evaluate patients for scoliosis:

- **Medical history:** The doctor talks to the patient and the patient's parent(s) and reviews the patient's records to look for medical problems that might be causing the spine to curve—for example, birth defects, trauma, or other disorders that can be associated with scoliosis.

- **Physical examination:** The doctor looks at the patient's back, chest, pelvis, legs, feet, and skin. The doctor checks if the patient's shoulders are level, whether the head is centered, and whether opposite sides of the body look level. The doctor also examines the back muscles while the patient is bending forward to see if one side of the rib cage is higher than the other. If there is a significant asymmetry (difference between opposite sides of the body), the doctor will refer the patient to an orthopedic spine specialist.

- **X-ray evaluation:** Patients with significant spinal curves, unusual back pain, or signs of involvement of the central nervous system such as bowel and bladder control problems need to have an X-ray.

- **Curve measurement:** The doctor measures the curve on the X-ray image. He or she finds the vertebrae at the beginning and end of the curve and measures the angle of the curve. Curves that are greater than 20 degrees require treatment.

Does scoliosis have to be treated? What are the treatments?

Many children who are sent to the doctor by a school scoliosis screening program have very mild spinal curves that do not need treatment. When treatment is needed, the doctor may send the child to an orthopedic spine specialist.

The doctor will suggest the best treatment for each patient based on the patient's age, how much more he or she is likely to grow, the degree and pattern of the curve, and the type of scoliosis. The doctor may recommend observation, bracing, or surgery.

- **Observation:** Doctors follow patients without treatment and re-examine them every four to six months when the patient is still growing (is skeletally immature) and has an idiopathic curve of less than 25 degrees.

- **Bracing:** Doctors advise patients to wear a brace to stop a curve from getting any worse when the patient has these characteristics:

  - Is still growing and has an idiopathic curve that is more than 25 to 30 degrees

  - Has at least two years of growth remaining, has an idiopathic curve that is between 20 and 29 degrees, and, if a girl, has not had her first menstrual period

  - Is still growing and has an idiopathic curve between 20 and 29 degrees that is getting worse

  As a child nears the end of growth, the indications for bracing will depend on how the curve affects the child's appearance, whether the curve is getting worse, and the size of the curve.

- **Surgery:** Doctors advise patients to have surgery to correct a curve or stop it from worsening when the patient is still growing, has a curve that is more than 45 degrees, and has a curve that is getting worse.

Are there other ways to treat scoliosis?

Some people have tried other ways to treat scoliosis, including manipulation by a chiropractor, electrical stimulation, dietary supplements, and corrective exercises. So far, studies of these treatments have not been shown to prevent curve progression, or worsening. Studies have shown that exercise alone will not stop progressive curves. However, patients may wish to exercise for the effects on their general health and well-being.

Which brace is best?

The decision about which brace to wear depends on the type of curve and whether the patient will follow the doctor's directions about how many hours a day to wear the brace.

There are two main types of braces. Braces can be custom-made or can be made from a prefabricated mold. All must be selected for the specific curve problem and fitted to each patient. To have their intended effect (to keep a curve from getting worse), braces must be worn every day for the full number of hours prescribed by the doctor until the child stops growing.

- **Milwaukee brace:** Patients can wear this brace to correct any curve in the spine. This brace has a neck ring.

- **Thoracolumbosacral orthosis (TLSO):** Patients can wear this brace to correct curves whose apex is at or below the eighth thoracic vertebra. The TLSO is an underarm brace, which means that it fits under the arm and around the rib cage, lower back, and hips.

If the doctor recommends surgery, which procedure is best?

Many surgical techniques can be used to correct the curves of scoliosis. The main surgical procedure is correction, stabilization, and fusion of the curve. Fusion is the joining of two or more vertebrae. Surgeons can choose different ways to straighten the spine and different implants to keep the spine stable after surgery. The decision about the type of implant will depend on the cost; the size of the implant, which depends on the size of the patient; the shape of the implant; its safety; and the experience of the surgeon. Each patient should discuss his or her options with at least two experienced surgeons.

Can people with scoliosis exercise?

Although exercise programs have not been shown to affect the natural history of scoliosis, exercise is encouraged in patients with scoliosis to minimize any potential decrease in functional ability over time. It is very important for all people, including those with scoliosis, to exercise and remain physically fit.

Chapter 26

Neurological Disorders in Children

Chapter Contents

Section 26.1

Brain Tumors

PDQ® Cancer Information Summary, National Cancer Institute; Bethesda, MD. Childhood Brain and Spinal Cord Tumors Treatment Overview (PDQ) – Patient Version. Updated 02/2012. Available at: http://www.cancer.gov. Accessed April 17, 2012.

A childhood brain or spinal cord tumor is a disease in which abnormal cells form in the tissues of the brain or spinal cord. There are many types of childhood brain and spinal cord tumors. The tumors are formed by the abnormal growth of cells and may begin in different areas of the brain or spinal cord.

The tumors may be benign (not cancer) or malignant (cancer). Benign brain tumors grow and press on nearby areas of the brain. They rarely spread into other tissues. Malignant brain tumors are likely to grow quickly and spread into other brain tissue. When a tumor grows into or presses on an area of the brain, it may stop that part of the brain from working the way it should. Both benign and malignant brain tumors can cause symptoms and need treatment.

Although cancer is rare in children, brain and spinal cord tumors are the third most common type of childhood cancer, after leukemia and lymphoma. Brain tumors can occur in both children and adults. Treatment for children is usually different than treatment for adults.

The cause of most childhood brain and spinal cord tumors is unknown.

Symptoms

The symptoms of childhood brain and spinal cord tumors are not the same in every child.

Headaches and other symptoms may be caused by childhood brain and spinal cord tumors. Other conditions may cause the same symptoms. Check with your child's doctor if any of the following problems occur:

Brain Tumor Symptoms

• Morning headache or headache that goes away after vomiting

- Frequent nausea and vomiting
- Vision, hearing, and speech problems
- Loss of balance and trouble walking
- Unusual sleepiness or change in activity level
- Unusual changes in personality or behavior
- Seizures
- Increase in head size (in infants)

Spinal Cord Tumor Symptoms

- Back pain or pain that spreads from the back toward the arms or legs
- A change in bowel habits or trouble urinating
- Weakness in the legs
- Trouble walking

In addition to these symptoms of brain and spinal cord tumors, some children are unable to reach certain growth and development milestones such as sitting up, walking, and talking in sentences.

Diagnosis

Tests that examine the brain and spinal cord are used to detect childhood brain and spinal cord tumors.

The following tests and procedures may be used:

- **Physical exam and history:** An exam of the body to check general signs of health, including checking for signs of disease, such as lumps or anything else that seems unusual. A history of the patient's health habits and past illnesses and treatments will also be taken.

- **Neurological exam:** A series of questions and tests to check the brain, spinal cord, and nerve function. The exam checks a person's mental status, coordination, and ability to walk normally, and how well the muscles, senses, and reflexes work.

- **Serum tumor marker test:** A procedure in which a sample of blood is examined to measure the amounts of certain substances released into the blood by organs, tissues, or tumor cells in the body.

- **MRI (magnetic resonance imaging) with gadolinium:** A procedure that uses a magnet, radio waves, and a computer to make a series of detailed pictures of the brain and spinal cord.

- **CT scan (CAT scan):** A procedure that makes a series of detailed pictures of areas inside the body, taken from different angles. The pictures are made by a computer linked to an X-ray machine.

- **Angiogram:** A procedure to look at blood vessels and the flow of blood in the brain.

- **PET scan (positron emission tomography scan):** A procedure to find malignant tumor cells in the body.

Most childhood brain tumors are diagnosed and removed in surgery. If doctors think there might be a brain tumor, a biopsy may be done to remove a sample of tissue. For tumors in the brain, the biopsy is done by removing part of the skull and using a needle to remove a sample of tissue. If cancer cells are found, the doctor may remove as much tumor as safely possible during the same surgery. A pathologist checks the cancer cells to find out the type and grade of brain tumor. The grade of the tumor is based on how abnormal the cancer cells look under a microscope and how quickly the tumor is likely to grow and spread.

Outlook

The prognosis (chance of recovery) depends on the following:

- Whether there are any cancer cells left after surgery

- The type of tumor

- Where the tumor is in the body

- The child's age

- Whether the tumor has just been diagnosed or has recurred (come back)

Treatment

Different types of treatment are available for children with brain and spinal cord tumors. Some treatments are standard (the currently used treatment), and some are being tested in clinical trials. A treatment clinical trial is a research study meant to help improve current treatments or obtain information on new treatments for patients with cancer.

Because cancer in children is rare, taking part in a clinical trial should be considered. Clinical trials are taking place in many parts of the country. Some clinical trials are open only to patients who have not started treatment.

Some cancer treatments cause side effects months or years after treatment has ended. These are called late effects. Late effects of cancer treatment may include the following:

• Physical problems

• Changes in mood, feelings, thinking, learning, or memory

• Second cancers (new types of cancer)

Some late effects may be treated or controlled. It is important to talk with your child's doctors about the effects cancer treatment can have on your child.

Three types of standard treatment are used:

Surgery: Surgery may be used to diagnose and treat childhood brain and spinal cord tumors.

Radiation therapy: Radiation therapy is a cancer treatment that uses high-energy X-rays or other types of radiation to kill cancer cells or keep them from growing. There are two types of radiation therapy. External radiation therapy uses a machine outside the body to send radiation toward the cancer. Internal radiation therapy uses a radioactive substance sealed in needles, seeds, wires, or catheters that are placed directly into or near the cancer.

Chemotherapy: Chemotherapy is a cancer treatment that uses drugs to stop the growth of cancer cells, either by killing the cells or by stopping them from dividing. When chemotherapy is taken by mouth or injected into a vein or muscle, the drugs enter the bloodstream and can reach cancer cells throughout the body (systemic chemotherapy). When chemotherapy is placed directly in the cerebrospinal fluid, an organ, or a body cavity such as the abdomen, the drugs mainly affect cancer cells in those areas (regional chemotherapy).

Anticancer drugs given by mouth or vein to treat brain and spinal cord tumors cannot cross the blood-brain barrier and enter the fluid that surrounds the brain and spinal cord. Instead, an anticancer drug is injected into the fluid-filled space to kill cancer cells there. This is called intrathecal chemotherapy.

Follow-Up

Some of the tests that were done to diagnose the cancer or to find out the stage of the cancer may be repeated. Some tests will be repeated in order to see how well the treatment is working. Decisions about whether to continue, change, or stop treatment may be based on the results of these tests. This is sometimes called re-staging.

Some of the tests will continue to be done from time to time after treatment has ended. The results of these tests can show if your condition has changed or if the cancer has recurred (come back). These tests are sometimes called follow-up tests or check-ups.

Section 26.2

Cerebral Palsy

This section excerpted from "Cerebral Palsy: Hope Through Research," National Institute of Neurological Disorders and Stroke (www.ninds.nih.gov), October 4, 2011.

What is cerebral palsy?

Doctors use the term cerebral palsy to refer to any one of a number of neurological disorders that appear in infancy or early childhood and permanently affect body movement and muscle coordination but aren't progressive—in other words, they don't get worse over time.

Even though cerebral palsy affects muscle movement, it isn't caused by problems in the muscles or nerves. It is caused by abnormalities inside the brain that disrupt the brain's ability to control movement and posture.

In some cases of cerebral palsy, the cerebral motor cortex hasn't developed normally during fetal growth. In others, the damage is a result of injury to the brain either before, during, or after birth. In either case, the damage is not repairable and the disabilities that result are permanent.

Children with cerebral palsy exhibit a wide variety of symptoms, including the following:

- Lack of muscle coordination when performing voluntary movements (ataxia)
- Stiff or tight muscles and exaggerated reflexes (spasticity)
- Walking with one foot or leg dragging
- Walking on the toes, a crouched gait, or a "scissored" gait
- Variations in muscle tone, either too stiff or too floppy
- Excessive drooling or difficulties swallowing or speaking
- Shaking (tremor) or random involuntary movements
- Difficulty with precise motions, such as writing or buttoning a shirt

The symptoms of cerebral palsy differ in type and severity from one person to the next, and may even change in an individual over time. Some people with cerebral palsy also have other medical disorders, including mental retardation, seizures, impaired vision or hearing, and abnormal physical sensations or perceptions.

Cerebral palsy doesn't always cause profound disabilities. While one child with severe cerebral palsy might be unable to walk and need extensive, lifelong care, another with mild cerebral palsy might be only slightly awkward and require no special assistance.

Cerebral palsy isn't contagious and can't be passed from one generation to the next. There is no cure for cerebral palsy, but supportive treatments, medications, and surgery can help many individuals improve their motor skills and ability to communicate with the world.

What are the early signs?

The signs of cerebral palsy usually appear in the early months of life, although specific diagnosis is usually delayed until later. Parents are often the first to suspect that their baby's motor skills aren't developing normally. Infants with cerebral palsy frequently have developmental delay, in which they are slow to reach developmental milestones such as learning to roll over, sit, crawl, smile, or walk. Some infants with cerebral palsy have abnormal muscle tone as infants. Decreased muscle tone (hypotonia) can make them appear relaxed, even floppy. Increased muscle tone (hypertonia) can make them seem stiff or rigid.

Parents who are concerned about their baby's development for any reason should contact their pediatrician. A doctor can determine the difference between a normal lag in development and a delay that could indicate cerebral palsy.

What causes cerebral palsy?

The majority of children with cerebral palsy are born with it, although it may not be detected until months or years later. This is called congenital cerebral palsy. Birth complications are estimated to account for only 5% to 10% of the babies born with congenital cerebral palsy.

A small number of children have acquired cerebral palsy, which means the disorder begins after birth. In these cases, doctors can often pinpoint a specific reason for the problem, such as brain damage in the first few months or years of life, brain infections such as bacterial meningitis or viral encephalitis, or head injury from a motor vehicle accident, a fall, or child abuse.

What causes the remaining 90% to 95%? There are multiple reasons why cerebral palsy happens—as the result of genetic abnormalities, maternal infections or fevers, or fetal injury, for example. But in all cases the disorder is the result of four types of brain damage that cause its characteristic symptoms:

Damage to the white matter of the brain (periventricular leukomalacia [PVL]): The white matter of the brain is responsible for transmitting signals inside the brain and to the rest of the body. PVL describes a type of damage that looks like tiny holes in the white matter of an infant's brain.

Abnormal development of the brain (cerebral dysgenesis): Any interruption of the normal process of brain growth during fetal development can cause brain malformations that interfere with the transmission of brain signals.

Bleeding in the brain (intracranial hemorrhage): Intracranial hemorrhage describes bleeding inside the brain caused by blocked or broken blood vessels. A common cause of this kind of damage is fetal stroke.

Brain damage caused by a lack of oxygen in the brain (hypoxic-ischemic encephalopathy or intrapartum asphyxia): Asphyxia, a lack of oxygen in the brain caused by an interruption in breathing or poor oxygen supply, is common in babies due to the stress of labor and delivery.

What are the risk factors?

Just as there are particular types of brain damage that cause cerebral palsy, there are also certain medical conditions or events that can happen during pregnancy and delivery that will increase a baby's risk of being born with cerebral palsy. If a mother or her baby has any of these risk factors, it doesn't mean that cerebral palsy is inevitable, but it does increase the chance for the kinds of brain damage that cause it.

Low birthweight and premature birth: The risk of cerebral palsy is higher among babies who weigh less than 5 1/2 pounds at birth or are born less than 37 weeks into pregnancy.

Multiple births: Twins, triplets, and other multiple births—even those born at term—are linked to an increased risk of cerebral palsy.

Infections during pregnancy: Infectious diseases caused by viruses, such as toxoplasmosis, rubella (German measles), cytomegalovirus, and herpes, can infect the womb and placenta.

Blood type incompatibility: Rh incompatibility is a condition that develops when a mother's Rh blood type (either positive or negative) is different from the blood type of her baby. Rh incompatibility is routinely tested for and treated in the United States, but conditions in other countries continue to keep blood type incompatibility a risk factor for cerebral palsy.

Exposure to toxic substances: Mothers who have been exposed to toxic substances during pregnancy, such as methyl mercury, are at a heightened risk of having a baby with cerebral palsy.

Mothers with thyroid abnormalities, mental retardation, or seizures: Mothers with any of these conditions are slightly more likely to have a child with cerebral palsy.

Can cerebral palsy be prevented?

Cerebral palsy related to genetic abnormalities is not preventable, but a few of the risk factors for congenital cerebral palsy can be managed or avoided. For example, rubella, or German measles, is preventable if women are vaccinated against the disease before becoming pregnant. Rh incompatibilities can also be managed early in pregnancy. But there are still risk factors that can't be controlled or avoided in spite of medical intervention. Interventions to treat prenatal causes of cerebral palsy haven't lowered the number of babies born with it.

Fortunately, acquired cerebral palsy, often due to head injury, is preventable using common safety tactics, such as using car seats for infants and toddlers, and making sure young children wear helmets when they ride bicycles.

What are the different forms?

The specific forms of cerebral palsy are determined by the extent, type, and location of a child's abnormalities. Doctors classify cerebral palsy according to the type of movement disorder involved—spastic (stiff muscles), athetoid (writhing movements), or ataxic (poor balance and coordination)—plus any additional symptoms. Doctors will often describe the type of cerebral palsy a child has based on which limbs are affected.

Spastic hemiplegia/hemiparesis: This type of cerebral palsy typically affects the arm and hand on one side of the body, but it can also include the leg. Children with spastic hemiplegia generally walk later and on tip-toe because of tight heel tendons. Speech will be delayed and, at best, may be competent, but intelligence is usually normal.

Spastic diplegia/diparesis: In this type of cerebral palsy, muscle stiffness is predominantly in the legs and less severely affects the arms and face, although the hands may be clumsy. Intelligence and language skills are usually normal.

Spastic quadriplegia/quadriparesis: This is the most severe form of cerebral palsy, often associated with moderate-to-severe mental retardation.

Dyskinetic cerebral palsy (also includes athetoid, choreoathetoid, and dystonic cerebral palsies): This type of cerebral palsy is characterized by slow and uncontrollable writhing movements of the hands, feet, arms, or legs. Intelligence is rarely affected in these forms of cerebral palsy.

Ataxic cerebral palsy: This rare type of cerebral palsy affects balance and depth perception. Children will often have poor coordination and walk unsteadily with a wide-based gait, placing their feet unusually far apart.

Mixed types: It is common for children to have symptoms that don't correspond to any single type of cerebral palsy. Their symptoms are a mix of types.

What other conditions are associated with cerebral palsy?

Many individuals with cerebral palsy have no additional medical disorders. However, because cerebral palsy involves the brain and the brain controls so many of the body's functions, cerebral palsy can also cause seizures, impair intellectual development, and affect vision, hearing, and behavior. Coping with these disabilities may be even more of a challenge than coping with the motor impairments of cerebral palsy.

How does a doctor diagnose cerebral palsy?

Early signs of cerebral palsy may be present from birth. Most children with cerebral palsy are diagnosed during the first two years of life. But if a child's symptoms are mild, it can be difficult for a doctor to make a reliable diagnosis before the age of four or five. Nevertheless, if a doctor suspects cerebral palsy, he or she will most likely schedule an appointment to observe the child and talk to the parents about their child's physical and behavioral development.

Doctors diagnose cerebral palsy by evaluating a child's motor skills and their medical history. In addition to checking for the most characteristic symptoms, a doctor also has to rule out other disorders that could cause similar symptoms. Most important, a doctor has to determine that the child's condition is not getting worse. Although symptoms may change over time, cerebral palsy by definition is not progressive.

How is cerebral palsy managed?

Cerebral palsy can't be cured, but treatment will often improve a child's capabilities. Many children go on to enjoy near-normal adult lives if their disabilities are properly managed. In general, the earlier treatment begins, the better chance children have of overcoming developmental disabilities or learning new ways to accomplish the tasks that challenge them.

There is no standard therapy that works for every individual with cerebral palsy. A comprehensive management plan will encompass the following:

- Physical therapy to improve walking and gait, stretch spastic muscles, and prevent deformities

- Occupational therapy to develop compensating tactics for everyday activities such as dressing, going to school, and participating in day-to-day activities

- Speech therapy to address swallowing disorders, speech impediments, and other obstacles to communication

- Counseling and behavioral therapy to address emotional and psychological needs and help children cope emotionally with their disabilities

- Drugs to control seizures, relax muscle spasms, and alleviate pain

- Surgery to correct anatomical abnormalities or release tight muscles

- Braces and other orthotic devices to compensate for muscle imbalance, improve posture and walking, and increase independent mobility

- Mechanical aids such as wheelchairs and rolling walkers for individuals who are not independently mobile

- Communication aids such as computers, voice synthesizers, or symbol boards to allow severely impaired individuals to communicate with others

Section 26.3

Epilepsy

If you have a child with epilepsy, you're not alone—2.5 million Americans have this disorder.

Anyone can get epilepsy at any age, but the majority of new diagnoses are in kids. About two-thirds of all kids with epilepsy outgrow the seizures that accompany it by the time they're teens.

About Epilepsy

Epilepsy is a disease of the central nervous system in which electrical signals of the brain to misfire. These disruptions cause temporary communication problems between nerve cells, leading to seizures. A seizure can be thought of as an "electrical storm" that causes the brain to do things that the person having the seizure doesn't intend.

Having a single or sometimes even several seizures is not necessarily considered epilepsy. Kids with epilepsy are prone to having multiple seizures over a fairly long period of time (months to years).

Epilepsy:

- is not the only cause of childhood seizures;

- is not a mental illness;

- does not necessarily affect intelligence;

- is not contagious;

- does not typically worsen over time.

Causes of Epilepsy

In less than half the cases of epilepsy, there is a specific identifiable brain problem that causes the seizures. These include:

- infectious illness (such as meningitis or encephalitis);

- brain malformation during pregnancy;

- trauma to the brain (including lack of oxygen) due to an accident before, during, or after birth or later in childhood;

- underlying metabolic disorders (chemical imbalances in the brain);

- brain tumors;

- blood vessel malformation;

- strokes;

- chromosome disorders.

In kids, more than half of epilepsy cases are idiopathic (meaning there's no other identifiable cause or visible problem in the brain). In most of these, there's a family history of epilepsy or the condition is believed to be genetic (kids with a parent or other close family member with epilepsy are more likely to have it, too). Researchers are working to determine what specific genetic factors are responsible for these forms of epilepsy.

Understanding Seizures

Seizures vary in severity, frequency, duration (from a few seconds to several minutes), and in their appearance. There are many different kinds of seizures, and what occurs during one depends on where in the brain the electrical signals are disrupted.

The two main categories of seizures are generalized seizures, which affect the whole brain all at once, and partial seizures, in which only part of the brain is mostly affected. Some people with epilepsy experience both kinds. Also, the electrical problem in a partial seizure can spread to cause a generalized seizure.

Seizures can be scary—a child may lose consciousness or jerk or thrash violently and may appear to stop breathing or have difficulty breathing. Milder seizures may leave a child momentarily confused or unaware of his or her surroundings. Some seizures are so brief and minor that only careful observation or an experienced eye will detect them—a child may simply blink or stare into space for a moment before resuming normal activity. Even in those cases, it is usually obvious to parents that a child is having episodes of concern.

After seizures that last more than 30 seconds, most kids are exhausted, tired, sleepy, disoriented, confused, or even combative and agitated for minutes to hours. This is known as the postictal phase.

During a seizure, it's very important to stay calm and keep your child safe. Be sure to:

- lay your child down away from furniture, stairs, radiators, or other hard or sharp objects;

- put something soft under his or her head;

- turn your child on his or her right side so fluid in the mouth can come out;

- never stick anything in your child's mouth or try to restrain him or her.

Do your best to note how often the seizures take place, what happens during them, and how long they last and report this to your doctor. Once a seizure is over, watch your child for signs of confusion or the postictal phase. He or she may want to sleep and you should allow that. Do not give extra medication unless the doctor has prescribed it.

Kids who experience partial seizures may be frightened or confused during or after the seizure. Offer plenty of comfort and reassure your child that you're there and everything is okay.

Most seizures are not life threatening, but if one lasts longer than five minutes or your child seems to have trouble breathing afterward, call 911 for immediate medical attention.

Diagnosis

Talk to your doctor if your child has seizures, staring spells, confusion spells, shaking spells, or unexplained deterioration in behavior or school performance. The doctor can refer you to a pediatric neurologist, who will take a patient medical history and examine your child, looking for findings that suggest problems with the brain or with the rest of the neurological system.

If the doctor suspects epilepsy, tests will be ordered, which may include:

- an electroencephalogram (EEG), which measures electrical activity of the brain via harmless sensors secured to the scalp while the child lays on a bed—usually the doctor will ask that a child be sleep-deprived (put to bed late and awakened early) before this painless test, which typically takes about one hour;

- an MRI test or a CAT scan of the brain, both of which look at images of the brain.

Treating Epilepsy

Your doctor will use the test and exam results to determine the best form of treatment. Medication to prevent seizures is usually the first type of treatment prescribed for epilepsy management. Most kids are successfully treated with one medication—and if the first doesn't work, the doctor will usually try a second or even a third before resorting to combinations of medications.

No medication for epilepsy is perfect and side effects are possible. The most common include tiredness, decreased alertness, and mood or behavioral concerns, so parents should watch for these and discuss concerns with the doctor.

Nowadays, many choices are available and most kids treated with antiseizure medications do not experience worrisome side effects. Nevertheless, discuss any concerns you have with the doctor so that dose adjustments or appropriate changes can be made if appropriate.

Rarely, blood tests might be needed to monitor a medication's level in the bloodstream or to watch for side effects.

If your child still has seizures after the second or third medication tried, it's less likely that subsequent medications will be fully effective. In this case, more complicated treatments may be recommended or tried. These include:

- combinations of medications;
- a special ketogenic diet (a high-fat, low-carbohydrate, low-protein diet that's often difficult to follow);
- implantation of a vagal nerve stimulator (an electrical pacemaker-like device placed in the chest and neck);
- surgery to remove the affected part of the brain, if possible (in the right situation, epilepsy surgery can be very effective or may even cure a child of seizures, but overall it is done in less than 10% of seizure patients, and only after an extensive screening and evaluation process).

Even people who respond successfully to medication sometimes have seizures (called "breakthrough seizures"). These don't mean the medication needs to be changed, although you should let the doctor know if they occur.

Living with Epilepsy

To help prevent seizures, make sure your child:

- takes medication(s) as prescribed;
- avoids triggers (such as fever and overtiredness);
- sees the neurologist as recommended—about one to four times a year—even if responding well to medication.

Keeping your child well fed, well rested, and reducing unnecessary stress are all key factors that can help manage epilepsy. Common-sense precautions to take (based on how controlled the epilepsy is) include:

- Younger kids should always be supervised in the bathtub (a responsible adult should always be within arm's reach) and older kids should take showers with the bathroom door unlocked—and only when there is someone else in the house. (It's also wise to lower the temperature of hot water so a child cannot be accidentally scalded during a seizure.)
- Swimming or biking alone are not good ideas for kids with epilepsy (although they can certainly enjoy these activities with other people). A responsible adult within arm's reach is recommended during swimming for kids with epilepsy. A helmet is required during bicycling, as it is for everyone.

With these simple safety precautions, your child should be able to play, participate in sports or other activities, and generally do what other kids like to do. State driving laws vary, but teens with epilepsy will probably be able to drive with some restrictions, as long as the seizures are controlled.

It's important to make sure that other adults who care for your child—family members, babysitters, teachers, coaches, etc.—know that your child has epilepsy, understand the condition, and know what to do in the event of a seizure.

Offer your child plenty of support, discuss epilepsy openly, and answer questions honestly. Kids with epilepsy might be embarrassed about the seizures or worry about having one at school or with friends.

Unfortunately, many kids with epilepsy have other neurological problems. In particular, learning and behavioral problems are common and can create more hardship for a child than the epilepsy itself. In some cases, the medication's side effects can aggravate these problems. Such difficulties might require the help of other specialists, teachers, and social workers. Consider having your child talk with a mental health counselor or psychologist if he or she struggles with these feelings or problems.

Parents caring for a child with epilepsy also might benefit from advice from specialists such as psychologists, social workers, or specialized educators. For those whose kids have more severe epilepsy, this help is critical. Specialists can help parents plan for the future (transition services) by identifying social, financial, and other community resources that will improve the child's well-being.

Section 26.4

Headache

This section excerpted from "Headache: Hope through Research,"
National Institute of Neurological Disorders and Stroke
(www.ninds.nih.gov), March 1, 2012.

Anyone can experience a headache. Nearly two out of three children will have a headache by age 15. More than 9 in 10 adults will experience a headache sometime in their life. Headache is our most common form of pain and a major reason cited for days missed at work or school as well as visits to the doctor. Without proper treatment, headaches can be severe and interfere with daily activities.

Certain types of headache run in families. Episodes of headache may ease or even disappear for a time and recur later in life. It's possible to have more than one type of headache at the same time.

Primary headaches occur independently and are not caused by another medical condition. It's uncertain what sets the process of a primary headache in motion. A cascade of events that affect blood vessels and nerves inside and outside the head causes pain signals to be sent to the brain. Brain chemicals called neurotransmitters are involved in creating head pain, as are changes in nerve cell activity. Migraine, cluster, and tension-type headache are the more familiar types of primary headache.

Secondary headaches are symptoms of another health disorder that causes pain-sensitive nerve endings to be pressed on or pulled or pushed out of place. They may result from underlying conditions including fever, infection, medication overuse, stress or emotional conflict, high blood pressure, psychiatric disorders, head injury or trauma, stroke, tumors, and nerve disorders.

Headaches can range in frequency and severity of pain. Some individuals may experience headaches once or twice a year, while others may experience headaches more than 15 days a month. Some headaches may recur or last for weeks at a time. Pain can range from mild to disabling and may be accompanied by symptoms such as nausea or increased sensitivity to noise or light, depending on the type of headache.

Diagnosing Your Headache

How and under what circumstances a person experiences a headache can be key to diagnosing its cause. Keeping a headache journal can help a physician better diagnose your type of headache and determine the best treatment. After each headache, note the time of day when it occurred; its intensity and duration; any sensitivity to light, odors, or sound; activity immediately prior to the headache; use of prescription and nonprescription medicines; amount of sleep the previous night; any stressful or emotional conditions; any influence from weather or daily activity; foods and fluids consumed in the past 24 hours; and any known health conditions at that time.

Once your doctor has reviewed your medical and headache history and conducted a physical and neurological exam, lab screening and diagnostic tests may be ordered to either rule out or identify conditions that might be the cause of your headaches. Blood tests and urinalysis can help diagnose brain or spinal cord infections, blood vessel damage, and toxins that affect the nervous system. Testing a sample of the fluid that surrounds the brain and spinal cord can detect infections, bleeding in the brain (called a brain hemorrhage), and measure any buildup of pressure within the skull. Diagnostic imaging, such as with CT and MRI, can detect irregularities in blood vessels and bones, certain brain tumors and cysts, brain damage from head injury, brain hemorrhage, inflammation, infection, and other disorders. Neuroimaging also gives doctors a way to see what's happening in the brain during headache attacks. An EEG measures brain wave activity and can help diagnose brain tumors, seizures, head injury, and inflammation that may lead to headaches.

Children and Headache

Headaches are common in children. Headaches that begin early in life can develop into migraines as the child grows older. Migraines in children or adolescents can develop into tension-type headaches at any time. In contrast to adults with migraine, young children often feel migraine pain on both sides of the head and have headaches that usually last less than two hours. Children may look pale and appear restless or irritable before and during an attack. Other children may become nauseous, lose their appetite, or feel pain elsewhere in the body during the headache.

Headaches in children can be caused by a number of triggers, including emotional problems such as tension between family members, stress from school activities, weather changes, irregular eating and sleep, dehydration, and certain foods and drinks. Of special concern among children are headaches that occur after head injury or those accompanied by rash, fever, or sleepiness.

It may be difficult to identify the type of headache because children often have problems describing where it hurts, how often the headaches occur, and how long they last. Asking a child with a headache to draw a picture of where the pain is and how it feels can make it easier for the doctor to determine the proper treatment.

Migraine in particular is often misdiagnosed in children. Parents and caretakers sometimes have to be detectives to help determine that a child has migraine. Clues to watch for include sensitivity to light and noise, which may be suspected when a child refuses to watch television or use the computer, or when the child stops playing to lie down in a dark room. Observe whether or not a child is able to eat during a headache. Very young children may seem cranky or irritable and complain of abdominal pain (abdominal migraine).

Headache treatment in children and teens usually includes rest, fluids, and over-the-counter pain relief medicines. Always consult with a physician before giving headache medicines to a child. Most tension-type headaches in children can be treated with over-the-counter medicines that are marked for children with usage guidelines based on the child's age and weight. Headaches in some children may also be treated effectively using relaxation/behavioral therapy. Children with cluster headache may be treated with oxygen therapy early in the initial phase of the attacks.

Coping with Headache

Headache treatment is a partnership between you and your doctor, and honest communication is essential. Finding a quick fix to your headache may not be possible. It may take some time for your doctor or specialist to determine the best course of treatment. Avoid using over-the-counter medicines more than twice a week, as they may actually worsen headache pain and the frequency of attacks. Relax whenever possible to ease stress and related symptoms, get enough sleep, regularly perform aerobic exercises, and eat a regularly scheduled and healthy diet that avoids food triggers. Gaining more control over your headache, stress, and emotions will make you feel better and let you embrace daily activities as much as possible.

Section 26.5

Neurofibromatosis

This section excerpted from "Neurofibromatosis Fact Sheet,"
National Institute of Neurological Disorders and Stroke
(www.ninds.nih.gov), January 13, 2012.

What are the neurofibromatoses?

The neurofibromatoses are a group of three genetically distinct disorders that cause tumors to grow in the nervous system. Tumors begin in the supporting cells that make up the nerve and the myelin sheath (the thin membrane that envelops and protects the nerves), rather than the cells that actually transmit information. The type of tumor that develops depends on the type of supporting cells involved.

Scientists have classified the disorders as neurofibromatosis type 1 (NF1, also called von Recklinghausen disease), neurofibromatosis type 2 (NF2), and a type that was once considered to be a variation of NF2 but is now called schwannomatosis.

The most common nerve-associated tumors in NF1 are neurofibromas (tumors of the peripheral nerves), whereas schwannomas (tumors that begin in Schwann cells that help form the myelin sheath) are most common in NF2 and schwannomatosis. Most tumors are benign, although occasionally they may become cancerous.

Why these tumors occur still isn't completely known, but it appears to be related mainly to mutations in genes that play key roles in suppressing cell growth in the nervous system.

What is NF1?

NF1 is the most common neurofibromatosis, occurring in 1 in 3,000 to 4,000 individuals in the United States. Although many affected people inherit the disorder, between 30% and 50% of new cases result from a spontaneous genetic mutation of unknown cause. Once this mutation has taken place, the mutant gene can be passed to succeeding generations.

What are the signs and symptoms of NF1?

To diagnose NF1, a doctor looks for two or more of the following:

- Six or more light brown spots on the skin (often called café-au-lait spots), measuring more than 5 millimeters in diameter in children or more than 15 millimeters across in adolescents and adults

- Two or more neurofibromas, or one plexiform neurofibroma (a neurofibroma that involves many nerves)

- Freckling in the area of the armpit or the groin

- Two or more growths on the iris of the eye (known as Lisch nodules or iris hamartomas)

- A tumor on the optic nerve (called an optic nerve glioma)

- Abnormal development of the spine (scoliosis), the temple (sphenoid) bone of the skull, or the tibia (one of the long bones of the shin)

- A parent, sibling, or child with NF1

What other symptoms or conditions are associated with NF1?

Many children with NF1 have larger than normal head circumference and are shorter than average. Hydrocephalus, the abnormal buildup of fluid in the brain, is a possible complication of the disorder. Headache and epilepsy are also more likely in individuals with NF1 than in the healthy population. Cardiovascular complications associated with NF1 include congenital heart defects, high blood pressure (hypertension), and constricted, blocked, or damaged blood vessels (vasculopathy). Children with NF1 may have poor language and visual-spatial skills, and perform less well on academic achievement tests, including those that measure reading, spelling, and math skills. Learning disabilities, such as attention deficit hyperactivity disorder (ADHD), are common in children with NF1.

When do symptoms appear?

Symptoms, particularly the most common skin abnormalities—café-au-lait spots, neurofibromas, Lisch nodules, and freckling in the armpit and groin—are often evident at birth or shortly afterwards, and almost always by the time a child is 10 years old. Because many features of these disorders are age dependent, a definitive diagnosis may take several years.

What is the prognosis for someone with NF1?

NF1 is a progressive disorder, which means most symptoms will worsen over time. In general, most people with NF1 will develop mild to moderate symptoms. Most people with NF1 have a normal life expectancy. Neurofibromas on or under the skin can increase with age and cause cosmetic and psychological issues.

How is NF1 treated?

Scientists don't know how to prevent neurofibromas from growing. Surgery is often recommended to remove tumors that become symptomatic and may become cancerous, as well as for tumors that cause significant cosmetic disfigurement. Several surgical options exist, but there is no general agreement among doctors about when surgery should be performed or which surgical option is best.

Treatments for other conditions associated with NF1 are aimed at controlling or relieving symptoms. Since children with NF1 have a higher than average risk for learning disabilities, they should undergo a detailed neurological exam before they enter school. Once these children are in school, teachers or parents who suspect there is evidence of one or more learning disabilities should request an evaluation.

What is NF2?

This rare disorder affects about 1 in 25,000 people. Approximately 50% of affected people inherit the disorder; in others the disorder is caused by a spontaneous genetic mutation of unknown cause. The hallmark finding in NF2 is the presence of slow-growing tumors on the eighth cranial nerves. These nerves have two branches: the acoustic branch helps people hear by transmitting sound sensations to the brain; and the vestibular branch helps people maintain their balance. The characteristic tumors of NF2 are called vestibular schwannomas because of their location and the types of cells involved. As these tumors grow, they may press against and damage nearby structures such as other cranial nerves and the brain stem, the latter which can cause serious disability. Schwannomas in NF2 may occur along any nerve in the body, including the spinal nerves, other cranial nerves, and peripheral nerves in the body. These tumors may be seen as bumps under the skin or can also be seen on the skin surface as small (less than one inch), dark, rough areas of hairy skin. In children, tumors may be smoother, less pigmented, and less hairy.

Although individuals with NF2 may have schwannomas that resemble small, flesh-colored skin flaps, they rarely have the café-au-lait spots that are seen in NF1.

Individuals with NF2 are at risk for developing other types of nervous system tumors, such as ependymomas and gliomas (two tumor types that grow in the spinal cord) and meningiomas (tumors that grow along the protective layers surrounding the brain and spinal cord).

When do symptoms appear?

Signs of NF2 may be present in childhood but are so subtle that they can be overlooked, especially in children who don't have a family history of the disorder. Typically, symptoms of NF2 are noticed between 18 and 22 years of age. The most frequent first symptom is hearing loss or ringing in the ears (tinnitus). Less often, the first visit to a doctor will be because of disturbances in balance, visual impairment (such as vision loss from cataracts), weakness in an arm or leg, seizures, or skin tumors.

What is the prognosis for someone with NF2?

Because NF2 is so rare, few studies have been done to look at the natural progression of the disorder. The course of NF2 varies greatly among individuals, although inherited NF2 appears to run a similar course among affected family members. Generally, vestibular schwannomas grow slowly, and balance and hearing deteriorate over a period of years.

How is NF2 treated?

NF2 is best managed at a specialty clinic with an initial screening and annual follow-up evaluations (more frequent if the disease is severe). Vestibular schwannomas grow slowly, but they can grow large enough to engulf one of the eighth cranial nerves and cause brain stem compression and damage to surrounding cranial nerves. Surgical options depend on tumor size and the extent of hearing loss. There is no general agreement among doctors about when surgery should be performed or which surgical option is best.

What is schwannomatosis?

Schwannomatosis is a rare form of neurofibromatosis that is genetically and clinically distinct from NF1 and NF2. Inherited forms of the disorder account for only 15% of all cases.

What are the signs and symptoms of schwannomatosis?

The distinguishing feature of schwannomatosis is the development of multiple schwannomas everywhere in the body except on the vestibular nerve. The dominant symptom is pain, which develops as a schwannoma enlarges, compresses nerves, or presses on adjacent tissue. Some people experience additional neurological symptoms, such as numbness, tingling, or weakness in the fingers and toes.

About one-third of individuals with schwannomatosis have tumors limited to a single part of the body, such as an arm, leg, or a segment of the spine. Some people develop many schwannomas, while others develop only a few.

What is the prognosis for someone with schwannomatosis?

Anyone with schwannomatosis experiences some degree of pain, but the intensity varies. A small number of people have such mild pain that they are never diagnosed with the disorder. Most people have significant pain, which can be managed with medications or surgery. In some extreme cases, pain will be so severe and disabling it will keep people from working or leaving the house.

How is schwannomatosis treated?

There is no currently accepted medical treatment or drug for schwannomatosis, but surgical management is often effective. Pain usually subsides when tumors are removed completely, although it may recur should new tumors form. When surgery isn't possible, ongoing monitoring and management of pain in a multidisciplinary pain clinic is advisable.

Are there prenatal tests for the neurofibromatoses?

Clinical genetic testing can confirm the presence of a mutation in the NF1 gene. Prenatal testing for the NF1 mutation is also possible using amniocentesis or chorionic villus sampling procedures. Genetic testing for the NF2 mutation is sometimes available, but is accurate only in about 65% of those individuals tested. Prenatal or genetic testing for schwannomatosis currently does not exist.

Section 26.6

Tourette Syndrome

"Facts about Tourette Syndrome," Centers for Disease Control
and Prevention (www.cdc.gov), September 6, 2011.

Tourette syndrome (TS) is a condition of the nervous system. TS causes
people to have "tics." Tics are sudden twitches, movements, or sounds that
people do repeatedly. People who have tics cannot stop their body from
doing these things. For example, a person might keep blinking over and
over again. Or, a person might make a grunting sound unwillingly.

Having tics is a little bit like having hiccups. Even though you
might not want to hiccup, your body does it anyway. Sometimes people
can stop themselves from doing a certain tic for awhile, but it's hard.
Eventually the person has to do the tic.

Types of Tics

There are two types of tics—motor and vocal:

Motor tics: Motor tics are movements of the body. Examples of motor tics include blinking, shrugging the shoulders, or jerking an arm.

Vocal tics: Vocal tics are sounds that a person makes with his or
her voice. Examples of vocal tics include humming, clearing the throat,
or yelling out a word or phrase.

Tics can be either simple or complex:

Simple tics: Simple tics involve just a few parts of the body. Examples of simple tics include squinting the eyes or sniffing.

Complex tics: Complex tics usually involve several different parts
of the body and can have a pattern. An example of a complex tic is bob-
bing the head while jerking an arm, and then jumping up.

Symptoms

The main symptoms of TS are tics. Symptoms usually begin when
a child is 5 to 10 years of age. The first symptoms often are motor tics
that occur in the head and neck area. Tics usually are worse during

times that are stressful or exciting. They tend to improve when a person is calm or focused on an activity.

The types of tics and how often a person has tics changes a lot over time. Even though the symptoms might appear, disappear, and reappear, these conditions are considered chronic.

In most cases, tics decrease during adolescence and early adulthood, and sometimes disappear entirely. However, many people with TS experience tics into adulthood and, in some cases, tics can become worse during adulthood.

Although the media often portray people with TS as involuntarily shouting out swear words (called coprolalia) or constantly repeating the words of other people (called echolalia), these symptoms are rare and are not required for a diagnosis of TS.

Diagnosis

There is no single test, like a blood test, to diagnose TS. Health professionals look at the person's symptoms to diagnose TS and other tic disorders. The tic disorders differ from each other in terms of the type of tic present (motor or vocal, or combination of the both), and how long the symptoms have lasted.

Treatments

Although there is no cure for TS, there are treatments available to help manage the tics. Many people with TS have tics that do not get in the way of their daily life and, therefore, do not need any treatment. However, medication and behavioral treatments are available if tics cause pain or injury; interfere with school, work, or social life; or cause stress.

Other Concerns and Conditions

TS often occurs with other conditions (called co-occurring conditions). Among children diagnosed with TS, 79% also have been diagnosed with at least one additional mental health, behavioral, or developmental condition. The two most common conditions are ADHD and obsessive-compulsive disorder (OCD). It is important to find out if a person with TS has any other conditions, and treat those conditions properly.

Risk Factors and Causes

Doctors and scientists do not know the exact cause of TS. Research suggests that it is an inherited genetic condition. That means it is passed on from parent to child through genes.

Chapter 27

Respiratory and Lung Conditions in Children

Chapter Contents

Section 27.1

Asthma

About Asthma

Asthma is a lung condition that causes difficulty breathing, and it's common among kids and teens. Symptoms include coughing, wheezing, and shortness of breath. Anyone can have asthma, even infants, and the tendency to develop the condition is often inherited.

Asthma affects the bronchial tubes, or airways. When someone breathes normally, air is taken in through the nose or mouth and then goes into the trachea (windpipe), passing through the bronchial tubes, into the lungs, and finally back out again.

But people with asthma have inflamed airways that produce lots of thick mucus. They're also overly sensitive, or hyperreactive, to certain things, like exercise, dust, or cigarette smoke. This hyperreactivity causes the smooth muscle that surrounds the airways to tighten up. The combination of airway inflammation and muscle tightening narrows the airways and makes it difficult for air to move through.

More than 23 million people have asthma in the United States. In fact, it's the number one reason kids chronically miss school. And flare-ups are the most common cause of pediatric emergency room visits due to a chronic illness.

Some kids have only mild, occasional symptoms or only show symptoms after exercising. Others have severe asthma that, left untreated, can dramatically limit how active they are and cause changes in lung function.

But thanks to new medications and treatment strategies, kids with asthma no longer need to sit on the sidelines, and parents no longer need to worry constantly about their child's well being.

With patient education and the right asthma management plan, families can learn to control symptoms and asthma flare-ups more independently, allowing kids to do just about anything they want.

About Asthma Flare-Ups

Many kids with asthma can breathe normally for weeks or months between asthma flare-ups (also called asthma attacks, flares, episodes, or exacerbations) that cause the airways to narrow and become obstructed, making it difficult for air to move through them. Although flare-ups often seem to happen without warning, they usually develop over time during a complicated process of increasing airway obstruction.

All children with asthma have airways that are inflamed, which means that they swell and produce lots of thick mucus. In addition, their airways are overly sensitive, or hyperreactive, to certain asthma triggers.

When exposed to these triggers, the muscles surrounding the airways tend to tighten, which makes the already clogged airways even narrower. Things that trigger flare-ups differ from person to person. Some common triggers are exercise, allergies, viral infections, and smoke.

So an asthma flare-up is caused by three important changes in the airways:

- Swelling of the lining of the airways

- Excess mucus that results in congestion and mucus "plugs" that get caught

- Bronchoconstriction, which refers to the tightening of the muscles surrounding the airways

Together, the swelling, excess mucus, and bronchoconstriction narrow the airways and make it difficult to move air through (like breathing through a straw). During an asthma flare-up, kids may experience coughing, wheezing (a breezy whistling sound in the chest when breathing), chest tightness, increased heart rate, sweating, and shortness of breath.

How Is Asthma Diagnosed?

Diagnosing asthma can be tricky and time-consuming because kids with asthma can have very different patterns of symptoms. For example, some kids cough constantly at night but seem fine during the day, while others seem to get frequent chest colds that linger. It's not uncommon for kids to have symptoms like these for months before being seen by a doctor.

When considering a diagnosis of asthma, a doctor rules out other possible causes of the symptoms. He or she asks questions about the family's asthma and allergy history, performs a physical exam, and might order a chest X-rays or lung function tests.

During this process, parents must provide the doctor with detailed information, such as:

- **Symptoms:** How severe they are, when and where they occur, how often they occur, and how long they last
- **Allergies:** The child's and the family's allergy history
- **Illnesses:** How often the child gets colds, how severe they are, and how long they last
- **Triggers:** Exposure to allergens and things in the air that can irritate the airways, recent life changes or stressful events, or other things that seem to lead to a flare-up

This information helps the doctor understand the pattern of symptoms, which can help determine what type of asthma the child has and how best to treat it.

To confirm the diagnosis of asthma, a breathing test may be done with a spirometer, a machine that analyzes airflow through the airways. A spirometer also can be used to see if the child's breathing problems can be helped with medication, a primary characteristic of asthma.

The doctor may take a spirometer reading, give the child an inhaled medication that opens the airways, and then take another reading to see if breathing improves with medication. If medication reverses airway narrowing significantly, as indicated by improved airflow, then there's a strong possibility that the child has asthma.

If your child is diagnosed with asthma, it's important to learn how to manage asthma so it won't control your family. Educate yourself about asthma and learn to identify and eliminate triggers.

Help your child keep an asthma diary, develop and follow an asthma action plan, and take medications as prescribed. In addition, a peak flow meter—a handheld tool that measures breathing ability—can be used at home. When peak flow readings drop, it's a sign of increasing airway inflammation.

Exercise-Induced Asthma

Kids who have exercise-induced asthma (EIA) develop asthma symptoms after vigorous activity, such as running, swimming, or biking. Some develop symptoms only after physical exertion, while others have additional asthma triggers. With the proper medications, most kids with EIA can play sports like any other child. In fact, asthma affects more than 20% of elite athletes, and one in every six Olympic athletes, according to the American Academy of Allergy, Asthma, and Immunology.

Usually, a doctor can diagnose EIA after taking a history alone. But sometimes further tests, including an exercise challenge in a lung function laboratory, are needed to confirm the diagnosis. The doctor might want to target a child's tolerance for a particular exercise, as not every type or intensity of exercise affects kids with EIA the same way.

If exercise is the only asthma trigger, the doctor may prescribe a medication for the child to take before exercising to prevent airways from tightening up. Of course, even after taking a preventive medication, asthma flare-ups can still occur.

Parents (or older kids) must carry the proper rescue medication to all games and activities. The school nurse, coaches, scout leaders, and teachers must be informed of a child's asthma plan of care to ensure that kids will take their medication as needed even when away from home.

Allergy-Triggered Asthma

An estimated 75% to 85% of people with asthma have some type of allergy. Even if the primary triggers are colds or exercise, allergies can sometimes play a minor role in aggravating the condition.

How do allergies cause flare-ups in kids with asthma? Kids inherit the tendency to have allergies from their parents. With any kind of allergy, the immune system overreacts to normally harmless allergens. Those substances, such as pollen, can cause allergic reactions in some people. As part of this overreaction, the body produces an antibody called immunoglobulin E (IgE) type, which specifically recognizes and attaches to the allergen when the body is exposed to it.

When this happens, it sets a process in motion resulting in the release of certain substances in the body. One of them is histamine, which causes allergic symptoms that can affect the eyes, nose, throat, skin, gastrointestinal tract, or lungs. When the airways in the lungs are affected, symptoms of asthma can occur.

The released histamine is what causes the familiar sneezing, runny nose, and itchy, watery eyes associated with some allergies—ways the body attempts to rid itself of the invading allergen. In kids with asthma, histamine can also trigger asthma symptoms and flare-ups.

An allergist can usually pinpoint allergies and, once identified, the best treatment is to avoid exposure to allergens whenever possible. Environmental control measures for the home can help reduce exposure to allergens. When avoidance isn't possible, antihistamine medications may be prescribed to block the release of histamine in the body.

Nasal steroids may be given to block allergic inflammation in the nose. In some cases, an allergist can prescribe immunotherapy, a series of allergy shots that gradually make the body unresponsive to specific allergens.

Asthma Categories

The severity of a child's asthma symptoms will fall into one of four main categories of asthma, each with different characteristics and requiring different treatment approaches:

- **Mild intermittent asthma:** A child who has brief episodes of wheezing, coughing, or shortness of breath occurring no more than twice a week is said to have mild intermittent asthma. Symptoms between flare-ups are rare, with the exception of one or two instances per month of mild symptoms at night.

- **Mild persistent asthma:** Kids with episodes of wheezing, coughing, or shortness of breath that occur more than twice a week but less than once a day are said to have mild persistent asthma. Symptoms usually occur at least twice a month at night and flare-ups may affect normal physical activity.

- **Moderate persistent asthma:** Kids with moderate persistent asthma have daily symptoms and require daily medication. Nighttime symptoms occur more than once a week. Flare-ups occur more than twice a week, last for several days, and usually affect normal physical activity.

- **Severe persistent asthma:** Kids with severe persistent asthma have symptoms continuously. They tend to have frequent flare-ups that may require emergency treatment and even hospitalization. Many children with severe persistent asthma have frequent symptoms at night and can handle only limited physical activity.

Asthma severity can both worsen and improve over time, placing a child in a new asthma category that requires different treatment.

All kids with asthma should follow a custom asthma action plan to control symptoms. And even mild asthma should never be ignored because airway inflammation is present even in between flare-ups.

Section 27.2

Bronchitis

"Bronchitis (Chest Cold)," Centers for Disease Control and Prevention (www.cdc.gov), September 1, 2010.

Acute bronchitis, or chest cold, is a condition that occurs when the bronchial tubes in the lungs become inflamed. The bronchial tubes swell and produce mucus, which causes a person to cough. This often occurs after an upper respiratory infection like a cold. Most symptoms of acute bronchitis (chest pain, shortness of breath, etc.) last for up to two weeks, but the cough can last for up to eight weeks in some people.

Chronic bronchitis lasts a long time and is more common among smokers. People with chronic bronchitis have a cough with mucus most days for three months a year for two consecutive years. If you have been diagnosed with chronic bronchitis, you should visit a specialist to be evaluated.

Another kind of lung infection that parents should know about is bronchiolitis. Infants can be diagnosed with bronchiolitis, a viral infection, which can obstruct the small airways and may require treatment.

Causes of Bronchitis

Bronchitis is caused by several types of viruses, most often the following:

- Respiratory syncytial virus (RSV)

- Adenovirus

- Influenza

- Parainfluenza

- Bacteria, in rare cases

- Pollutants (airborne chemicals or irritants)

Signs and Symptoms of Bronchitis

- Cough that produces mucus (may be without mucus the first few days)

- Soreness in the chest

- Fatigue

- Mild headache

- Mild body aches

- Low-grade fever (less than 102° F)

- Watery eyes

- Sore throat

See a health care provider if you or your child has any of the following symptoms:

- Temperature higher than 100.4° F

- A fever and cough with thick or bloody mucus

- A chronic heart or lung problem

- Shortness of breath or trouble breathing

- Symptoms that last more than three weeks

- Repeated episodes of bronchitis/bronchiolitis

If your child is younger than three months of age and has a fever, it's important to always call your health care provider right away.

Your health care provider can determine if you or your child has acute bronchitis, chronic bronchitis, bronchiolitis, or another type of respiratory infection. Then a decision can be made about possible needed treatment.

When Antibiotics are Needed

Antibiotics will rarely be needed since acute bronchitis and bronchiolitis are almost always caused by a virus and chronic bronchitis requires other therapies. However, treatment may be prescribed to relieve symptoms. If your health care provider diagnoses you or your child with another type of respiratory infection such as pneumonia or whooping cough, antibiotics will most likely be prescribed.

When Antibiotics Will Not Help

When bronchitis is caused by a virus or irritation in the air (like cigarette smoke), antibiotic treatment will not help it get better. Since acute bronchitis almost always gets better on its own, it is better to wait and take antibiotics only when they are needed. Taking antibiotics when they are not needed can be harmful.

How to Feel Better

Rest, over-the-counter medicines, and other self-care methods may help you or your child feel better. Talk to your health care provider or pharmacist. Remember, always use over-the-counter products as directed. Many over-the-counter products are not recommended for children younger than certain ages.

Preventing Acute Bronchitis

- Avoid smoking.

- Avoid exposure to secondhand smoke and do not expose children to secondhand smoke.

- Practice good hand hygiene.

- Keep you and your child up to date with recommended immunizations.

Section 27.3

Cystic Fibrosis

This section excerpted from "What Is Cystic Fibrosis?" National Heart, Lung, and Blood Institute (www.nhlbi.nih.gov), June 1, 2011.

Cystic fibrosis, or CF, is an inherited disease of the secretory glands. Secretory glands include glands that make mucus and sweat. CF mainly affects the lungs, pancreas, liver, intestines, sinuses, and sex organs.

Mucus is a substance made by tissues that line some organs and body cavities, such as the lungs and nose. Normally, mucus is a slippery, watery substance. It keeps the linings of certain organs moist and prevents them from drying out or getting infected.

If you have CF, your mucus becomes thick and sticky. It builds up in your lungs and blocks your airways. The buildup of mucus makes it easy for bacteria to grow. This leads to repeated, serious lung infections. Over time, these infections can severely damage your lungs.

The thick, sticky mucus also can block tubes, or ducts, in your pancreas. This can cause vitamin deficiency and malnutrition because nutrients pass through your body without being used.

CF also causes your sweat to become very salty. This can upset the balance of minerals in your blood and cause many health problems.

If you or your child has CF, you're also at higher risk for diabetes or a bone-thinning condition called osteoporosis.

CF also causes infertility in men, and the disease can make it harder for women to get pregnant.

Outlook

The symptoms and severity of CF vary. If you or your child has the disease, you may have serious lung and digestive problems. If the disease is mild, symptoms may not show up until the teen or adult years.

The symptoms and severity of CF also vary over time. Sometimes you'll have few symptoms. Other times, your symptoms may become more severe. As the disease gets worse, you'll have more severe symptoms more often.

Lung function often starts to decline in early childhood in people who have CF. Over time, damage to the lungs can cause severe breathing problems. Respiratory failure is the most common cause of death in people who have CF.

As treatments for CF continue to improve, so does life expectancy for those who have the disease. Today, some people who have CF are living into their forties or fifties, or longer.

Causes

A defect in the CFTR gene causes CF. This gene makes a protein that controls the movement of salt and water in and out of your body's cells. In people who have CF, the gene makes a protein that doesn't work well.

More than a thousand known defects can affect the CFTR gene. The type of defect you or your child has may affect the severity of CF.

Every person inherits two CFTR genes—one from each parent. Children who inherit a faulty CFTR gene from each parent will have CF. Children who inherit one faulty gene and one normal gene are "CF carriers." CF carriers usually have no symptoms of CF and live normal lives. However, they can pass the faulty CFTR gene to their children.

Signs and Symptoms

The signs and symptoms of CF vary from person to person and over time. One of the first signs of CF that parents may notice is that their baby's skin tastes salty when kissed, or the baby doesn't pass stool when first born.

Most of the other signs and symptoms of CF happen later. They're related to how CF affects the respiratory, digestive, or reproductive systems of the body.

Respiratory System Signs and Symptoms

People who have CF have thick, sticky mucus that builds up in their airways. This buildup of mucus makes it easier for bacteria to grow and cause infections. Infections can block the airways and cause frequent coughing that brings up thick sputum (spit) or mucus that's sometimes bloody.

People who have CF tend to have lung infections caused by unusual germs that don't respond to standard antibiotics. People who have CF have frequent bouts of sinusitis, an infection of the sinuses. Frequent bouts of bronchitis and pneumonia also can occur. These infections can cause long-term lung damage.

Digestive System Signs and Symptoms

In CF, mucus can block tubes, or ducts, in your pancreas. These blockages prevent enzymes from reaching your intestines. As a result, your intestines can't fully absorb fats and proteins. This can cause ongoing diarrhea or bulky, foul-smelling, greasy stools. Intestinal blockages also may occur, especially in newborns. Too much gas or severe constipation in the intestines may cause stomach pain and discomfort.

A hallmark of CF in children is poor weight gain and growth. These children are unable to get enough nutrients from their food because of the lack of enzymes to help absorb fats and proteins.

As CF gets worse, other problems may occur, such as the following:

- Pancreatitis, a condition in which the pancreas become inflamed, causing pain

- Rectal prolapse, in which frequent coughing or problems passing stools may cause rectal tissue from inside you to move out of your rectum

- Liver disease due to inflamed or blocked bile ducts

- Diabetes

- Gallstones

Reproductive System Signs and Symptoms

Men who have CF are infertile because they're born without a vas deferens. The vas deferens is a tube that delivers sperm from the testes to the penis.

Women who have CF may have a hard time getting pregnant because of mucus blocking the cervix or other CF complications.

Other Signs, Symptoms, and Complications

Other signs and symptoms of CF are related to an upset of the balance of minerals in your blood.

CF causes your sweat to become very salty. As a result, your body loses large amounts of salt when you sweat. This can cause dehydration (a lack of fluid in your body), increased heart rate, fatigue (tiredness), weakness, decreased blood pressure, heat stroke, and, rarely, death.

CF also can cause clubbing and low bone density. Clubbing is the widening and rounding of the tips of your fingers and toes. This sign develops late in CF because your lungs aren't moving enough oxygen into your bloodstream. Low bone density also tends to occur late in CF. It can lead to a bone-thinning disorder called osteoporosis.

Diagnosis

Doctors diagnose CF based on the results from various tests.

Newborn Screening

All states screen newborns for CF using a genetic test or a blood test. The genetic test shows whether a newborn has faulty CFTR genes. The blood test shows whether a newborn's pancreas is working properly.

Sweat Test

If a genetic test or blood test suggests CF, a doctor will confirm the diagnosis using a sweat test. This test is the most useful test for diagnosing CF. High salt levels confirm a diagnosis of CF.

Other Tests

If you or your child has CF, your doctor may recommend other tests, such as the following:

- Genetic tests help find out what type of CFTR defect is causing your CF.

- A chest X-ray creates pictures of the structures in your chest and can show whether your lungs are inflamed or scarred, or whether they trap air.

- A sinus X-ray may show signs of sinusitis, a complication of CF.

- Lung function tests measure how much air you can breathe in and out, how fast you can breathe air out, and how well your lungs deliver oxygen to your blood.

- In a sputum culture, your doctor will take a sample of your sputum (spit) to see whether bacteria are growing in it.

Prenatal Screening and Carrier Testing

If you're pregnant, prenatal genetic tests can show whether your fetus has CF. These tests include amniocentesis and chorionic villus sampling (CVS).

If you have a family history of CF or a partner who has CF (or a family history of it) and you're planning a pregnancy, you may want to find out whether you're a CF carrier. A genetics counselor can test a blood or saliva sample to find out whether you have a faulty CF gene. This type of testing can detect faulty CF genes in 9 out of 10 cases.

Treatment

CF has no cure. However, treatments have greatly improved in recent years.

If you or your child has CF, you may be treated by a CF specialist. The United States also has more than 100 CF Care Centers. These centers have teams of doctors, nurses, dietitians, respiratory therapists, physical therapists, and social workers who have special training related to CF care. Most CF Care Centers have pediatric and adult programs or clinics.

For more information about CF Care Centers, go to the Cystic Fibrosis Foundation's Care Center Network webpage [at http://www.cff .org/LivingWithCF/CareCenterNetwork].

Treatment for Lung Problems

The main treatments for lung problems in people who have CF are chest physical therapy (CPT), exercise, and medicines. Your doctor also may recommend a pulmonary rehabilitation (PR) program.

Chest physical therapy: CPT also is called chest clapping or percussion. It involves pounding your chest and back over and over with your hands or a device to loosen the mucus from your lungs so that you can cough it up.

Exercise: Aerobic exercise that makes you breathe harder can help loosen the mucus in your airways so you can cough it up. Exercise also helps improve your overall physical condition. However, in CF, your body loses large amounts of salt when you sweat. Thus, your doctor may recommend a high-salt diet or salt supplements to maintain the balance of minerals in your blood.

Medicines: If you have CF, you doctor may prescribe antibiotics, anti-inflammatory medicines, bronchodilators, or mucus-thinning medicines. These medicines help treat or prevent lung infections, reduce swelling, open up the airways, and thin mucus.

Treatments for advanced lung disease: If you have advanced lung disease, you may need oxygen therapy. Oxygen usually is given through nasal prongs or a mask. If other treatments haven't worked, a lung transplant may be an option if you have severe lung disease.

Pulmonary rehabilitation: Your doctor may recommend PR as part of your treatment plan. PR is a broad program that helps improve the well-being of people who have chronic (ongoing) breathing problems.

Treatment for Digestive Problems

CF can cause many digestive problems, such as bulky stools, intestinal gas, a swollen belly, severe constipation, and pain or discomfort.

Nutritional therapy can improve your strength and ability to stay active. It also can improve growth and development in children. Nutritional therapy also may make you strong enough to resist some lung infections.

Other treatments for digestive problems may include enemas and mucus-thinning medicines to treat intestinal blockages. Sometimes surgery is needed to remove an intestinal blockage.

Your doctor also may prescribe medicines to reduce your stomach acid and help oral pancreatic enzymes work better.

Chapter 28

Skin Conditions in Children

Chapter Contents

Section 28.1

Eczema (Atopic Dermatitis)

This section excerpted from "Handout on Health: Atopic Dermatitis,"
National Institute of Arthritis and Musculoskeletal and Skin Diseases
(www.niams.nih.gov), August 2011.

Atopic dermatitis is a chronic disease that affects the skin. It is not contagious. In atopic dermatitis, the skin becomes extremely itchy. Scratching leads to redness, swelling, cracking, "weeping" clear fluid, and, finally, crusting and scaling. In most cases, there are periods of time when the disease is worse (called exacerbations or flares) followed by periods when the skin improves or clears up entirely (called remissions). As some children with atopic dermatitis grow older, their skin disease improves or disappears altogether, although their skin often remains dry and easily irritated. In others, atopic dermatitis continues to be a significant problem in adulthood.

Atopic dermatitis is often referred to as "eczema," which is a general term for the several types of inflammation of the skin.

Atopic dermatitis is very common. Scientists estimate that 65% of patients develop symptoms in the first year of life, and 85% develop symptoms before the age of five.

Causes of Atopic Dermatitis

The cause of atopic dermatitis is not known, but the disease seems to result from a combination of genetic (hereditary) and environmental factors.

Children are more likely to develop this disorder if a parent has had it or another atopic disease like asthma or hay fever. If both parents have an atopic disease, the likelihood increases. Although some people outgrow skin symptoms, approximately half of children with atopic dermatitis go on to develop hay fever or asthma. Environmental factors can bring on symptoms of atopic dermatitis at any time in individuals who have inherited the atopic disease trait.

Atopic dermatitis is also associated with malfunction of the body's immune system, the system that recognizes and helps fight bacteria and viruses that invade the body. The immune system can become misguided and create inflammation in the skin even in the absence of a major infection.

Symptoms of Atopic Dermatitis

The most common symptoms are dry, itchy skin and rashes on the face, inside the elbows and behind the knees, and on the hands and feet. Itching is the most important symptom of atopic dermatitis. Scratching and rubbing in response to itching irritates the skin, increases inflammation, and actually increases itchiness.

The appearance of the skin that is affected by atopic dermatitis depends on the amount of scratching and the presence of secondary skin infections. The skin may be red and scaly, be thick and leathery, contain small raised bumps, or leak fluid and become crusty and infected.

In infants, atopic dermatitis typically begins around 6 to 12 weeks of age. It may first appear around the cheeks and chin as a patchy facial rash, which can progress to red, scaling, oozing skin. Once the infant becomes more mobile and begins crawling, exposed areas, such as the inner and outer parts of the arms and legs, may also be affected.

In childhood, the rash tends to occur behind the knees and inside the elbows; on the sides of the neck; around the mouth; and on the wrists, ankles, and hands. Often, the rash begins with papules that become hard and scaly when scratched. The skin around the lips may be inflamed, and constant licking of the area may lead to small, painful cracks in the skin around the mouth.

In some children, the disease goes into remission for a long time, only to come back at the onset of puberty when hormones, stress, and the use of irritating skin care products or cosmetics may cause the disease to flare.

Diagnosing Atopic Dermatitis

The doctor will base a diagnosis on the symptoms the patient experiences and may need to see the patient several times to make an accurate diagnosis and to rule out other diseases and conditions. In some cases, the family doctor or pediatrician may refer the patient to a dermatologist or allergist for further evaluation.

The doctor may ask about family history of allergic disease; whether the patient also has diseases such as hay fever or asthma; and about exposure to irritants, sleep disturbances, any foods that seem to be related to skin flares, previous treatments for skin-related symptoms, and use of steroids or other medications.

Currently, there is no single test to diagnose atopic dermatitis. However, there are some tests that can give the doctor an indication of allergic sensitivity.

Treatment of Atopic Dermatitis

The doctor will suggest a treatment plan based on the patient's age, symptoms, and general health. Most patients will notice improvement with proper skin care and lifestyle changes.

The doctor has two main goals in treating atopic dermatitis: healing the skin and preventing flares. These may be assisted by developing skin care routines and avoiding substances that lead to skin irritation and trigger the immune system and the itch-scratch cycle. It is important for the patient and family members to note any changes in the skin's condition in response to treatment, and to be persistent in identifying the treatment that seems to work best.

New medications known as immunomodulators have been developed that help control inflammation and reduce immune system reactions when applied to the skin. They can be used in patients older than two years of age and have few side effects.

Corticosteroid creams and ointments have been used for many years to treat atopic dermatitis and other autoimmune diseases affecting the skin. Sometimes over-the-counter preparations are used, but in many cases the doctor will prescribe a stronger corticosteroid cream or ointment. When topical corticosteroids are not effective, the doctor may prescribe a systemic corticosteroid, which is taken by mouth or injected instead of being applied directly to the skin.

Antibiotics to treat skin infections may be applied directly to the skin in an ointment, but are usually more effective when taken by mouth.

Certain antihistamines that cause drowsiness can reduce nighttime scratching and allow more restful sleep when taken at bedtime. This effect can be particularly helpful for patients whose nighttime scratching makes the disease worse.

Treating Atopic Dermatitis in Infants and Children

- Give lukewarm baths.
- Apply lubricant immediately following the bath.
- Keep child's fingernails filed short.
- Select soft cotton fabrics when choosing clothing.

- Consider using sedating antihistamines to promote sleep and reduce scratching at night.

- Keep the child cool; avoid situations where overheating occurs.

- Learn to recognize skin infections and seek treatment promptly.

- Attempt to distract the child with activities to keep him or her from scratching.

- Identify and remove irritants and allergens.

Section 28.2

Psoriasis

"Fast Facts about Psoriasis," National Institute of Arthritis and Musculoskeletal and Skin Diseases (www.niams.nih.gov), September 2009.

Psoriasis is a skin disease that causes scaling and inflammation (pain, swelling, heat, and redness). Most psoriasis causes patches of thick, red skin with silvery scales. These patches can itch or feel sore. They are often found on the elbows, knees, other parts of the legs, scalp, lower back, face, palms, and soles of the feet. But they can show up other places such as fingernails, toenails, genitals, and inside the mouth.

What causes psoriasis?

Psoriasis begins in the immune system, mainly with a type of white blood cell called a T cell. T cells help protect the body against infection and disease. With psoriasis, T cells are put into action by mistake. They become so active that they set off other immune responses. This leads to swelling and fast turnover of skin cells. People with psoriasis may notice that sometimes the skin gets better and sometimes it gets worse. Things that can cause the skin to get worse include the following:

- Infections

- Stress

- Changes in weather that dry the skin

- Certain medicines

How is psoriasis diagnosed?

Psoriasis can be hard to diagnose because it can look like other skin diseases. The doctor might need to look at a small skin sample under a microscope.

How is psoriasis treated?

All treatments don't work the same for everyone. Doctors may switch treatments if one doesn't work, if there is a bad reaction, or if the treatment stops working.

Topical treatment: Treatments applied right on the skin (creams, ointments) may help. These treatments can do the following:

- Help reduce inflammation and skin cell turnover
- Suppress the immune system
- Help the skin peel and unclog pores
- Soothe the skin

Light therapy: Natural ultraviolet light from the sun and artificial ultraviolet light are used to treat psoriasis.

Systemic treatment: If the psoriasis is severe, doctors might prescribe drugs or give medicine through a shot. Antibiotics are not used to treat psoriasis unless bacteria make the psoriasis worse.

Combination therapy: When you combine topical, light, and systemic treatments, you can often use lower doses of each. Combination therapy can also lead to better results.

Section 28.3

Warts

About Warts

Many of us have had a wart somewhere on our bodies at some time.
Other than being a nuisance, most warts are harmless and go away
on their own.

More common in kids than in adults, warts are skin infections
caused by viruses of the human papillomavirus (HPV) family. They
can affect any area of the body, but tend to invade warm, moist places,
like small cuts or scratches on the fingers, hands, and feet. Warts are
usually painless unless they're on the soles of the feet or another part
of the body that gets bumped or touched all the time.

Kids can pick up HPV—and get warts—from touching anything
someone with a wart has used, like towels and surfaces. Kids who bite
their fingernails or pick at hangnails tend to get warts more often than
kids who don't because they can expose less-protected skin and create
open areas for a virus to enter and cause the wart.

Types of warts include:

- **Common warts:** Usually found on fingers, hands, knees, and elbows, a common wart is a small, hard bump that's dome-shaped
  and usually grayish-brown. It has a rough surface that may look
  like the head of a cauliflower, with black dots inside.

- **Flat warts:** These are about the size of a pinhead, are smoother
  than other kinds of warts, and have flat tops. Flat warts may be
  pink, light brown, or yellow. Most kids who get flat warts have
  them on their faces, but they can also grow on arms, knees, or
  hands and can appear in clusters.

- **Plantar warts:** Found on the bottom of the foot, plantar warts
  can be very uncomfortable—like walking on a small stone.

- **Filiform warts:** These have a finger-like shape, are usually flesh-colored, and often grow on or around the mouth, eyes, or nose.

Sometimes warts are sexually transmitted and appear in the genital area, but most warts appear on the fingers, hands, and feet.

Are Warts Contagious?

Simply touching a wart on someone doesn't guarantee that you'll get one, too. But the viruses that cause warts are passed from person to person by close physical contact or from a surface that a person with a wart touches, like a bathmat or a shower floor. (You can't, however, get a wart from holding a frog or toad, as kids sometimes think!)

A tiny cut or scratch can make any area of skin more vulnerable to warts. Also, picking at a wart can spread warts to other parts of the body.

The length of time between when someone is exposed to the virus that causes warts and when a wart appears varies. Warts can grow very slowly and may take weeks or longer, in some cases, to develop.

Preventing Warts

Although there's no way to prevent warts, it's always a good idea to encourage kids to wash their hands and skin regularly and well. If your child has a cut or scratch, use soap and water to clean the area because open wounds are more susceptible to warts and other infections.

It's also wise to have kids wear waterproof sandals or flip-flops in public showers, locker rooms, and around public pools (this can help protect against plantar warts and other infections, like athlete's foot).

Treating Warts

Warts don't generally cause any problems, so it's not always necessary to have them removed. Without treatment, it can take anywhere from six months to two years for a wart to go away. A doctor might decide to remove a wart if it's painful or interferes with activities because of the discomfort.

Doctors have different ways of removing warts, including:

- using over-the-counter or prescription medications to put on the wart;

- burning the wart off using a light electrical current;

- freezing the wart with liquid nitrogen (called cryosurgery);

- using laser treatment (with recalcitrant warts).

Within a few days after the doctor's treatment, the wart may fall off, but several treatments might be necessary. Doctors don't usually cut off a wart because it can cause scarring and the wart may return.

If an older child has a simple wart on the finger, ask the doctor about using an over-the-counter wart remedy that can help remove the wart. This treatment can take several weeks or months before you see results, but eventually the wart should crumble away from the healthy skin. Wart medicines contain strong chemicals and should be used with care because they can also damage the areas of healthy skin. Talk with your doctor before using any over-the-counter wart medicine on the face or genitals.

Also make sure that your child:

- soaks the wart in warm water and removes dead skin on the surface of the wart with an emery board (that's never going to be used for nails) before applying the medicine (be careful not to file into it);

- keeps the area of the wart covered while the medicine works;

- knows not to rub, scratch, or pick at it to avoid spreading the virus to another part of the body or causing the wart to become infected.

You might also have heard that you can use duct tape to remove a wart. Talk to your doctor about whether this type of home treatment is okay for your child.

When to Call the Doctor

Before you try to remove a wart with a store-bought remedy, call your doctor if:

- you have a young child or infant with a wart anywhere on the body;

- your child (of any age) has a wart on the face, genitals, or rectum.

Also call the doctor if a wart or surrounding skin is:

- painful;

- red;

- bleeding;

- swollen;

- oozing pus.

Although they can be a nuisance, warts are common in childhood and unlikely to cause serious problems.

Chapter 29

Vision and Eye Problems in Children

Chapter Contents

Section 29.1

Amblyopia (Lazy Eye)

This section excerpted from "Facts about Amblyopia,"
National Eye Institute (www.nei.nih.gov), September 2009.

What is amblyopia?

The brain and the eye work together to produce vision. Light enters the eye and is changed into nerve signals that travel along the optic nerve to the brain. Amblyopia is the medical term used when the vision in one of the eyes is reduced because the eye and the brain are not working together properly. The eye itself looks normal, but it is not being used normally because the brain is favoring the other eye. This condition is also sometimes called lazy eye.

How common is amblyopia?

Amblyopia is the most common cause of visual impairment in childhood. The condition affects approximately 2 to 3 out of every 100 children. Unless it is successfully treated in early childhood, amblyopia usually persists into adulthood and is the most common cause of monocular (one eye) visual impairment among children and young and middle-aged adults.

What causes amblyopia?

Amblyopia may be caused by any condition that affects normal visual development or use of the eyes. Amblyopia can be caused by strabismus, an imbalance in the positioning of the two eyes. Strabismus can cause the eyes to cross in (esotropia) or turn out (exotropia). Sometimes amblyopia is caused when one eye is more nearsighted, farsighted, or astigmatic than the other eye. Occasionally, amblyopia is caused by other eye conditions such as cataract.

How is amblyopia treated in children?

Treating amblyopia involves making the child use the eye with the reduced vision (weaker eye). Currently, there are two ways used to do this:

Atropine: A drop of a drug called atropine is placed in the stronger eye once a day to temporarily blur the vision so that the child will prefer to use the eye with amblyopia. Treatment with atropine also stimulates vision in the weaker eye and helps the part of the brain that manages vision develop more completely.

Patching: An opaque, adhesive patch is worn over the stronger eye for weeks to months. This therapy forces the child to use the eye with amblyopia. Patching stimulates vision in the weaker eye and helps the part of the brain that manages vision develop more completely.

Previously, eye care professionals often thought that treating amblyopia in older children would be of little benefit. However, surprising results from a nationwide clinical trial show that many children age 7 through 17 with amblyopia may benefit from treatments that are more commonly used on younger children. This study shows that age alone should not be used as a factor to decide whether or not to treat a child for amblyopia.

Can amblyopia be treated in adults?

Studies are very limited at this time and scientists don't know what the success rate might be for treating amblyopia in adults. During the first six to nine years of life, the visual system develops very rapidly. Complicated connections between the eye and the brain are created during that period of growth and development. Scientists are exploring whether treatment for amblyopia in adults can improve vision.

Section 29.2

Conjunctivitis (Pinkeye)

This section excerpted from "Conjunctivitis (Pink Eye),"
Centers for Disease Control and Prevention (www.cdc.gov), June 4, 2010.

Causes

Conjunctivitis is a common eye condition worldwide. It causes inflammation (swelling) of the conjunctiva—the thin layer that lines the inside of the eyelid and covers the white part of the eye. Conjunctivitis is often called "pink eye" or "red eye" because it can cause the white of the eye to take on a pink or red color.

The most common causes of conjunctivitis are viruses, bacteria, and allergens. But there are other causes, including chemicals, fungi, certain diseases, and contact lens use.

Viral Conjunctivitis

Viral conjunctivitis is caused by infection of the eye with a virus. Viral conjunctivitis has the following characteristics:

- Can be caused by a number of different viruses, many of which are associated with an upper respiratory tract infection, cold, or sore throat

- Usually begins in one eye and may progress to the second eye within days

- Spreads easily and rapidly between people and can result in epidemics

- Is typically mild, with symptoms being the worst on days 3–5 of infection; the condition usually clears up in 7–14 days without treatment and resolves without any long-term effects

Bacterial Conjunctivitis

Bacterial conjunctivitis is caused by infection of the eye with certain bacteria. Bacterial conjunctivitis has these characteristics:

- Usually begins in one eye and may sometimes progress to the second eye

- Is a leading cause of children being absent from day care or school

- Cases are typically mild and can last as few as two to three days or up to two to three weeks; many cases improve in two to five days without treatment

Allergic Conjunctivitis

Allergic conjunctivitis is caused by the body's reaction to certain substances to which it is allergic, such as pollen from trees, plants, grasses, and weeds; dust mites; molds; dander from animals; contact lenses and lens solution; and cosmetics. Allergic conjunctivitis shows these signs:

- Occurs more frequently among people with other allergic conditions, such as hay fever, asthma, and eczema

- Usually occurs in both eyes

- Can occur seasonally, when pollen counts are high

- Can occur year-round due to indoor allergens

- May result from exposure to certain drugs and cosmetics

- Clears up once the allergen or irritant is removed or after treatment with allergy medications

Signs and Symptoms

It can be hard to determine the exact cause of every case of conjunctivitis. This is because some signs and symptoms of the condition can differ depending on the cause, and other signs and symptoms are similar no matter what caused the conjunctivitis.

Symptoms of conjunctivitis can include the following:

- Pink or red color in the white of the eye(s)

- Swelling of the conjunctiva (the thin layer that lines the white part of the eye and the inside of the eyelid) and/or eyelids

- Increased tearing

- Discharge of pus, especially yellow-green (more common in bacterial conjunctivitis)

- Itching, irritation, and/or burning

- Feeling like a foreign body is in the eye(s) or an urge to rub the eye(s)

- Crusting of eyelids or lashes, especially in the morning

- Symptoms of a cold, flu, or other respiratory infection

- Sensitivity to bright light

- Enlargement and/or tenderness of the lymph node in front of the ear

- Symptoms of allergy, such as an itchy nose, sneezing, a scratchy throat, or asthma, in cases of allergic conjunctivitis

Diagnosis

Viral Conjunctivitis

Viral conjunctivitis can often be diagnosed from signs and symptoms and patient history. For example, if conjunctivitis accompanies a common cold or respiratory tract infection and if discharge from the eye is watery rather than thick, the cause is likely a virus.

Laboratory tests are not usually needed to diagnose viral conjunctivitis. However, testing may be done if a more severe form of viral conjunctivitis is suspected, such as conjunctivitis caused by herpes simplex virus or varicella-zoster virus. This testing is done using a sample of the discharge from an infected eye.

Bacterial Conjunctivitis

Bacterial conjunctivitis can usually be diagnosed by a doctor, nurse, or other health care provider from signs and symptoms and patient history. For example, if conjunctivitis accompanies an ear infection and if discharge from the eye is thick rather than watery, the cause may be a bacterium. Although not routinely done, your health care provider may obtain a sample of eye discharge from the conjunctiva for laboratory analysis to determine which form of infection you have and how best to treat it.

Allergic Conjunctivitis

Allergic conjunctivitis can be diagnosed from signs and symptoms and patient history; for example, allergic conjunctivitis may occur seasonally when pollen counts are high, and it can cause the patient's eyes to itch intensely. This type of conjunctivitis is a common occurrence in people who have other signs of allergic disease, such as hay fever, asthma, or eczema.

Prevention

Conjunctivitis caused by allergens is not contagious; however, viral and bacterial conjunctivitis can be easily spread from person to person and can cause epidemics. You can greatly reduce the risk of getting conjunctivitis or of passing it on to someone else by following some simple good hygiene steps.

- Wash your hands often with soap and warm water. If soap and water are not available, use an alcohol-based hand rub.

- Avoid touching or rubbing your eyes.

- Wash any discharge from around the eyes several times a day. Hands should be washed first and then a clean washcloth or fresh cotton ball or tissue can be used to cleanse the eye area. Wash your hands with soap and warm water when done.

- Wash hands after applying eye drops or ointment.

- Do not use the same eye drop dispenser/bottle for infected and noninfected eyes—even for the same person.

- Wash pillowcases, sheets, washcloths, and towels in hot water and detergent; hands should be washed after handling such items.

- Avoid sharing articles like towels, blankets, and pillowcases.

- Clean eyeglasses, being careful not to contaminate items (like towels) that might be shared by other people.

- Do not share eye makeup, face makeup, makeup brushes, contact lenses and containers, or eyeglasses.

- Do not use swimming pools.

In addition, if you have infectious conjunctivitis, there are steps you can take to avoid reinfection once the infection goes away:

- Throw away and replace any eye or face makeup you used while infected.

- Replace contact lens solutions that you used while your eyes were infected.

- Throw away disposable contact lenses and cases that were used while your eyes were infected.

- Clean extended-wear lenses as directed.

- Clean eyeglasses and cases that were used while infected.

There is no vaccine that prevents all types of conjunctivitis. However, there are vaccines to protect against a few viral and bacterial diseases—rubella, measles, chickenpox, shingles, pneumococcal and *Haemophilus influenzae* type b (Hib) disease—that are associated with conjunctivitis.

Treatment

Viral Conjunctivitis

Most cases of viral conjunctivitis are mild. Days 3–5 of infection are often the worst, but the infection will usually clear up in 7–14 days without treatment and without any long-term consequences.

Artificial tears and cold packs may be used to relieve the dryness and inflammation (swelling) caused by conjunctivitis. Antiviral medication can be prescribed by a physician to treat more serious forms of conjunctivitis, such as those caused by herpes simplex virus or varicella-zoster virus.

Bacterial Conjunctivitis

Mild bacterial conjunctivitis may get better without antibiotic treatment. However, antibiotics can help shorten the illness and reduce the spread of infection to others. Many topical antibiotics (drugs given as eye drops or ointment) are effective for treating bacterial conjunctivitis. Artificial tears and cold compresses may be used to relieve some of the dryness and inflammation.

Allergic Conjunctivitis

Conjunctivitis caused by an allergy usually improves when the allergen (such as pollen or animal dander) is removed. Allergy medications and certain eye drops (topical antihistamine and vasoconstrictors), including some prescription eye drops, can also provide relief from allergic conjunctivitis.

When to Seek Medical Care

A health care provider should be seen in the following scenarios:

- Conjunctivitis is accompanied by moderate to severe pain in the eye(s).

- Conjunctivitis is accompanied by vision problems, such as sensitivity to light or blurred vision, that does not improve when any discharge that is present is wiped from the eye(s).

- Conjunctivitis is accompanied by intense redness in the eye(s).

- Conjunctivitis symptoms become worse or persist when a patient is suspected of having a severe form of viral conjunctivitis.

- Conjunctivitis occurs in a patient who is immunocompromised (has a weakened immune system) from HIV infection, cancer treatment, or other medical conditions or treatments.

- Bacterial conjunctivitis is being treated with antibiotics and does not begin to improve after 24 hours of treatment.

Section 29.3

Refractive Disorders

This section excerpted from "Facts about Refractive Errors," National Eye Institute (www.nei.nih.gov), October 2010.

What are refractive errors?

Refractive errors occur when the shape of the eye prevents light from focusing directly on the retina. The length of the eyeball (longer or shorter), changes in the shape of the cornea, or aging of the lens can cause refractive errors.

Refraction is the bending of light as it passes through one object to another. Vision occurs when light rays are bent (refracted) as they pass through the cornea and the lens.

What are the different types of refractive errors?

The most common types of refractive errors are myopia, hyperopia, presbyopia, and astigmatism.

Myopia (nearsightedness) is a condition where objects up close appear clearly, while objects far away appear blurry. With myopia, light comes to focus in front of the retina instead of on the retina.

Hyperopia (farsightedness) is a common type of refractive error where distant objects may be seen more clearly than objects that are near. However, people experience hyperopia differently. Some people may not notice any problems with their vision, especially when they are young. For people with significant hyperopia, vision can be blurry for objects at any distance, near or far.

Astigmatism is a condition in which the eye does not focus light evenly onto the retina, the light-sensitive tissue at the back of the eye. This can cause images to appear blurry and stretched out.

Presbyopia is an age-related condition in which the ability to focus up close becomes more difficult. As the eye ages, the lens can no longer change shape enough to allow the eye to focus close objects clearly.

Who is at risk for refractive errors?

Presbyopia affects most adults over age 35. Other refractive errors can affect both children and adults. Individuals who have parents with certain refractive errors may be more likely to get one or more refractive errors.

What are the signs and symptoms of refractive errors?

Blurred vision is the most common symptom of refractive errors. Other symptoms may include the following:

- Double vision

- Haziness

- Glare or halos around bright lights

- Squinting

- Headaches

- Eye strain

How are refractive errors diagnosed?

An eye care professional can diagnose refractive errors during a comprehensive dilated eye examination. People with a refractive error often visit their eye care professional with complaints of visual discomfort or blurred vision. However, some people don't know they aren't seeing as clearly as they could.

How are refractive errors treated?

Refractive errors can be corrected with eyeglasses, contact lenses, or surgery.

Eyeglasses are the simplest and safest way to correct refractive errors. Your eye care professional can prescribe appropriate lenses to correct your refractive error and give you optimal vision.

Contact lenses work by becoming the first refractive surface for light rays entering the eye, causing a more precise refraction or focus. In many cases, contact lenses provide clearer vision, a wider field of vision, and greater comfort. They are a safe and effective option if fitted and used properly.

Refractive surgery aims to change the shape of the cornea permanently. There are many types of refractive surgeries. Your eye care professional can help you decide if surgery is an option for you.

Section 29.4

Retinitis Pigmentosa

What Is Retinitis Pigmentosa (RP)?

Retinitis pigmentosa (RP) is the name given to a group of hereditary retinal diseases characterized by progressive loss of visual field, night blindness, and reduced or absent electroretinogram (ERG test) recording, which indicates that a large portion of the retina is damaged.

RP causes the degeneration of photoreceptor cells in the retina. Photoreceptor cells capture and process light helping us to see. As these cells degenerate and die, patients experience progressive vision loss.

There are two types of photoreceptor cells: rod cells and cone cells. Rod cells are concentrated along the outer perimeter of the retina. Rod cells help us to see images that come into our peripheral or side vision. They also help us to see in dark and dimly lit environments. Cone cells are concentrated in the macula, the center of the retina, and allow us to see fine visual detail in the center of our vision. Cone cells also allow us to perceive color. Together, rods and cones are the cells responsible for converting light into electrical impulses that are transmitted to the brain where "seeing" actually occurs.

What Are the Different Types of Retinitis Pigmentosa?

Genetics of RP

Within the nucleus of every human cell reside a host of genes. Genes are the fundamental building blocks of life. Inherited from our parents, genes carry family traits like eye and hair color, the shape of our face, and even diseases like RP.

Genes are like computer programs containing sets of coded instructions. Each gene instructs the cell to create a specialized protein that performs a specific task for the cell. In retinal cells, some genes encode proteins that allow the cell to process light. Other genes encode proteins that uptake nutrients and eliminate waste. Still other genes encode proteins that form the cell walls and other structures within the cell.

Sometimes, the coded instructions within a gene become altered. These alterations, known as mutations, can confer a benefit, allowing the organism to better adapt to its environment. However, mutations can also interfere with the proper encoding of a protein. The resulting protein cannot perform its job within the cell, thereby hampering the cell's well being and leading to disease.

Retinal cells are among the most specialized cells in the human body and depend on a number of unique genes to create vision. A disease-causing mutation in any one of these genes can lead to vision loss. To date, Foundation Fighting Blindness researchers have discovered over 100 genes that can contain mutations leading to RP.

RP can be passed to succeeding generations by one of three genetic inheritance patterns—autosomal dominant, autosomal recessive, or X-linked inheritance.

Each type of inheritance causes a different pattern of affected and unaffected family members. For example, in families with autosomal recessive RP, unaffected parents can have both affected and unaffected children. In recessive RP, there is often no prior family history. In families with the autosomal dominant RP, an affected parent can have both affected and unaffected children. In families with the X-linked type, only males are affected, while females carry the genetic trait but do not experience serious vision loss.

It is very important to remember that because RP is an inherited disorder, it can potentially affect another member of the family. If one member of a family is diagnosed with a hereditary retinal degeneration, it is strongly advised that all members of that family contact an ophthalmologist.

Related Diseases

Other inherited diseases share some of the clinical symptoms of RP. Some of these conditions are complicated by other symptoms besides loss of vision. The most common of these is Usher syndrome, which causes both hearing and vision loss. Other rare syndromes include Bardet-Biedl (Laurence-Moon) syndrome, rod-cone dystrophy, choroideremia, gyrate-atrophy, Leber congenital amaurosis, and Stargardt's disease.

RP and related diseases are rare and difficult to accurately diagnose. Only a specialist can properly distinguish between the subtle clinical features of these diseases. Therefore, it is important that patients who are symptomatic see an ophthalmologist who specializes in retinal degenerative diseases.

Symptoms

- Normal visual acuity in early stages, possibly—but not usually— progressing to no light perception
- Donut-shaped visual field loss progressing to severe constriction (loss of peripheral vision)
- Night blindness
- Decreased response to magnification
- Need for more light

The most common feature of all forms of RP is a gradual degeneration of the rods and cones. Most forms of RP first cause the degeneration of rod cells. These forms of RP, sometimes called rod-cone dystrophy, usually begin with night blindness. Night blindness is somewhat like the experience normally sighted individuals encounter when entering a dark movie theatre on a bright, sunny day. However, patients with RP cannot adjust well to dark and dimly lit environments.

As the disease progresses and more rod cells degenerate, patients lose their peripheral vision. Patients with RP often experience a ring of vision loss in their mid-periphery with small islands of vision in their very far periphery. Others report the sensation of tunnel vision, as though they see the world through the opening of a straw. Many patients with RP retain a small degree of central vision throughout their life.

Other forms of RP, sometimes called cone-rod dystrophy, first affect central vision. Patients first experience a loss of central vision that cannot be corrected with glasses or contact lenses. With the loss of cone cells also comes disturbances in color perception. As the disease progresses, rod cells also degenerate causing night blindness and loss of peripheral vision.

Symptoms of RP are most often recognized in children, adolescents, and young adults, with progression of the disease continuing throughout the individual's life. The pattern and degree of visual loss are variable.

Diagnosis

These special tests can be used to help diagnose RP:

Acuity tests: These tests measure the accuracy of your central vision at specific distances in specific lighting situations.

Color testing: This can help determine the status of your cone cells, the retinal cells that interpret color.

Visual field test: This test uses a machine to measure how much peripheral vision you have.

Dark adaptation test: This test will measure how well your eyes adjust to changes in lighting and can help the doctor better understand the current function of your rod cells, which are the retinal cells responsible for night vision.

ERG test: The ERG records the electrical currents produced by the retina due to a light stimulus. The intensity and speed of the electrical signal becomes reduced as the photoreceptor cells degenerate.

Risk Factors

Recent research findings suggest that in some forms of RP, prolonged, unprotected exposure to sunlight may accelerate vision loss.

Some women feel that their vision loss progressed more rapidly during pregnancy. However, the effect of pregnancy on RP has not been clinically studied.

RP is an inherited, genetic disease. It is caused by mutations in genes that are active in retinal cells. Gene mutations are programmed into your cells at the time of conception. RP is not caused by injury, infection or exposure to any toxic substance.

What You Can Do to Reduce Risk

Reducing your exposure to sunlight is important for keeping the eye protected. However, since RP is an inherited disorder and it runs in families, the disease is not preventable. If someone in your family is diagnosed with a retinal degeneration, it is strongly advised that all members of the family contact an eye care professional.

Treatment

As yet, there is no known cure for RP. However, intensive research is currently under way to discover the cause, prevention, and treatment of RP.

Researchers have identified some of the genes that cause RP. It is now possible, in some families with X-linked RP or autosomal dominant RP, to perform a test on genetic material from blood and other cells to determine if members of an affected family have one of several RP genes.

Section 29.5

Strabismus (Crossed Eye)

Strabismus, also known as crossed or turned eye, is the medical term used when the two eyes are not straight. It occurs in approximately 2% to 4% of the population.

What Are the Different Types of Strabismus?

There are three common types of strabismus:

Crossed eyes: A child may be born with this condition, or it may develop within a few months of birth or around two years of age. This is also called esotropia, or convergent strabismus.

Walleye, or divergent eyes: A child may be born with this condition, or it may develop later. This is also called exotropia, or divergent strabismus.

Vertical strabismus: The eyes are out of alignment vertically.

Symptoms

- Turned or crossed eye
- Squinting
- Head tilting or turning
- Double vision (in some cases)

Diagnosis

Even if a child's eyes appear to be straight, the child should be examined by an ophthalmologist—a medically qualified eye specialist—by the age of one year. It is possible to examine a child of any age for strabismus and determine whether the eyes are properly focused. If you are not sure whether your child's eyes are straight, consult your family doctor, who may advise referring the child to an ophthalmologist.

The ophthalmologist may use special tests, such as prism testing, to evaluate the alignment of the eyes.

Risk Factors

Most commonly, a tendency to have some type of strabismus is inherited. If any members of your family have had strabismus, the condition is more likely to develop in your child.

Sometimes the condition is due to the eyes being far-sighted and the need for corrective eyeglasses or, occasionally, to some muscle abnormality. Very rarely, strabismus may be secondary to a serious abnormality inside the eye, such as a cataract or tumor.

What You Can Do to Reduce Risk

According to Joseph H. Calhoun, MD, director, Pediatric Ophthalmology & Strabismum, Wills Eye Hospital in Philadelphia, Pennsylvania, "Any cause for poor vision in one eye in a child may lead to strabismum. There are many causes for poor vision in one eye, but a major concern of ophthalmologists is retinoblastoma, a malignant tumor of the retina. Although it is very rare, in the range of one in

20,000 children, this possibility is why every child with strabismus should have a pupil dilated examination of the retina as soon as strabismus is recognized."

And, to detect poor vision in one eye or the other, parents should take children for regular eye examinations. The American Academy of Ophthalmology recommends regular eye exams according to the following timetable:

- Newborn to three months
- Six months to one year
- Three years (approximately)
- Five years (approximately)

However, if you or your child notices problems with his or her vision, visit the eye doctor immediately.

What Happens to Sight in Eyes with Strabismus?

Defective binocular vision: The eyes need to be straight for fusion in the brain of the images of the two eyes. This gives accurate vision and stereopsis, or 3-D vision; 3-D vision is used to judge depth.

Reduction of vision in the turned eye (amblyopia): A reduction of vision may occur in one eye in strabismus, especially under certain circumstances, such as late treatment.

One such circumstance is if a child is born with straight eyes, but one eye turns in around age two. If this condition is not treated urgently, vision may be reduced to partial sight (legal blindness) in the turned eye. If treatment is begun immediately, however, perfect vision can often be restored.

Treatment

The aim of treatment is to restore good vision to each eye and good binocular vision. Treatment usually includes patching the eye that is always straight to bring the vision up to normal in the turned eye. Glasses may be used, particularly for eyes that are out of focus. Glasses and special drops (phospholine iodide) may also help straighten the eyes. Surgery on the eye muscles is sometimes necessary.

The results of treatment are good and may be excellent, but may depend on how quickly treatment is begun. This applies particularly to children who are born with straight eyes but manifest a turned eye around age two. If treatment is unduly delayed, vision may not be restored. This type of legal blindness can be completely prevented. Do not delay if your child has strabismus. Seek professional advice from your family doctor.

Part Four

Developmental and Pediatric Mental Health Concerns

Chapter 30

Autism Spectrum Disorders

What is autism?

Autism spectrum disorder (ASD) is a range of complex neurodevelopment disorders, characterized by social impairments, communication difficulties, and restricted, repetitive, and stereotyped patterns of behavior. Autistic disorder, sometimes called autism or classical ASD, is the most severe form of ASD, while other conditions along the spectrum include a milder form known as Asperger syndrome and childhood disintegrative disorder and pervasive developmental disorder not otherwise specified (usually referred to as PDD-NOS). Although ASD varies significantly in character and severity, it occurs in all ethnic and socioeconomic groups and affects every age group. Experts estimate that 6 children out of every 1,000 will have an ASD. Males are four times more likely to have an ASD than females.

What are some common signs of autism?

The hallmark feature of ASD is impaired social interaction. As early as infancy, a baby with ASD may be unresponsive to people or focus intently on one item to the exclusion of others for long periods of time. A child with ASD may appear to develop normally and then withdraw and become indifferent to social engagement.

This chapter excerpted from "Autism Fact Sheet," National Institute of Neurological Disorders and Stroke (www.ninds.nih.gov), January 18, 2012.

Children with an ASD may fail to respond to their names and often avoid eye contact with other people. They have difficulty interpreting what others are thinking or feeling because they can't understand social cues, such as tone of voice or facial expressions, and don't watch other people's faces for clues about appropriate behavior. They lack empathy.

Many children with an ASD engage in repetitive movements such as rocking and twirling, or in self-abusive behavior such as biting or head-banging. They also tend to start speaking later than other children and may refer to themselves by name instead of "I" or "me." Children with an ASD don't know how to play interactively with other children. Some speak in a sing-song voice about a narrow range of favorite topics, with little regard for the interests of the person to whom they are speaking.

Children with characteristics of an ASD may have co-occurring conditions, including Fragile X syndrome (which causes mental retardation), tuberous sclerosis, epileptic seizures, Tourette syndrome, learning disabilities, and attention deficit disorder. About 20% to 30% of children with an ASD develop epilepsy by the time they reach adulthood.

How is autism diagnosed?

ASD varies widely in severity and symptoms and may go unrecognized, especially in mildly affected children or when it is masked by more debilitating handicaps. Very early indicators that require evaluation by an expert include the following:

- No babbling or pointing by age one
- No single words by 16 months or two-word phrases by age two
- No response to name
- Loss of language or social skills
- Poor eye contact
- Excessive lining up of toys or objects
- No smiling or social responsiveness

Later indicators include these symptoms:

- Impaired ability to make friends with peers
- Impaired ability to initiate or sustain a conversation with others
- Absence or impairment of imaginative and social play
- Stereotyped, repetitive, or unusual use of language

- Restricted patterns of interest that are abnormal in intensity or focus

- Preoccupation with certain objects or subjects

- Inflexible adherence to specific routines or rituals

Health care providers will often use a questionnaire or other screening instrument to gather information about a child's development and behavior. Some screening instruments rely solely on parent observations, while others rely on a combination of parent and doctor observations. If screening instruments indicate the possibility of an ASD, a more comprehensive evaluation is usually indicated.

A comprehensive evaluation requires a multidisciplinary team, including a psychologist, neurologist, psychiatrist, speech therapist, and other professionals who diagnose children with ASDs. The team members will conduct a thorough neurological assessment and in-depth cognitive and language testing. Because hearing problems can cause behaviors that could be mistaken for an ASD, children with delayed speech development should also have their hearing tested.

Children with some symptoms of an ASD but not enough to be diagnosed with classical autism are often diagnosed with PDD-NOS. Children with autistic behaviors but well-developed language skills are often diagnosed with Asperger syndrome. Much rarer are children who may be diagnosed with childhood disintegrative disorder, in which they develop normally and then suddenly deteriorate between the ages of 3 to 10 years and show marked autistic behaviors.

What causes autism?

Scientists aren't certain about what causes ASD, but it's likely that both genetics and environment play a role. Researchers have identified a number of genes associated with the disorder. Studies of people with ASD have found irregularities in several regions of the brain. Other studies suggest that people with ASD have abnormal levels of serotonin or other neurotransmitters in the brain. These abnormalities suggest that ASD could result from the disruption of normal brain development early in fetal development caused by defects in genes that control brain growth and that regulate how brain cells communicate with each other, possibly due to the influence of environmental factors on gene function. While these findings are intriguing, they are preliminary and require further study. The theory that parental practices are responsible for ASD has long been disproved.

What role does inheritance play?

Twin and family studies strongly suggest that some people have a genetic predisposition to autism. Identical twin studies show that if one twin is affected, there is up to a 90% chance the other twin will be affected. There are a number of studies in progress to determine the specific genetic factors associated with the development of ASD. In families with one child with ASD, the risk of having a second child with the disorder is approximately 5%, or one in 20. This is greater than the risk for the general population. Researchers are looking for clues about which genes contribute to this increased susceptibility. In some cases, parents and other relatives of a child with ASD show mild impairments in social and communicative skills or engage in repetitive behaviors. Evidence also suggests that some emotional disorders, such as bipolar disorder, occur more frequently than average in the families of people with ASD.

Do symptoms of autism change over time?

For many children, symptoms improve with treatment and with age. Children whose language skills regress early in life—before the age of three—appear to have a higher than normal risk of developing epilepsy or seizure-like brain activity. During adolescence, some children with an ASD may become depressed or experience behavioral problems, and their treatment may need some modification as they transition to adulthood. People with an ASD usually continue to need services and supports as they get older, but many are able to work successfully and live independently or within a supportive environment.

How is autism treated?

There is no cure for ASDs. Therapies and behavioral interventions are designed to remedy specific symptoms and can bring about substantial improvement. The ideal treatment plan coordinates therapies and interventions that meet the specific needs of individual children. Most health care professionals agree that the earlier the intervention, the better.

- **Educational/behavioral interventions:** Therapists use highly structured and intensive skill-oriented training sessions to help children develop social and language skills, such as Applied Behavioral Analysis. Family counseling for the parents and siblings of children with an ASD often helps families cope with the particular challenges of living with a child with an ASD.

- **Medications:** Doctors may prescribe medications for treatment of specific autism-related symptoms, such as anxiety, depression, or obsessive-compulsive disorder. Antipsychotic medications are used to treat severe behavioral problems. Seizures can be treated with one or more anticonvulsant drugs. Medication used to treat people with attention deficit disorder can be used effectively to help decrease impulsivity and hyperactivity.

- **Other therapies:** There are a number of controversial therapies or interventions available, but few, if any, are supported by scientific studies. Parents should use caution before adopting any unproven treatments. Although dietary interventions have been helpful in some children, parents should be careful that their child's nutritional status is carefully followed.

Chapter 31

Attention Deficit Hyperactivity Disorder

Attention deficit hyperactivity disorder (ADHD) is one of the most common childhood disorders and can continue through adolescence and adulthood. Symptoms include difficulty staying focused and paying attention, difficulty controlling behavior, and hyperactivity (overactivity).

ADHD has three subtypes:

- **Predominantly hyperactive-impulsive:** Most symptoms (six or more) are in the hyperactivity-impulsivity categories. Fewer than six symptoms of inattention are present, although inattention may still be present to some degree.

- **Predominantly inattentive:** The majority of symptoms (six or more) are in the inattention category and fewer than six symptoms of hyperactivity-impulsivity are present, although hyperactivity-impulsivity may still be present to some degree.

  Children with this subtype are less likely to act out or have difficulties getting along with other children. They may sit quietly, but they are not paying attention to what they are doing. Therefore, the child may be overlooked, and parents and teachers may not notice that he or she has ADHD.

- **Combined hyperactive-impulsive and inattentive:** Six or more symptoms of inattention and six or more symptoms of

This chapter excerpted from "Attention Deficit Hyperactivity Disorder (ADHD)," National Institute of Mental Health (www.nimh.nih.gov), 2008.

hyperactivity-impulsivity are present. Most children have the combined type of ADHD.

Treatments can relieve many of the disorder's symptoms, but there is no cure. With treatment, most people with ADHD can be successful in school and lead productive lives. Researchers are developing more effective treatments and interventions, and using new tools such as brain imaging, to better understand ADHD and to find more effective ways to treat and prevent it.

Symptoms in Children

Inattention, hyperactivity, and impulsivity are the key behaviors of ADHD. It is normal for all children to be inattentive, hyperactive, or impulsive sometimes, but for children with ADHD, these behaviors are more severe and occur more often. To be diagnosed with the disorder, a child must have symptoms for six or more months and to a degree that is greater than other children of the same age.

Children who have symptoms of inattention show these symptoms:

- Be easily distracted, miss details, forget things, and frequently switch from one activity to another

- Have difficulty focusing on one thing

- Become bored with a task after only a few minutes, unless they are doing something enjoyable

- Have difficulty focusing attention on organizing and completing a task or learning something new

- Have trouble completing or turning in homework assignments, often losing things (e.g., pencils, toys, assignments) needed to complete tasks or activities

- Do not seem to listen when spoken to

- Daydream, become easily confused, and move slowly

- Have difficulty processing information as quickly and accurately as others

- Struggle to follow instructions

Children who have symptoms of hyperactivity may show these signs:

- Fidget and squirm in their seats

- Talk nonstop

- Dash around, touching or playing with anything and everything in sight

- Have trouble sitting still during dinner, school, and story time

- Be constantly in motion

- Have difficulty doing quiet tasks or activities

Children who have symptoms of impulsivity may show these characteristics:

- Be very impatient

- Blurt out inappropriate comments, show their emotions without restraint, and act without regard for consequences

- Have difficulty waiting for things they want or waiting their turns in games

- Often interrupt conversations or others' activities

Causes

Scientists are not sure what causes ADHD, although many studies suggest that genes play a large role. Like many other illnesses, ADHD probably results from a combination of factors. In addition to genetics, researchers are looking at possible environmental factors, and are studying how brain injuries, nutrition, and the social environment might contribute to ADHD.

Genes: Inherited from our parents, genes are the "blueprints" for who we are. Results from several international studies of twins show that ADHD often runs in families. Researchers are looking at several genes that may make people more likely to develop the disorder. Knowing the genes involved may one day help researchers prevent the disorder before symptoms develop. Learning about specific genes could also lead to better treatments.

Environmental factors: Studies suggest a potential link between cigarette smoking and alcohol use during pregnancy and ADHD in children. In addition, preschoolers who are exposed to high levels of lead, which can sometimes be found in plumbing fixtures or paint in old buildings, may have a higher risk of developing ADHD.

Brain injuries: Children who have suffered a brain injury may show some behaviors similar to those of ADHD. However, only a small percentage of children with ADHD have suffered a traumatic brain injury.

Sugar: The idea that refined sugar causes ADHD or makes symptoms worse is popular, but more research discounts this theory than supports it. In one study, researchers gave children foods containing either sugar or a sugar substitute every other day. The children who received sugar showed no different behavior or learning capabilities than those who received the sugar substitute.

In another study, children who were considered sugar-sensitive by their mothers were given the sugar substitute aspartame, also known as NutraSweet. Although all the children got aspartame, half their mothers were told their children were given sugar, and the other half were told their children were given aspartame. The mothers who thought their children had gotten sugar rated them as more hyperactive than the other children and were more critical of their behavior, compared to mothers who thought their children received aspartame.

Food additives: Recent British research indicates a possible link between consumption of certain food additives like artificial colors or preservatives and an increase in activity. Research is under way to confirm the findings and to learn more about how food additives may affect hyperactivity.

Diagnosis

Children mature at different rates and have different personalities, temperaments, and energy levels. Most children get distracted, act impulsively, and struggle to concentrate at one time or another. Sometimes, these normal factors may be mistaken for ADHD. ADHD symptoms usually appear early in life, often between the ages of three and six, and because symptoms vary from person to person, the disorder can be hard to diagnose. Parents may first notice that their child loses interest in things sooner than other children or seems constantly "out of control." Often, teachers notice the symptoms first, when a child has trouble following rules or frequently "spaces out" in the classroom or on the playground.

No single test can diagnose a child as having ADHD. Instead, a licensed health professional needs to gather information about the child and his or her behavior and environment. A family may want to first talk with the child's pediatrician. Some pediatricians can assess the child themselves, but many will refer the family to a mental health specialist with experience in childhood mental disorders such as ADHD. The pediatrician or mental health specialist will first try to rule out other possibilities for the symptoms. For example, certain situations, events, or health conditions may cause temporary behaviors in a child that seem like ADHD.

Between them, the referring pediatrician and specialist will determine if a child exhibits any of these characteristics:

- Is experiencing undetected seizures that could be associated with other medical conditions

- Has a middle ear infection that is causing hearing problems

- Has any undetected hearing or vision problems

- Has any medical problems that affect thinking and behavior

- Has any learning disabilities

- Has anxiety or depression, or other psychiatric problems that might cause ADHD-like symptoms

- Has been affected by a significant and sudden change, such as the death of a family member, a divorce, or parent's job loss

A specialist will also check school and medical records for clues, to see if the child's home or school settings appear unusually stressful or disrupted, and gather information from the child's parents and teachers. Coaches, babysitters, and other adults who know the child well also may be consulted.

The specialist pays close attention to the child's behavior during different situations. Some situations are highly structured, some have less structure. Others would require the child to keep paying attention. Most children with ADHD are better able to control their behaviors in situations where they are getting individual attention and when they are free to focus on enjoyable activities.

Finally, if after gathering all this information the child meets the criteria for ADHD, he or she will be diagnosed with the disorder.

Treatment

Currently available treatments focus on reducing the symptoms of ADHD and improving functioning. Treatments include medication, various types of psychotherapy, education, or training, or a combination of treatments.

Medications

The most common type of medication used for treating ADHD is called a "stimulant." Although it may seem unusual to treat ADHD with a medication considered a stimulant, it actually has a calming effect on children with ADHD. Many types of stimulant medications are available. A few other ADHD medications are non-stimulants and work differently than stimulants. For many children, ADHD medications reduce hyperactivity and impulsivity and improve their ability to focus, work, and learn. Medication also may improve physical coordination.

However, a one-size-fits-all approach does not apply for all children with ADHD. What works for one child might not work for another. Sometimes several different medications or dosages must be tried before finding one that works for a particular child.

The most commonly reported side effects are decreased appetite, sleep problems, anxiety, and irritability. Some children also report mild stomachaches or headaches. Most side effects are minor and disappear over time or if the dosage level is lowered.

Psychotherapy

Different types of psychotherapy are used for ADHD. Behavioral therapy aims to help a child change his or her behavior. It might involve practical assistance, such as help organizing tasks or completing schoolwork, or working through emotionally difficult events. Behavioral therapy also teaches a child how to monitor his or her own behavior. Learning to give oneself praise or rewards for acting in a desired way, such as controlling anger or thinking before acting, is another goal of behavioral therapy. Parents and teachers also can give positive or negative feedback for certain behaviors. In addition, clear rules, chore lists, and other structured routines can help a child control his or her behavior.

Therapists may teach children social skills, such as how to wait their turn, share toys, ask for help, or respond to teasing. Learning to read facial expressions and the tone of voice in others, and how to respond appropriately, can also be part of social skills training.

The Role of Parents

Children with ADHD need guidance and understanding from their parents and teachers to reach their full potential and to succeed in school. Before a child is diagnosed, frustration, blame, and anger may have built up within a family. Parents and children may need special help to overcome bad feelings. Mental health professionals can educate parents about ADHD and how it impacts a family. They also will help the child and his or her parents develop new skills, attitudes, and ways of relating to each other.

Parenting skills training helps parents learn how to use a system of rewards and consequences to change a child's behavior. Parents are taught to give immediate and positive feedback for behaviors they want to encourage, and ignore or redirect behaviors they want to discourage.

Parents are also encouraged to share a pleasant or relaxing activity with the child, to notice and point out what the child does well, and to praise the child's strengths and abilities. They may also learn to structure situations in more positive ways.

Sometimes, the whole family may need therapy. Therapists can help family members find better ways to handle disruptive behaviors and to encourage behavior changes. Finally, support groups help parents and families connect with others who have similar problems and concerns.

Coexisting Conditions

Some children with ADHD also have other illnesses or conditions. For example, they may have one or more of the following:

- **A learning disability:** A child in preschool with a learning disability may have difficulty understanding certain sounds or words or have problems expressing himself or herself in words. A school-aged child may struggle with reading, spelling, writing, and math.

- **Oppositional defiant disorder:** Kids with this condition, in which a child is overly stubborn or rebellious, often argue with adults and refuse to obey rules.

- **Conduct disorder:** This condition includes behaviors in which the child may lie, steal, fight, or bully others. He or she may destroy property, break into homes, or carry or use weapons

- **Anxiety and depression:** Treating ADHD may help to decrease anxiety or some forms of depression.

- **Bipolar disorder:** Some children with ADHD may also have this condition in which extreme mood swings go from mania (an extremely high elevated mood) to depression in short periods of time.

- **Tourette syndrome:** Very few children have this brain disorder, but among those who do, many also have ADHD. Some people with Tourette syndrome have nervous tics and repetitive mannerisms, such as eye blinks, facial twitches, or grimacing. Others clear their throats, snort, or sniff frequently, or bark out words inappropriately. These behaviors can be controlled with medication.

ADHD also may coexist with a sleep disorder, bedwetting, substance abuse, or other disorders or illnesses.

Chapter 32

Conduct and Oppositional Disorders

Conduct Disorder

Conduct disorder is a disorder of childhood and adolescence that involves long-term (chronic) behavior problems, such as:

- defiant or impulsive behavior;
- drug use;
- criminal activity.

Causes

Conduct disorder has been associated with:

- child abuse;
- drug addiction or alcoholism in the parents;
- family conflicts;
- genetic defects;
- poverty.

The diagnosis is more common among boys.

It is hard to know how common the disorder is, because many of the qualities needed to make the diagnosis (such as "defiance" and "rule breaking") can be hard to define. For an accurate diagnosis, the behavior must be far more extreme than simple adolescent rebellion or boyish enthusiasm.

Conduct disorder is often associated with attention-deficit disorder. Both conditions carry a risk for alcohol or other drug addiction.

Conduct disorder also can be an early sign of depression or bipolar disorder.

Symptoms

Children with conduct disorder tend to be impulsive, hard to control, and not concerned about the feelings of other people.

Symptoms may include:

- breaking rules without obvious reason;
- cruel or aggressive behavior toward people or animals (for example: bullying, fighting, using dangerous weapons, forcing sexual activity, and stealing);
- failure to attend school (truancy— beginning before age 13);
- heavy drinking and/or heavy illicit drug use;
- intentionally setting fires;
- lying to get a favor or avoid things they have to do;
- running away;
- vandalizing or destroying property.

These children often make no effort to hide their aggressive behaviors. They may have a hard time making real friends.

Exams and Tests

There is no real test for diagnosing conduct disorder. The diagnosis is made when a child or adolescent has a history of conduct disorder behaviors.

A physical examination and blood tests can help rule out medical conditions that are similar to conduct disorder. Rarely, a brain scan may also help rule out other disorders.

Treatment

For treatment to be successful, the child's family needs to be closely involved. Parents can learn techniques to help manage their child's problem behavior.

In cases of abuse, the child may need to be removed from the family and placed in a less chaotic home. Treatment with medications or talk therapy may be used for depression and attention-deficit disorder, which commonly occur with conduct disorder.

Many "behavioral modification" schools, "wilderness programs," and "boot camps" are sold to parents as solutions for conduct disorder. These programs may use a form of "attack therapy" or "confrontation," which can actually be harmful. There is no research to support these techniques. Research suggests that treating children at home, along with their families, is more effective.

If you are considering an inpatient program, be sure to check it out thoroughly. Serious injuries and deaths have occurred with some programs. They are not regulated in many states.

Possible Complications

Children with conduct disorder may go on to develop personality disorders as adults, particularly antisocial personality disorder. As their behaviors worsen, these individuals may also develop drug and legal problems.

Depression and bipolar disorder may develop in adolescence and early adulthood. Suicide and violence toward others are also possible complications of this disorder.

When to Contact a Medical Professional

See your health care provider if your child:

- regularly gets in trouble;
- has mood swings;
- is bullying others or cruel to animals;
- is being victimized;
- seems to be overly aggressive.

Early treatment may help.

Oppositional Defiant Disorder

Oppositional defiant disorder is a pattern of disobedient, hostile, and defiant behavior toward authority figures.

Causes

This disorder is more common in boys than in girls. Some studies have shown that it affects 20% of school-age children. However, most experts believe this figure is high due to changing definitions of normal childhood behavior, and possible racial, cultural, and gender biases.

This behavior typically starts by age eight, but it may start as early as the preschool years. This disorder is thought to be caused by a combination of biological, psychological, and social factors.

Symptoms

- Actively does not follow adults' requests

- Angry and resentful of others

- Argues with adults

- Blames others for own mistakes

- Has few or no friends or has lost friends

- Is in constant trouble in school

- Loses temper

- Spiteful or seeks revenge

- Touchy or easily annoyed

To fit this diagnosis, the pattern must last for at least six months and must be more than normal childhood misbehavior.

The pattern of behaviors must be different from those of other children around the same age and developmental level. The behavior must lead to significant problems in school or social activities.

Exams and Tests

Children with symptoms of this disorder should be evaluated by a psychiatrist or psychologist. In children and adolescents, the following conditions can cause similar behavior problems and should be considered as possibilities:

- Anxiety disorders

- Attention-deficit /hyperactivity disorder (ADHD)

- Bipolar disorder

- Depression

- Learning disorders

- Substance abuse disorders

Treatment

The best treatment for the child is to talk with a mental health professional in individual and possibly family therapy. The parents should also learn how to manage the child's behavior.

Medications may also be helpful, especially if the behaviors occur as part of another condition (such as depression, childhood psychosis, or ADHD).

Possible Complications

In many cases, children with oppositional defiant disorder grow up to have conduct disorder as teenagers or adults. In some cases children may grow up to have antisocial personality disorder.

When to Contact a Medical Professional

Call your health care provider if you have concerns about your child's development or behavior.

Prevention

Be consistent about rules and consequences at home. Don't make punishments too harsh or inconsistent.

Model the right behaviors for your child. Abuse and neglect increase the chances that this condition will occur.

Chapter 33

Developmental Disorders and Disorders that Affect Learning

Chapter Contents

Section 33.1

Auditory Processing Disorder

This section excerpted from "Auditory Processing Disorder in Children,"
National Institute on Deafness and Other Communication Disorders
(www.nidcd.nih.gov), June 7, 2010.

What is auditory processing?

Auditory processing is a term used to describe what happens when
your brain recognizes and interprets the sounds around you. Humans
hear when energy that we recognize as sound travels through the ear
and is changed into electrical information that can be interpreted by
the brain. The "disorder" part of auditory processing disorder means
that something is adversely affecting the processing or interpretation
of the information.

Children with auditory processing disorder (APD) often do not recognize subtle differences between sounds in words, even though the
sounds themselves are loud and clear. For example, the request "Tell me
how a chair and a couch are alike" may sound to a child with APD like
"Tell me how a couch and a chair are alike." It can even be understood
by the child as "Tell me how a cow and a hair are alike." These kinds of
problems are more likely to occur when a person with APD is in a noisy
environment or when he or she is listening to complex information.

What causes auditory processing difficulty?

We are not sure. Human communication relies on taking in complicated perceptual information from the outside world through the senses, such as hearing, and interpreting that information in a meaningful
way. Human communication also requires certain mental abilities, such
as attention and memory. Scientists still do not understand exactly
how all of these processes work and interact or how they malfunction
in cases of communication disorders. Even though your child seems
to "hear normally," he or she may have difficulty using those sounds
for speech and language.

594

The cause of APD is often unknown. In children, auditory processing difficulty may be associated with conditions such as dyslexia, attention deficit disorder, autism spectrum disorder, specific language impairment, pervasive developmental disorder, or developmental delay.

What are the symptoms of possible auditory processing difficulty?

Children with auditory processing difficulty typically have normal hearing and intelligence. However, they have also been observed to do the following:

- Have trouble paying attention to and remembering information presented orally

- Have problems carrying out multistep directions

- Have poor listening skills

- Need more time to process information

- Have low academic performance

- Have behavior problems

- Have language difficulty (e.g., they confuse syllable sequences and have problems developing vocabulary and understanding language)

- Have difficulty with reading, comprehension, spelling, and vocabulary

How is suspected auditory processing difficulty diagnosed in children?

You, a teacher, or a day care provider may be the first person to notice symptoms of auditory processing difficulty in your child. So talking to your child's teacher about school or preschool performance is a good idea. Many health professionals can also diagnose APD in your child.

Much of what will be done by these professionals will be to rule out other problems. A pediatrician or a family doctor can help rule out possible diseases that can cause some of these same symptoms. If there is a disease or disorder related to hearing, you may be referred to an otolaryngologist—a physician who specializes in diseases and disorders of the head and neck.

To determine whether your child has a hearing function problem, an audiologic evaluation is necessary. An audiologist will give tests that can determine the softest sounds and words a person can hear and other tests to see how well people can recognize sounds in words and sentences.

A speech-language pathologist can find out how well a person understands and uses language. A mental health professional can give you information about cognitive and behavioral challenges that may contribute to problems in some cases, or he or she may have suggestions that will be helpful.

What treatments are available for auditory processing difficulty?

Much research is still needed to understand APD problems, related disorders, and the best intervention for each child or adult. Several strategies are available to help children with auditory processing difficulties. Any strategy selected should be used under the guidance of a team of professionals, and the effectiveness of the strategy needs to be evaluated. Researchers are currently studying a variety of approaches to treatment. Several strategies you may hear about include the following:

- Auditory trainers are electronic devices that allow a person to focus attention on a speaker and reduce the interference of background noise. They are often used in classrooms, where the teacher wears a microphone to transmit sound and the child wears a headset to receive the sound.

- Environmental modifications such as classroom acoustics, placement, and seating may help. An audiologist may suggest ways to improve the listening environment, and he or she will be able to monitor any changes in hearing status.

- Exercises to improve language-building skills can increase the ability to learn new words and increase a child's language base.

- Auditory memory enhancement, a procedure that reduces detailed information to a more basic representation, may help. Also, informal auditory training techniques can be used by teachers and therapists to address specific difficulties.

- Auditory integration training may be promoted by practitioners as a way to retrain the auditory system and decrease hearing distortion. However, current research has not proven the benefits of this treatment.

Section 33.2

Developmental Apraxia of Speech

This section excerpted from "Apraxia of Speech,"
National Institute on Deafness and Other Communication Disorders
(www.nidcd.nih.gov), June 7, 2010.

What is apraxia of speech?

Apraxia of speech, also known as verbal apraxia or dyspraxia, is a speech disorder in which a person has trouble saying what he or she wants to say correctly and consistently. It is not due to weakness or paralysis of the speech muscles (the muscles of the face, tongue, and lips). The severity of apraxia of speech can range from mild to severe.

What are the types and causes of apraxia?

There are two main types of speech apraxia: acquired apraxia of speech and developmental apraxia of speech. Acquired apraxia of speech can affect a person at any age, although it most typically occurs in adults. It is caused by damage to the parts of the brain that are involved in speaking and involves the loss or impairment of existing speech abilities. The disorder may result from a stroke, head injury, tumor, or other illness affecting the brain.

Developmental apraxia of speech (DAS) occurs in children and is present from birth. It appears to affect more boys than girls. DAS is different from what is known as a developmental delay of speech, in which a child follows the "typical" path of speech development but does so more slowly than normal.

The cause or causes of DAS are not yet known. Some scientists believe that DAS is a disorder related to a child's overall language development. Others believe it is a neurological disorder that affects the brain's ability to send the proper signals to move the muscles involved in speech. However, brain imaging and other studies have not found evidence of specific brain lesions or differences in brain structure in children with DAS. Children with DAS often have family members who have a history of communication disorders or learning disabilities. This observation and recent research findings suggest that genetic factors may play a role in the disorder.

What are the symptoms?

People with either form of apraxia of speech may have a number of different speech characteristics, or symptoms. One of the most notable symptoms is difficulty putting sounds and syllables together in the correct order to form words. Longer or more complex words are usually harder to say than shorter or simpler words. People with apraxia of speech also tend to make inconsistent mistakes when speaking. For example, they may say a difficult word correctly but then have trouble repeating it, or they may be able to say a particular sound one day and have trouble with the same sound the next day. People with apraxia of speech often appear to be groping for the right sound or word, and may try saying a word several times before they say it correctly. Another common characteristic of apraxia of speech is the incorrect use of "prosody"—that is, the varying rhythms, stresses, and inflections of speech that are used to help express meaning.

Children with developmental apraxia of speech generally can understand language much better than they are able to use language to express themselves. Some children with the disorder may also have other problems. These can include other speech problems, such as dysarthria; language problems such as poor vocabulary, incorrect grammar, and difficulty in clearly organizing spoken information; problems with reading, writing, spelling, or math; coordination or "motor-skill" problems; and chewing and swallowing difficulties.

The severity of both acquired and developmental apraxia of speech varies from person to person. Apraxia can be so mild that a person has trouble with very few speech sounds or only has occasional problems pronouncing words with many syllables. In the most severe cases, a person may not be able to communicate effectively with speech and may need the help of alternative or additional communication methods.

How is it diagnosed?

Professionals known as speech-language pathologists play a key role in diagnosing and treating apraxia of speech. There is no single factor or test that can be used to diagnose apraxia. In addition, speech-language experts do not agree about which specific symptoms are part of developmental apraxia. Ruling out other contributing factors, such as muscle weakness or language-comprehension problems, can also help with the diagnosis.

To diagnose developmental apraxia of speech, parents and professionals may need to observe a child's speech over a period of time. In formal testing for both acquired and developmental apraxia, the speech-language pathologist may ask the person to perform speech tasks such as repeating a particular word several times or repeating a list of words of increasing length (for example, love, loving, lovingly).

How is it treated?

In some cases, people with acquired apraxia of speech recover some or all of their speech abilities on their own. This is called spontaneous recovery. Children with developmental apraxia of speech will not outgrow the problem on their own. Speech-language therapy is often helpful for these children and for people with acquired apraxia who do not spontaneously recover all of their speech abilities.

Speech-language pathologists use different approaches to treat apraxia of speech, and no single approach has been proven to be the most effective. Therapy is tailored to the individual and is designed to treat other speech or language problems that may occur together with apraxia. Each person responds differently to therapy, and some people will make more progress than others. People with apraxia of speech usually need frequent and intensive one-on-one therapy. Support and encouragement from family members and friends are also important.

In severe cases, people with acquired or developmental apraxia of speech may need to use other ways to express themselves. These might include formal or informal sign language, a language notebook with pictures or written words that the person can show to other people, or an electronic communication device such as a portable computer that writes and produces speech.

Section 33.3

Developmental Delay

What is a developmental delay?

Child development refers to the process in which children go through changes in skill development during predictable time periods, called developmental milestones. Developmental delay occurs when children have not reached these milestones by the expected time period. For example, if the normal range for learning to walk is between 9 and 15 months, and a 20-month-old child has still not begun walking, this would be considered a developmental delay.

Developmental delays can occur in all five areas of development or may just happen in one or more of those areas. Additionally, growth in each area of development is related to growth in the other areas. So if there is a difficulty in one area (e.g., speech and language), it is likely to influence development in other areas (e.g., social and emotional).

What are the risk factors for developmental delay?

Risk factors for developmental problems fall into two categories:

- Genetic

- Environmental

Children are placed at genetic risk by being born with a genetic or chromosomal abnormality. A good example of a genetic risk is Down syndrome, a disorder that causes developmental delay because of an abnormal chromosome. Environmental risk results from exposure to harmful agents either before or after birth, and can include things like poor maternal nutrition or exposure to toxins (e.g., lead or drugs) or infections that are passed from a mother to her baby during pregnancy (e.g., measles or HIV). Environmental risk also includes a child's life experiences. For example, children who are born prematurely, face severe poverty, mother's depression, poor nutrition, or lack of care are at increased risk for developmental delays.

Risk factors have a cumulative impact upon development. As the number of risk factors increases, a child is put at greater risk for developmental delay.

What are the warning signs of a developmental delay?

There are several general "warning signs" of possible delay. These include:

- Behavioral warning signs:
  - Does not pay attention or stay focused on an activity for as long a time as other children of the same age
  - Focuses on unusual objects for long periods of time; enjoys this more than interacting with others
  - Avoids or rarely makes eye contact with others
  - Gets unusually frustrated when trying to do simple tasks that most children of the same age can do
  - Shows aggressive behaviors and acting out and appears to be very stubborn compared with other children
  - Displays violent behaviors on a daily basis
  - Stares into space, rocks body, or talks to self more often than other children of the same age
  - Does not seek love and approval from a caregiver or parent

- Gross motor warning signs:
  - Has stiff arms and/or legs
  - Has a floppy or limp body posture compared to other children of the same age
  - Uses one side of body more than the other
  - Has a very clumsy manner compared with other children of the same age
- Vision warning signs:

601

- Seems to have difficulty following objects or people with her eyes
- Rubs eyes frequently
- Turns, tilts, or holds head in a strained or unusual position when trying to look at an object
- Seems to have difficulty finding or picking up small objects dropped on the floor (after the age of 12 months)
- Has difficulty focusing or making eye contact
- Closes one eye when trying to look at distant objects
- Eyes appear to be crossed or turned
- Brings objects too close to eyes to see
- One or both eyes appear abnormal in size or coloring
- Hearing warning signs:
  - Talks in a very loud or very soft voice
  - Seems to have difficulty responding when called from across the room, even when it is for something interesting
  - Turns body so that the same ear is always turned toward sound
  - Has difficulty understanding what has been said or following directions after she has turned three years of age
  - Doesn't startle to loud noises
  - Ears appear small or deformed
  - Fails to develop sounds or words that would be appropriate at her age

In addition, because children usually acquire developmental milestones or skills during a specific time frame or "window," we can predict when most children will learn different skills. If a child is not learning a skill that other children are learning at the same age, that may be a "warning sign" that the child may be at risk for developmental delay. If a child has not learned these skills during a specific time frame, it does not mean your child is delayed. We would recommend, though, that you let your child's doctor know about your concerns.

How is a developmental delay identified?

Developmental delay is identified through two types of play-based assessments:

- Developmental screening

- Developmental evaluation

A developmental screening test is a quick and general measurement of skills. Its purpose is to identify children who are in need of further evaluation. A screening test can be in one of two formats, either a questionnaire that is handed to a parent or child care provider that asks about developmental milestones or a test that is given to your child by a health or educational professional.

A screening test is only meant to identify children who might have a problem. The screening test may either over-identify or under-identify children with delay. As a result, a diagnosis cannot be made simply by using a screening test. If the results of a screening test suggest a child may have a developmental delay, the child should be referred for a developmental evaluation.

A developmental evaluation is a long, in-depth assessment of a child's skills and should be administered by a highly trained professional, such as a psychologist. Evaluation tests are used to create a profile of a child's strengths and weaknesses in all developmental areas. The results of a developmental evaluation are used to determine if the child is in need of early intervention services and/or a treatment plan.

What are early intervention services?

Early intervention services include a variety of different resources and programs that provide support to families to enhance a child's development. These services are specifically tailored to meet a child's individual needs. Services include:

- assistive technology (devices a child might need);

- audiology or hearing services;

- counseling and training for a family;

- educational programs;

- medical services;

- nursing services;

- nutrition services;

- occupational therapy;

- physical therapy;

- psychological services;

- respite services;
- speech/language.

These services are provided by public agencies and private organizations for children who are found to be eligible for these services after a developmental evaluation.

Why is early intervention important?

If a child is found on a developmental evaluation to have some developmental delays, it is important that intervention occurs early on in childhood for a number of reasons. Generally, children need to learn these developmental skills in a consecutive fashion. For example, a child needs to learn to sit up on her own before she will be able to stand up.

Also, early intervention helps a child advance in all areas of development. Sometimes if a child has a delay in one area (i.e., speech), it can affect other developmental areas (i.e., social and emotional). Therefore, it is vital that a child receive early intervention as soon as possible.

Finally, early intervention is critical for the child to develop good self-esteem. Without early intervention, a child's self-image may suffer and they may become avoidant of school. For example, a child who has a language delay may feel embarrassed to speak in front of their peers and teacher at school. Early intervention can help prevent these embarrassing moments for a child before they begin school.

What can I do if I am concerned that my child may have a developmental delay?

If you are concerned that your child may have a developmental delay, it is important to talk with your child's doctor. Your child's doctor can talk with you, examine your child, and refer you to agencies that help to screen or evaluate children for developmental delay. If your child's doctor does not know of such an agency or if you are more worried than your doctor, you can seek help on your own.

What is an Individualized Education Program (IEP)?

An IEP is a written document, ordered by federal law, that defines a child's disabilities, states current levels of academic performance, describes educational needs, and specifies annual goals and objectives. The unique needs of each child determine what specific programs and services are required. The IEP planning process can be very confusing for both parents and professionals. Here you will find answers to commonly asked questions about the IEP process.

How does the IEP process start and what can I expect?

- Talk about requesting an IEP with the child's teacher or doctor.

- Learn about the IEP process on the internet.

- Write a letter to the special education office or to the child's school principal requesting an assessment (and date your request). Even if the child is in private school, he or she can be evaluated by the school district.

- You should receive an assessment plan from the school within 15 days.

- You have 15 more days in which to agree to the school's assessment plan or request a different one.

- You should be invited to participate in an IEP meeting within 50 days. All testing must be completed by the meeting date.

What is an assessment plan?

- An assessment plan is a description of the various tests (cognitive, motor/perceptual, communication, social/emotional, and educational) to be used in a student's assessment in preparation for his or her IEP meeting. The assessment plan should:

  - be specific regarding which tests will be given (these should be individualized tests and NOT standardized tests given in a group situation);

  - match your child's perceived disabilities with a test or subtest that clearly assesses that area;

  - consider all information, including parental input and classroom performance.

How do I prepare for the IEP meeting?

- Talk to your child's teacher and doctor about their observations.

- Request copies of school and medical records at least 7 days before the IEP meeting. Parents are legally entitled to these results.

- Understand the test results describing your child's current levels of educational performance, including how your child compares to other children his or her age.

- Define for yourself your child's problem areas and strengths.

What will happen at the IEP planning meeting?

- At the planning meeting, the team will review the test results to determine if your child is eligible for an IEP. If your child qualifies for an IEP, the team will be developing educational and behavioral goals for your child at this meeting. Make sure to ask any questions you may have and pay attention to what is written on the IEP form.

- Remember this is a legal document. You are not required to sign it if you don't understand it or are not sure you agree with it.

What should the IEP include?

- An outline of your child's educational needs, including learning styles, teaching methods, and student-teacher ratio

- Written goals that match your child's specific needs with benchmarks to determine if an IEP is working on a yearly basis

- Standardized measurement criteria for assessing objectives

- Decision on the appropriate school placement and educational strategies for your child

- Stated plan for how often IEP reviews will occur

What is an Individualized Family Service Plan (IFSP)?

An IFSP is the coordination of services that are family centered. It is based on your child's strengths, as well as your concerns and priorities for your child. You can participate in the process of assessment by gathering information concerning your child's medical and developmental history, and also by making observations about his or her strengths and difficulties. The IFSP planning process can be very confusing for parents and professionals. Here you will find answers to commonly asked questions about the IFSP.

Who develops the IFSP?

- Along with your service coordinator, you have an active role in developing the service plan. You help decide which family members, friends, teachers, physicians, and other professionals should be included, and who will help to write the plan. You let the team know what you want for your child and for your family, and the team will work with you to achieve those goals.

- The IFSP should focus on your family's concerns and priorities, and should be supportive of your family's routine, values, and culture. It should also be clearly explained to you, and written in your family's language, if possible.

How do I prepare for the IFSP planning meeting?

- To prepare for an IFSP planning meeting, you can talk with other parents, learn more about your child's diagnosis, and list your questions and concerns to discuss with your service coordinator. It is especially important to identify needs for transportation, child care, and/or interpreters. Certain questions you may want to consider asking yourself and/or your service coordinator include:

  - What is needed for my child, and how will this be decided?

  - What services are available?

  - What are the options?

  - What will my family's new rights and responsibilities include?

What can I do during the planning meeting?

- Share information that you think is important. This could include medical records, a baby book, a growth chart, or other evaluations.

- Talk about your child, and discuss any concerns or questions you may have about his or her development.

- Consider how you will be involved in the processes of evaluation, assessment, and service planning.

- Decide who should be involved, including specific family members as well as others, such as another parent, a friend, or a child care provider.

- Consider which service delivery environment is best suited to meet your child's needs: home, child care setting, infant development program, etc.

What should the IFSP include?

- A statement of your child's level of development, from your own observations and from formal assessment measures (if necessary)

- A "family assessment," which is a statement of your family's resources and concerns as they relate to your child's development (with your permission)

- A statement of the outcomes you expect for your child and family, including how and when they will be achieved

- A statement of which early intervention services will be provided, and in what environments they will occur (such as your home, child care setting, or a school program)

- A statement of when services will begin, how often they will be provided, and how long they will continue

- A plan for transitions as your child's needs change (this must be included when your child approaches three years of age)

- The name of your service coordinator

How can I help my child meet these developmental milestones?

- Remember that the IFSP is not a finalized document. It is an ongoing process. Your child's needs may change quickly, so your family's IFSP should be reviewed at least every six months, and revised when necessary. If you think your services need to be changed, contact your service coordinator for an IFSP review.

- In early intervention, transitions happen whenever your child's services change to better meet both of your needs. Planning for transition requires your participation. Decisions concerning your child cannot be made without you, and no change can be made to the IFSP without your consent.

Section 33.4

Dyslexia

As with other learning disabilities, dyslexia is a lifelong challenge
that people are born with. This language processing disorder can hin-
der reading, writing, spelling, and sometimes even speaking. Dyslexia
is not a sign of poor intelligence or laziness. It is also not the result
of impaired vision. Children and adults with dyslexia simply have a
neurological disorder that causes their brains to process and interpret
information differently.

Dyslexia occurs among people of all economic and ethnic backgrounds. Often more than one member of a family has dyslexia. According to the National Institute of Child and Human Development,
as many as 15% of Americans have major troubles with reading.

Much of what happens in a classroom is based on reading and writing. So it's important to identify dyslexia as early as possible. Using alternate learning methods, people with dyslexia can achieve success.

What are the effects of dyslexia?

Dyslexia can affect people differently. This depends, in part, upon the
severity of the learning disability and the success of alternate learning
methods. Some with dyslexia can have trouble with reading and spelling,
while others struggle to write, or to tell left from right. Some children
show few signs of difficulty with early reading and writing. But later on,
they may have trouble with complex language skills, such as grammar,
reading comprehension, and more in-depth writing.

Dyslexia can also make it difficult for people to express themselves
clearly. It can be hard for them to use vocabulary and to structure their
thoughts during conversation. Others struggle to understand when people speak to them. This isn't due to hearing problems. Instead, it's from
trouble processing verbal information. It becomes even harder with abstract thoughts and non-literal language, such as jokes and proverbs.

All of these effects can have a big impact on a person's self-image. Without help, children often get frustrated with learning. The stress of dealing with schoolwork often makes children with dyslexia lose the motivation to continue and overcome the hurdles they face.

What are the warning signs?

The following are common signs of dyslexia in people of different ages. If you or someone you know displays these signs, it doesn't necessarily mean you have a learning disability. But if troubles continue over time, consider testing for dyslexia.

Young children have trouble with:

- recognizing letters, matching letters to sounds, and blending sounds into speech;
- pronouncing words, for example saying "mawn lower" instead of "lawn mower";
- learning and correctly using new vocabulary words;
- learning the alphabet, numbers, and days of the week or similar common word sequences;
- rhyming.

School-age children have trouble with:

- mastering the rules of spelling;
- remembering facts and numbers;
- handwriting or with gripping a pencil;
- learning and understanding new skills—instead, relying heavily on memorization;
- reading and spelling, such as reversing letters (d, b) or moving letters around (left, felt);
- following a sequence of directions;
- trouble with word problems in math.

Teenagers and adults have trouble with:

- reading at the expected level;
- understanding non-literal language, such as idioms, jokes, or proverbs;

- reading aloud;

- organizing and managing time;

- trouble summarizing a story;

- learning a foreign language;

- memorizing.

How is dyslexia identified?

Trained professionals can identify dyslexia using a formal evaluation. This looks at a person's ability to understand and use spoken and written language. It looks at areas of strength and weakness in the skills that are needed for reading. It also takes into account many other factors. These include family history, intellect, educational background, and social environment.

How is dyslexia treated?

It helps to identify dyslexia as early in life as possible. Adults with unidentified dyslexia often work in jobs below their intellectual capacity. But with help from a tutor, teacher, or other trained professional, almost all people with dyslexia can become good readers and writers. Use the following strategies to help to make progress with dyslexia.

- Expose your child to early oral reading, writing, drawing, and practice to encourage development of print knowledge, basic letter formation, recognition skills, and linguistic awareness (the relationship between sound and meaning).

- Have your child practice reading different kinds of texts. This includes books, magazines, ads, and comics.

- Include multi-sensory, structured language instruction. Practice using sight, sound, and touch when introducing new ideas.

- Seek modifications in the classroom. This might include extra time to complete assignments, help with note taking, oral testing, and other means of assessment.

- Use books on tape and assistive technology. Examples are screen readers and voice recognition computer software.

- Get help with the emotional issues that arise from struggling to overcome academic difficulties.

Reading and writing are key skills for daily living. However, it is important to also emphasize other aspects of learning and expression. Like all people, those with dyslexia enjoy activities that tap into their strengths and interests. For example, people with dyslexia may be attracted to fields that do not emphasize language skills. Examples are design, art, architecture, engineering, and surgery.

Section 33.5

Learning Disabilities

This section excerpted from "Learning Disabilities (LD),"
National Dissemination Center for Children with Disabilities
(nichcy.org), January 2011.

What are learning disabilities?

Learning disability is a general term that describes specific kinds of learning problems. A learning disability can cause a person to have trouble learning and using certain skills. The skills most often affected are: reading, writing, listening, speaking, reasoning, and doing math.

"Learning disabilities" is not the only term used to describe these difficulties:

- **Dyslexia** refers to difficulties in reading.

- **Dysgraphia** refers to difficulties in writing.

- **Dyscalculia** refers to difficulties in math.

All of these are considered learning disabilities.

Learning disabilities (LD) vary from person to person. One person with LD may not have the same kind of learning problems as another person with LD. Researchers think that learning disabilities are caused by differences in how a person's brain works and how it processes information. Children with learning disabilities are not "dumb" or "lazy." In fact, they usually have average or above average intelligence. Their brains just process information differently.

There is no "cure" for learning disabilities. They are life-long. However, children with LD can be high achievers and can be taught ways to get around the learning disability. With the right help, children with LD can and do learn successfully.

How common are learning disabilities?

Very common! As many as one out of every five people in the United States has a learning disability. Almost 1 million children (ages 6 through 21) have some form of a learning disability and receive special education in school. In fact, one-third of all children who receive special education have a learning disability.

What are the signs of a learning disability?

While there is no one "sign" that a person has a learning disability, there are certain clues. Most relate to elementary school tasks, because learning disabilities tend to be identified in elementary school. This is because school focuses on the very things that may be difficult for the child—reading, writing, math, listening, speaking, reasoning. A child probably won't show all of these signs, or even most of them. However, if a child shows a number of these problems, then parents and the teacher should consider the possibility that the child has a learning disability.

When a child has a learning disability, he or she may show these signs:

- May have trouble learning the alphabet, rhyming words, or connecting letters to their sounds
- May make many mistakes when reading aloud, and repeat and pause often
- May not understand what he or she reads
- May have real trouble with spelling
- May have very messy handwriting or hold a pencil awkwardly
- May struggle to express ideas in writing
- May learn language late and have a limited vocabulary
- May have trouble remembering the sounds that letters make or hearing slight differences between words
- May have trouble understanding jokes, comic strips, and sarcasm
- May have trouble following directions

- May mispronounce words or use a wrong word that sounds similar

- May have trouble organizing what he or she wants to say or not be able to think of the word he or she needs for writing or conversation

- May not follow the social rules of conversation, such as taking turns, and may stand too close to the listener

- May confuse math symbols and misread numbers

- May not be able to retell a story in order (what happened first, second, third)

- May not know where to begin a task or how to go on from there

If a child has unexpected problems learning to read, write, listen, speak, or do math, then teachers and parents may want to investigate more. The same is true if the child is struggling to do any one of these skills. The child may need to be evaluated to see if he or she has a learning disability.

The Evaluation Process

If you are concerned that your child may have a learning disability, contact his or her school and request that the school conduct an individualized evaluation under IDEA (Individuals with Disabilities Education Act, the nation's special education law) to see if, in fact, a learning disability is causing your child difficulties in school. Visit the National Dissemination Center for Children with Disabilities (NICHCY)'s website and read more about the evaluation process, beginning at: http://www.nichcy.org/schoolage/evaluation.

What if the school system declines to evaluate your child?

If the school doesn't think that your child's learning problems are caused by a learning disability, it may decline to evaluate your child. If this happens, there are specific actions you can take:

- Contact your state's Parent Training and Information Center (PTI) for assistance. Find your PTI by visiting http://www.parent centernetwork.org/parentcenterlisting.html.

- Consider having your child evaluated by an independent evaluator. You may have to pay for this evaluation, or you can ask that the school pay for it. To learn more about independent evaluations, visit NICHCY at http://www.nichcy.org/schoolage/parental -rights/iee.

- Ask for mediation, or use one of IDEA's other dispute resolution options. Parents have the right to disagree with the school's decision not to evaluate their child and be heard. To find out more about dispute resolution options, visit NICHCY at http://www .nichcy.org/schoolage/disputes/overview.

What is IDEA's definition of "specific learning disability"?

(10) Specific learning disability—(i) General. Specific learning disability means a disorder in one or more of the basic psychological processes involved in understanding or in using language, spoken or written, that may manifest itself in the imperfect ability to listen, think, speak, read, write, spell, or to do mathematical calculations, including conditions such as perceptual disabilities, brain injury, minimal brain dysfunction, dyslexia, and developmental aphasia.

(ii) Disorders not included. Specific learning disability does not include learning problems that are primarily the result of visual, hearing, or motor disabilities, of mental retardation, of emotional disturbance, or of environmental, cultural, or economic disadvantage. [34 CFR §300.8(c)(10)]

What are the additional evaluation procedures for LD?

The ways in which children are identified as having a learning disability have changed over the years. Until recently, the most common approach was to use a "severe discrepancy" formula. This referred to the gap, or discrepancy, between the child's intelligence or aptitude and his or her actual performance. However, IDEA now requires that school systems may provide the student with a research-based intervention and keep close track of the student's performance. Analyzing the student's response to that intervention may then be considered by school districts in the process of identifying that a child has a learning disability.

There are also other aspects required when evaluating children for LD. These include observing the student in his or her learning environment (including the regular education setting) to document academic performance and behavior in the areas of difficulty.

What about school?

Once a child is evaluated and found eligible for special education and related services, school staff and parents meet and develop what is known as an Individualized Education Program, or IEP. This document is very important in the educational life of a child with learning disabilities. It describes the child's needs and the services that the public school system will provide free of charge to address those needs. Learn more about the IEP, what it includes, and how it is developed, at http://www.nichcy.org/schoolage/iep.

Supports or changes in the classroom (called accommodations) help most students with LD. Accessible instructional materials (AIM) are among the most helpful to students whose LD affects their ability to read and process printed language. Assistive technology can also help many students work around their learning disabilities.

Tips and Resources for Parents

A child with learning disabilities may need help at home as well as in school. Here are a number of suggestions and considerations for parents.

- Learn about LD. The more you know, the more you can help yourself and your child.

- Praise your child when he or she does well. Children with LD are often very good at a variety of things. Find out what your child really enjoys doing, such as dancing, playing soccer, or working with computers. Give your child plenty of opportunities to pursue his or her strengths and talents.

- Find out the ways your child learns best. Does he or she learn by hands-on practice, looking, or listening? Help your child learn through his or her areas of strength.

- Let your son or daughter help with household chores. These can build self-confidence and concrete skills. Keep instructions simple, break down tasks into smaller steps, and reward your child's efforts with praise.

- Make homework a priority.

- Pay attention to your child's mental health (and your own!). Be open to counseling, which can help your child deal with frustration, feel better about himself or herself, and learn more about social skills.

- Talk to other parents whose children have LD. Parents can share practical advice and emotional support.

- Meet with school personnel and help develop an IEP to address your child's needs.

- Establish a positive working relationship with your child's teacher. Through regular communication, exchange information about your child's progress at home and at school.

Section 33.6

Stuttering

This section excerpted from "Stuttering," National Institute on Deafness and Other Communication Disorders (www.nidcd.nih.gov), March 2010.

What is stuttering?

Stuttering is a speech disorder in which sounds, syllables, or words are repeated or prolonged, disrupting the normal flow of speech. These speech disruptions may be accompanied by struggling behaviors, such as rapid eye blinks or tremors of the lips. Stuttering can make it difficult to communicate with other people, which often affects a person's quality of life.

Symptoms of stuttering can vary significantly throughout a person's day. In general, speaking before a group or talking on the telephone may make a person's stuttering more severe, while singing, reading, or speaking in unison may temporarily reduce stuttering.

Who stutters?

Roughly three million Americans stutter. Stuttering affects people of all ages. It occurs most often in children between the ages of two and five as they are developing their language skills. Approximately 5% of all children will stutter for some period in their life, lasting from a few weeks to several years. Boys are twice as likely to stutter as girls; as they get older, however, the number of boys who continue to stutter is three to four times larger than the number of girls. Most children outgrow stuttering. About 1% or less of adults stutter.

How is speech normally produced?

We make speech sounds through a series of precisely coordinated muscle movements involving breathing, phonation (voice production), and articulation (movement of the throat, palate, tongue, and lips). Muscle movements are controlled by the brain and monitored through our senses of hearing and touch.

What causes stuttering?

Although the precise mechanisms are not understood, there are two types of stuttering that are more common. (A third type of stuttering, called psychogenic stuttering, can be caused by emotional trauma or problems with thought or reasoning. At one time, all stuttering was believed to be psychogenic, but today we know that psychogenic stuttering is rare.)

Developmental stuttering: Developmental stuttering occurs in young children while they are still learning speech and language skills. It is the most common form of stuttering. Some scientists and clinicians believe that developmental stuttering occurs when children's speech and language abilities are unable to meet the child's verbal demands. Developmental stuttering also runs in families.

Neurogenic stuttering: Neurogenic stuttering may occur after a stroke, head trauma, or other type of brain injury. With neurogenic stuttering, the brain has difficulty coordinating the different components involved in speaking because of signaling problems between the brain and nerves or muscles.

How is stuttering diagnosed?

Stuttering is usually diagnosed by a speech-language pathologist (SLP), a health professional who is trained to test and treat individuals with voice, speech, and language disorders. The speech-language pathologist will consider a variety of factors, including the child's case history (such as when the stuttering was first noticed and under what circumstances), an analysis of the child's stuttering behaviors, and an evaluation of the child's speech and language abilities and the impact of stuttering on his or her life.

When evaluating a young child for stuttering, a speech-language pathologist will try to predict if the child is likely to continue his or her stuttering behavior or outgrow it. To determine this difference, the speech-language pathologist will consider such factors as the family's history of stuttering, whether the child's stuttering has lasted six months or longer, and whether the child exhibits other speech or language problems.

How is stuttering treated?

Although there is currently no cure for stuttering, there are a variety of treatments available. The nature of the treatment will differ based upon a person's age, communication goals, and other factors.

For very young children, early treatment may prevent developmental stuttering from becoming a lifelong problem. Certain strategies can help children learn to improve their speech fluency while developing positive attitudes toward communication. Health professionals generally recommend that a child be evaluated if he or she has stuttered for three to six months, exhibits struggle behaviors associated with stuttering, or has a family history of stuttering or related communication disorders. Some researchers recommend that a child be evaluated every three months to determine if the stuttering is increasing or decreasing. Treatment often involves teaching parents about ways to support their child's production of fluent speech. Parents may be encouraged to do the following:

- Provide a relaxed home environment that allows many opportunities for the child to speak. This includes setting aside time to talk to one another, especially when the child is excited and has a lot to say.

- Refrain from reacting negatively when the child stutters. Instead, parents should react to the stuttering as they would any other difficulty the child may experience in life. This may involve gentle corrections of the child's stuttering and praise for the child's fluent speech.

- Be less demanding on the child to speak in a certain way or to perform verbally for people, particularly if the child experiences difficulty during periods of high pressure.

- Speak in a slightly slowed and relaxed manner. This can help reduce time pressures the child may be experiencing.

- Listen attentively when the child speaks and wait for him or her to say the intended word. Don't try to complete the child's sentences. Also, help the child learn that a person can communicate successfully even when stuttering occurs.

- Talk openly and honestly to the child about stuttering if he or she brings up the subject. Let the child know that it is okay for some disruptions to occur.

Stuttering therapy: Many of the current therapies for teens and adults who stutter focus on learning ways to minimize stuttering when they speak, such as by speaking more slowly, regulating their breathing, or gradually progressing from single-syllable responses to longer words and more complex sentences. Most of these therapies also help address the anxiety a person who stutters may feel in certain speaking situations.

Drug therapy: The U.S. Food and Drug Administration (FDA) has not approved any drug for the treatment of stuttering. However, some drugs that are approved to treat other health problems—such as epilepsy, anxiety, or depression—have been used to treat stuttering. These drugs often have side effects that make them difficult to use over a long period of time. In a recent study, researchers concluded that drug therapy has been largely ineffective in controlling stuttering. Clinical trials of other possible drug treatments are currently underway.

Electronic devices: Some people who stutter use electronic devices to help control fluency. For example, one type of device fits into the ear canal, much like a hearing aid, and digitally replays a slightly altered version of the wearer's voice into the ear so that it sounds as if he or she is speaking in unison with another person. In some people, electronic devices help improve fluency in a relatively short period of time. Nevertheless, questions remain about how long such effects may last and whether people are able to easily use these devices in real-world situations. For these reasons, researchers are continuing to study the long-term effectiveness of these devices.

Self-help groups: Many people find that they achieve their greatest success through a combination of self-study and therapy. Self-help groups provide a way for people who stutter to find resources and support as they face the challenges of stuttering.

Chapter 34

Fragile X Syndrome

Facts about Fragile X Syndrome

Fragile X syndrome (FXS) is a genetic disorder. A genetic disorder means that there are changes to the person's genes. FXS is caused by changes in the fragile X mental retardation 1 (FMR1) gene. The FMR1 gene usually makes a protein called fragile X mental retardation protein (FMRP). FMRP is needed for normal brain development. People who have FXS do not make this protein. People who have other fragile X–associated disorders have changes in their FMR1 gene but usually make some of the protein.

FXS affects both males and females. However, females often have milder symptoms than males. The exact number of people who have FXS is unknown, but it has been estimated that about 1 in 5,000 males are born with the disorder.

Signs and Symptoms

Some, but not all, people with FXS have facial features that may become more noticeable with age. These features include the following:

- A large head
- A long face
- Prominent ears, chin, and forehead

This chapter excerpted from "Fragile X Syndrome (FXS), Facts about Fragile X Syndrome" and "Fragile X Syndrome (FXS): Data and Statistics," Centers for Disease Control and Prevention (www.cdc.gov), July 20, 2011.

Other signs that a child might have FXS include these symptoms:

- Developmental delays (not sitting, walking, or talking at the same time as other children the same age)

- Learning disabilities (trouble learning new skills)

- Social and behavior problems (such as not making eye contact, anxiety, trouble paying attention, hand flapping, acting and speaking without thinking, and being very active)

Males who have FXS usually have some degree of intellectual disability that can range from mild to severe. Females with FXS can have normal intelligence or some degree of intellectual disability with or without learning disabilities. Autism spectrum disorders (ASDs) also occur more frequently in people with FXS.

Diagnosis

FXS can be diagnosed by testing a person's DNA from a blood test. A doctor or genetic counselor can order the test. Testing also can be done to find changes in the FMR1 gene that can lead to fragile X–associated disorders.

A diagnosis of FXS can be helpful to the family because it can provide a reason for a child's intellectual disabilities and behavior problems. This allows the family and other caregivers to learn more about the disorder and manage care so that the child can reach his or her full potential. However, the results of DNA tests can affect other family members and raise many issues. So, anyone who is thinking about FXS testing should consider having genetic counseling prior to getting tested.

Treatments

There is no cure for FXS. However, treatment services can help people learn important skills. Services can include therapy to learn to talk, walk, and interact with others. In addition, medicine can be used to help control some issues, such as behavior problems. To develop the best treatment plan, people with FXS, parents, and health care providers should work closely with one another, and with everyone involved in treatment and support—which may include teachers, child care providers, coaches, therapists, and other family members. Taking advantage of all the resources available will help guide success.

Early intervention services help children from birth to three years old (36 months) learn important skills. These services may improve a child's development. Even if the child has not been diagnosed with FXS, he or she may be eligible for services. These services are provided through an early intervention system in each state. Through this system, you can ask for an evaluation. In addition, treatment for particular symptoms, such as speech therapy for language delays, often does not need to wait for a formal diagnosis. While early intervention is extremely important, treatment services at any age can be helpful.

Finding Support

Having support and community resources can help increase confidence in managing FXS, enhance quality of life, and assist in meeting the needs of all family members. It might be helpful for parents of children with FXS to talk with one another. One parent might have learned how to address some of the same concerns another parent has. Often, parents of children with special needs can give advice about good resources for these children.

Remember that the choices of one family might not be best for another family, so it's important that parents understand all options and discuss them with their child's health care providers.

- Contact the National Fragile X Foundation at 800-688-8765 or Treatment@FragileX.org to get information about treatments, educational strategies, therapies, and intervention.

- Parent to Parent (www.p2pusa.org) programs provide information and emotional support to families of children who have special needs.

Data and Statistics

Diagnosis

- The average age of FXS diagnosis of boys is 35 to 37 months. Girls are diagnosed at an average age of 42 months.

- Parents are usually the first to notice symptoms of FXS at about 12 months of age for boys and 16 months of age for girls.

  - Parents reported having to visit a physician repeatedly before the physician confirmed a developmental delay at an average age of 20 months of age for boys and 26 months of age for girls.

  - About 16 months typically passed between professional confirmation of a delay and the diagnosis of FXS.

- More than one third (37.6%) of families reported that more than 10 visits were required before the diagnosis of FXS.

Co-Occurring Conditions and Characteristics

A national parent survey found that a significant percentage of males and females with FXS had been diagnosed or treated for other co-occurring conditions.

Co-occurring conditions for males include the following:

- Developmental delay or intellectual disability: 96%

- Attention problems: 84%

- Anxiety: 70%

- Hyperactivity: 66%

- Autism: 46%

- Self-injury: 41%

- Aggressiveness: 38%

- Seizures: 18%

- Depression: 12%

Co-occurring conditions for females include the following:

- Attention problems: 67%

- Developmental delay or intellectual disability: 64%

- Anxiety: 56%

- Hyperactivity: 30%

- Depression: 22%

- Autism: 16%

- Aggressiveness: 14%

- Self-injury: 10%

- Seizures: 7%

Parents reported that 32% of the children with FXS currently experience sleep difficulties. Male children with FXS also have higher rates of obesity (31%) when compared with typically developing same-aged peers (18%).

Premutation

People with a fragile X premutation do not have fragile X syndrome but might have another fragile X–associated disorder. Some people with fragile X premutations have noticeable symptoms, and others do not.

- The exact number of people who have a fragile X premutation is unknown. It has been estimated that about 1 in 259 females and 1 in 813 males may be affected by a fragile X premutation.

Chapter 35

Mental Health
Disorders in Children

Chapter Contents

Section 35.1

Anxiety and Panic Disorders

What Is Anxiety?

Anxiety disorders are one of the most common mental health conditions in children and adolescents. While everyone may have occasional moments of feeling anxious or worried, an anxiety disorder is a medical condition that causes people to feel persistently, uncontrollably worried over an extended period of time. The disorder may result in significant distress in a number of settings, such as school, peer relationships, and home life, and it may dramatically affect people's lives by limiting their ability to engage in a variety of activities.

Anxiety that occurs in multiple settings, involving excessive apprehension about a number of situations on most days, is known as a generalized anxiety disorder. Generalized anxiety disorder (sometimes known as GAD) affects approximately 3% to 4% of children. Other anxiety disorders, which are triggered by more specific situations, include:

- social phobia or social anxiety—fear of meeting new people or of embarrassing oneself in social situations;

- specific phobia—fear of a particular object (for example, spider) or situation (for example, airplane travel);

- separation anxiety disorder—fear of separating from home or primary caregiver;

- panic disorder—unpredictable and repeated panic attacks unrelated to surrounding circumstances;

- obsessive-compulsive disorder—uncontrollable, repetitive thoughts and fears, often accompanied by repetitive behaviors intended to prevent the fears from being realized;

- selective mutism—persistent failure to speak in specific social situations (despite the physical ability to speak in other situations), most likely due to severe social anxiety.

The tendency to develop any anxiety disorder involves complex genetic and environmental factors, and it is possible for one person to have more than one anxiety disorder.

What Does Generalized Anxiety Disorder Look Like in Children and Adolescents?

Children with generalized anxiety disorder are often preoccupied with worries about their success in activities and their ability to obtain the approval of others. These children may have persistent thoughts of self-doubt that they are unable to control, and they constantly criticize themselves. Children may be preoccupied with being on time to events and insist on doing a task "perfectly." In contrast to the ordinary, occasional worries or fears experienced in childhood, generalized anxiety disorder persists for at least six months and affects children throughout the day (at home, at school, and with friends).

Children may appear inflexible or excessively worried about conforming to rules, or they may not be able to enjoy hobbies or other recreational activities. Some children may appear shy when, in fact, they are preoccupied with significant worries. Even if children are aware that their worries are more intense than is warranted by a situation, they may not be able to stop the worry. A trained clinician (such as a child psychiatrist, child psychologist, or pediatric neurologist) should integrate information from home, school, and the clinical visit to make a diagnosis.

At Home

At home, children with generalized anxiety disorder may have a combination of the symptoms listed here.

- Excessive worry and anxiety about a variety of matters on most days for at least six months; children may worry about school tasks, interactions with peers, being on time, and following rules (Worry about receiving approval is common. Children may worry about future activities, new experiences, or many other matters.)

- Frequent self-doubt and self-critical comments

- Inability to stop the worry despite parental reassurance

- Physical problems, including headaches, stomach ache, fatigue, and muscle tensions

- Signs of persistent anxiety, including restlessness, feeling "on edge," difficulty concentrating or relaxing, or mind going blank

- Irritability, which often increases with increased worry

- Sleep problems, which may include waking up early, waking up feeling unrested, or trouble falling asleep or staying asleep

- Experimentation with alcohol or drugs as a way to reduce suffering (Drugs and alcohol can themselves produce or worsen anxiety.)

- Depression or thoughts of not wanting to be alive in some situations if children believe there is no hope of reducing their symptoms

At School

At school, a child with generalized anxiety disorder may have a combination of the symptoms listed here.

- Excessive worry and anxiety about a variety of matters

- Repeated seeking of teacher approval

- An inability to explain the worries; children may not understand why they are so anxious

- Inability to stop the worry; despite adult reassurance, the worries continue

- Difficulty transitioning from home to school; children may develop difficulty entering school in the morning if they associate more worries with school (This may lead to late arrival times, long and tearful morning drop-offs, or tearful episodes at school.)

- Refusal or reluctance to attend school; anxiety may lead a child to insist on staying at home

- Avoidance of academic and peer activities

- Self-criticism and low self-esteem

- Difficulty concentrating due to persistent worry, which may affect a variety of school activities, from following directions and completing assignments to paying attention

- Other conditions, such as attention deficit hyperactivity disorder (ADHD), may also be present, compounding learning difficulties;

having one mental health condition does not "inoculate" the child from having other conditions as well

- Other anxiety disorders, such as social phobia, separation anxiety, or panic disorder; anxiety disorders may not be recognized both because children may try to hide symptoms and because their symptoms are experienced internally and may not be easily seen

- Learning disorders may co-exist and should not be overlooked in this population (A child's difficulties in school should not be presumed to be due entirely to anxiety. If the child still has academic difficulty after symptoms are treated, an educational evaluation for a learning disorder should be considered. A child's repeated reluctance to attend school may be an indicator of an undiagnosed learning disability.)

- Side effects from medications (Medications may have cognitive or behavioral effects or physically uncomfortable side effects that interfere with school performance. After a child begins receiving medical treatment for symptoms, any mood changes or new behaviors should be discussed with parents, as they can reflect medication side effects.)

At the Doctor's Office

A child's symptoms of generalized anxiety may be evident during an office visit when a child is reluctant to meet the clinician. This feature alone does not indicate a child has anxiety, since children routinely are nervous during office visits.

Clinicians may benefit from talking with parents, school staff, and other important caregivers to evaluate a child's functioning in each area to determine the underlying cause of the child's symptoms. Clinicians may encounter some of the following challenges in diagnosing and treating a child or adolescent with generalized anxiety.

- Symptoms vary over time and their appearance changes as a child grows. A clinician may need to see a child over time to determine the appropriate diagnosis.

- Other anxiety disorders may look like generalized anxiety disorder.

- Symptoms of mood disorders, such as depression and bipolar disorder, and behavior disorders, such as attention deficit hyperactivity disorder, can resemble the symptoms of anxiety. Depression is often identified in these children.

- Certain medical conditions can cause anxiety. These conditions include hyperthyroidism, hyperparathyroidism, hypoglycemia, cardiac disorders, seizure disorders, gastrointestinal problems, and vestibular or inner-ear disorders. Relevant laboratory tests and physical examinations may be helpful when a child has anxiety.

- Caffeine and other substances, such as stimulants, can produce anxiety. Consequently, evaluation for caffeine use and other substance use, especially with adolescents, is important.

- Physical complaints such as stomach aches, headaches, and dizziness often occur in children with anxiety. The clinician must determine whether these complaints warrant further medical investigation.

- Children may have difficulty talking about their worries. Phrasing questions with particular sensitivity and compassion may allow a more complete picture of symptoms to emerge.

- Children may be unaware, or unwilling to admit, that their feelings or behavior may indicate symptoms of a disorder.

- Families may need to be coached about what they can reasonably expect from their child. Children who suffer from any anxiety disorder will benefit if their family understands that therapy and medicines may reduce, but may not cure, symptoms.

How Is Generalized Anxiety Disorder Treated?

Generalized anxiety disorder is treatable through ongoing interventions provided by a child's medical practitioners, therapists, school staff, and family. These treatments include psychological interventions (counseling), biological interventions (medicines), and interventions at home and at school to reduce sources of stress for the child. Open, collaborative communication between a child's family, school, and treatment professionals optimizes the care and quality of life for the child with anxiety.

Psychological Interventions (Counseling)

Counseling can help children with anxiety, and everyone around them, to understand that their symptoms are caused by a disorder with complex genetic and environmental origins—not by flawed attitude or personality. Counseling also can reduce the impact of symptoms on daily life. Relaxation training can teach the child how to reduce both the worries and the accompanying physical symptoms. A variety of psychological interventions can be helpful, and parents should discuss their child's particular needs with their clinician to determine which psychological treatments could be most beneficial for their child.

- Individual psychotherapy is generally recommended as the first line of treatment for children and adolescents with generalized anxiety disorder. Children with anxiety may carry a sense of failure, as if the disorder was their fault. Individual psychotherapy can help reduce symptoms, and can help young people to become aware of and address their feelings of failure and self-blame.

- Cognitive behavior therapy (CBT) can teach young people new skills to reduce anxiety. In CBT, a child or adolescent is helped to become aware of and to describe anxiety-laden thought patterns. A trained clinician guides the child to think of new, more positive patterns of thinking. The young person is then given a chance to practice using these new thought patterns outside the clinical visit, and to discuss his or her experiences with the clinician afterwards. These methods are based upon well-researched practices that have helped many children and adolescents.

- Parent guidance sessions can help parents to manage their child's illness, identify effective parenting skills, learn how to function as a family despite the illness, and to address complex feelings that can arise when raising a child with a psychiatric disorder. Family therapy may be beneficial when issues are affecting the family as a whole.

- Group psychotherapy can be valuable to a child by providing a safe place to talk with other children who face adversity or allowing a child to practice social skills or symptom-combating skills in a carefully structured setting.

- School-based counseling can be effective in helping a child with anxiety navigate the social, behavioral, and academic demands of the school setting.

Biological Interventions (Medicines)

While psychotherapy may be sufficient to treat some children with anxiety, other children's symptoms do not improve significantly with psychotherapy alone. These children may benefit from medications.

The U.S. Food and Drug Administration (FDA) has not approved specific medications for the treatment of generalized anxiety disorder in children and adolescents. However, medications approved by the FDA for other uses and age groups are prescribed for young people with generalized anxiety disorder. The FDA allows doctors to use their best judgment to prescribe medication for conditions for which the medication has not specifically been approved.

The antidepressants Celexa, Lexapro, Luvox, Paxil, Prozac (fluoxetine), and Zoloft are commonly prescribed to treat the symptoms of anxiety. These medicines belong to a group of medications called selective serotonin reuptake inhibitors, or SSRIs.

In most cases these medicines begin to be effective in reducing symptoms after the child or adolescent has taken them for at least 2–4 weeks. Fully 12 weeks may be required in order to determine whether the medication is going to be effective for a particular individual. Medications should only be started, stopped, or adjusted under the direct supervision of a trained clinician.

There is no "best" medicine to treat generalized anxiety disorder, and it is important to remember that medicines usually reduce rather than eliminate symptoms. Different medicines or dosages may be needed at different times in a child's life or to address the emergence of particular symptoms. Successful treatment requires taking medicine daily as prescribed, allowing time for the medicine to work, and monitoring for both effectiveness and side effects. The family, clinician, and school should maintain frequent communication to ensure that medications are working as intended and to monitor and manage side effects.

The following cautions should be observed when any child or adolescent is treated with antidepressants.

- Benefits and risks should be evaluated. Questions have arisen about whether antidepressants can cause some children or adolescents to have suicidal thoughts. The evidence to date shows that antidepressants, when carefully monitored, have safely helped many children and adolescents. The latest reports on this issue from the U.S. Food and Drug Administration can be found on its website at www.fda.gov. Consideration of any medicine deserves a discussion with the prescribing clinician about its risks and benefits.

- Careful monitoring is recommended for any child receiving medication. Though most side effects occur soon after starting a medicine, adverse reactions can occur months after medicines are introduced. Agitation, restlessness, increased irritability, or comments about self-harm should be addressed immediately with the clinician if any of these symptoms emerge after the child starts an antidepressant. Frequent follow-up (weekly for the first month) is now advocated by the FDA for children starting an antidepressant.

- Some children who have generalized anxiety disorder may also have bipolar disorder. In some individuals with bipolar disorder, antidepressants may initially improve depressive symptoms but can sometimes worsen manic symptoms. While antidepressants do not "cause" bipolar disorder, they can unmask or worsen manic symptoms.

Helpful information about specific medications can be found at www.medlineplus.gov (click on "Drug Information") and in the book *Straight Talk about Psychiatric Medications for Kids (Revised Edition)* by Timothy E. Wilens, MD.

Interventions at Home

At home, as well as at school, providing a sympathetic and tolerant environment and making some adaptations may be helpful to aid a child or adolescent with anxiety.

- Understand the illness. Understanding the nature of anxiety and how it is experienced by the child will help parents sympathize with a child's struggles.

- Listen to the child's feelings. Isolation can foster low self-esteem and depression in children struggling with anxiety. The simple experience of being listened to empathically, without receiving advice, may have a powerful and helpful effect.

- Keep calm when a child becomes anxious about an event or matter. If a child sees a parent is able to remain calm, the child can model the parent's attitude.

- Reassure the child and gently note that he or she survived prior situations that caused anxiety.

- Teach relaxation techniques, including deep breathing, counting to 10, or visualizing a soothing place. Teaching children how to relax can empower them to develop mastery over symptoms and improve a sense of control over their body.

- Plan for transitions. Getting to school in the morning or preparing for bed in the evening may be complicated by fears and anxieties. Anticipating and planning for these transition times may be helpful for family members.

- Support the child's quick return to school, in the case of school refusal. The best way to reduce anxiety about school is to address specific causes of anxiety and help the child return to school as quickly as possible. A shorter school day may help until symptoms improve. Children's symptoms are more likely to decrease when they discover that they can survive the anxiety. Long absences are likely to cause higher levels of anxiety upon returning.

- Encourage the child's participation in activities that may provide a reprieve from worries.

- Praise the child's efforts to address symptoms. Young people often feel that they only hear about their mistakes. Even if improvements are small, every good effort deserves to be praised.

- Encourage the child to help develop interventions. Enlisting the child in the task will lead to more successful strategies and will foster the child's ability to problem-solve.

Interventions at School

There are many ways that schools can help a child with generalized anxiety disorder succeed in the classroom. Meetings between parents and school staff, such as teachers, guidance counselors, or nurses, will allow for collaboration to develop helpful school structure for the child. The child may need particular changes (accommodations/modifications) within a classroom. Examples of some accommodations, modifications, and school strategies include the following:

- Establish check-ins on arrival to facilitate transition into school.

- Accommodate late arrival due to difficulty with transitions.

- Because transitions may be particularly difficult for these children, allow extra time for moving to another activity or location. When a child with anxiety refuses to follow directions, for example, the reason may be symptoms of anxiety rather than intentional oppositionality.

- If the child is avoiding school, determine the cause of the child's reluctance and address it, initiate a plan to for him or her to return to school as quickly as possible. It may help ease anxiety if the child attends for a shorter school day temporarily.

- Identify a "safe" place where the child may go to reduce anxiety during stressful periods. Developing guidelines for appropriate use of the safe place will help both the student and staff.

- Develop relaxation techniques to help reduce anxiety at school. Employing the techniques developed at home can be useful.

- Provide alternative activities to distract the child from physical symptoms. Calming activities may be helpful.

- Encourage small group interactions to develop increased areas of competency.

- Provide assistance with peer interactions. An adult's help may be very beneficial for both the child and his or her peers.

- Encourage the child to help develop interventions. Enlisting the child in the task will lead to more successful strategies and will foster the child's ability to problem-solve.

- Reward a child's efforts. Every good effort deserves to be praised.

Flexibility and a supportive environment are essential for a student with generalized anxiety disorder to achieve success in school. School faculty and parents together may be able to identify patterns of difficulty and develop remedies to reduce a child's challenges at these times.

Section 35.2

Bipolar Disorder

This section excerpted from "Bipolar Disorder in Children and Teens: A Parent's Guide," National Institute of Mental Health (www.nimh.nih.gov), August 31, 2010.

Bipolar disorder, also known as manic-depressive illness, is a brain disorder that causes unusual shifts in mood and energy. It can also make it hard for someone to carry out day-to-day tasks, such as going to school or hanging out with friends. Symptoms of bipolar disorder are severe. They are different from the normal ups and downs that everyone goes through from time to time. They can result in damaged relationships, poor school performance, and even suicide. But bipolar disorder can be treated, and people with this illness can lead full and productive lives.

Bipolar disorder often develops in a person's late teens or early adult years, but some people have their first symptoms during childhood. At least half of all cases start before age 25.

Symptoms of Bipolar Disorder in Children and Teens

Youth with bipolar disorder experience unusually intense emotional states that occur in distinct periods called "mood episodes." An overly joyful or overexcited state is called a manic episode, and an extremely sad or hopeless state is called a depressive episode. Sometimes, a mood episode includes symptoms of both mania and depression. This is called a mixed state. People with bipolar disorder also may be explosive and irritable during a mood episode. Extreme changes in energy, activity, sleep, and behavior go along with these changes in mood.

Symptoms of mania include the following changes:

- Being in an overly silly or joyful mood that's unusual for your child

- Different from times when he or she might usually get silly and have fun

- Having an extremely short temper (an irritable mood that is unusual)

638

- Sleeping little but not feeling tired

- Talking a lot and having racing thoughts

- Having trouble concentrating, attention jumping from one thing to the next in an unusual way

- Talking and thinking about sex more often

- Behaving in risky ways more often, seeking pleasure a lot, and doing more activities than usual

Symptoms of depression include these changes:

- Being in a sad mood that lasts a long time

- Losing interest in activities they once enjoyed

- Feeling worthless or guilty

- Complaining about pain more often, such as headaches, stomach aches, and muscle pains

- Eating a lot more or less and gaining or losing a lot of weight

- Sleeping or oversleeping when these were not problems before

- Losing energy

- Recurring thoughts of death or suicide

It's normal for almost every child or teen to have some of these symptoms sometimes. These passing changes should not be confused with bipolar disorder. Bipolar symptoms are more extreme and tend to last for most of the day, nearly every day, for at least one week. Also, depressive or manic episodes include moods very different from a child's normal mood, and the behaviors may start at the same time. Sometimes the symptoms of bipolar disorder are so severe that the child needs to be treated in a hospital.

In addition to mania and depression, bipolar disorder can cause a range of moods. One side includes severe depression, moderate depression, and mild low mood. Moderate depression may cause less extreme symptoms, and mild low mood is called dysthymia when it is chronic or long-term. In the middle of the scale is normal or balanced mood.

Sometimes, a child may have more energy and be more active than normal but not show the severe signs of a full-blown manic episode. When this happens, it is called hypomania, and it generally lasts for at least four days in a row. Hypomania causes noticeable changes in behavior but does not harm a child's ability to function in the way mania does.

Risk of Getting Bipolar Disorder

Bipolar disorder tends to run in families. Children with a parent or sibling who has bipolar disorder are four to six times more likely to develop the illness, compared with children who do not have a family history of bipolar disorder. However, most children with a family history of bipolar disorder will not develop the illness. Compared with children whose parents do not have bipolar disorder, children whose parents have bipolar disorder may be more likely to have symptoms of anxiety disorders and ADHD.

Several studies show that youth with anxiety disorders are more likely to develop bipolar disorder than youth without anxiety disorders. However, anxiety disorders are very common in young people. Most children and teens with anxiety disorders do not develop bipolar disorder.

Early-Onset Bipolar Disorder

Bipolar disorder that starts during childhood or during the teen years is called early-onset bipolar disorder. Early-onset bipolar disorder seems to be more severe than the forms that first appear in older teens and adults. Youth with bipolar disorder are different from adults with bipolar disorder. Young people with the illness appear to have more frequent mood switches, are sick more often, and have more mixed episodes.

Watch out for any sign of suicidal thinking or behaviors. Take these signs seriously. On average, people with early-onset bipolar disorder have greater risk for attempting suicide than those whose symptoms start in adulthood. One large study on bipolar disorder in children and teens found that more than one-third of study participants made at least one serious suicide attempt. Some suicide attempts are carefully planned, and others are not. Either way, it is important to understand that suicidal feelings and actions are symptoms of an illness that must be treated.

Diagnosis

No blood tests or brain scans can diagnose bipolar disorder. However, a doctor may use tests like these to help rule out other possible causes for your child's symptoms. For example, the doctor may recommend testing for problems in learning, thinking, or speech and language. A careful medical exam may also detect problems that commonly co-occur with bipolar disorder and need to be treated, such as substance abuse.

Doctors who have experience with diagnosing early-onset bipolar disorder, such as psychiatrists, psychologists, or other mental health specialists, will ask questions about changes in your child's mood. They will also ask about sleep patterns, activity or energy levels, and if your child has had any other mood or behavioral disorders. The doctor may also ask whether there is a family history of bipolar disorder or other psychiatric illnesses, such as depression or alcoholism.

Treatment

To date, there is no cure for bipolar disorder. However, treatment with medications, psychotherapy (talk therapy), or both may help people get better.

To treat children and teens with bipolar disorder, doctors often rely on information about treating adults. This is because there haven't been many studies on treating young people with the illness, although several have been started recently.

One large study with adults found that treating adults with medications and intensive psychotherapy for about nine months helped them get better. These adults got better faster and stayed well longer than adults treated with less intensive psychotherapy for six weeks. Combining medication treatment and psychotherapies may help young people with early-onset bipolar disorder as well. However, it's important for you to know that children sometimes respond differently to psychiatric medications than adults do.

Medications

Before starting medication, the doctor will want to determine your child's physical and mental health. This is called a "baseline" assessment. Your child will need regular follow-up visits to monitor treatment progress and side effects. Most children with bipolar disorder will also need long-term or even lifelong medication treatment. This is often the best way to manage symptoms and prevent relapse, or a return of symptoms.

It's better to limit the number and dose of medications. A good way to remember this is "start low, go slow." Talk to the psychiatrist about using the smallest amount of medication that helps relieve your child's symptoms. To judge a medication's effectiveness, your child may need to take a medication for several weeks or months. The doctor needs this time to decide whether to switch to a different medication. Because children's symptoms are complex, it's not unusual for them to need more than one type of medication.

To date, lithium (sometimes known as Eskalith), risperidone (Risperdal), and aripiprazole (Abilify) are the only medications approved by the U.S. Food and Drug Administration (FDA) to treat bipolar disorder in young people.

Lithium is a type of medication called a mood stabilizer. It can help treat and prevent manic symptoms in children ages 12 and older. In addition, there is some evidence that lithium might act as an antidepressant and help prevent suicidal behavior. However, FDA's approval of lithium was based on treatment studies in adults. In fact, some experts say the FDA might not approve giving lithium to bipolar youth if the agency were to review this treatment today.

Risperidone and aripiprazole are a type of medication called an atypical, or second-generation, antipsychotic. These medications are called "atypical" to set them apart from earlier types of medications, called conventional or first-generation antipsychotics. Short-term treatment with risperidone can help reduce symptoms of mania or mixed mania in children ages 10 and up. Aripiprazole is approved to treat these symptoms in children 10–17 years old who have bipolar I.

Your child's psychiatrist may recommend other types of medication. Studies in adults with bipolar disorder show these medications may be helpful. However, these medications have not been approved by the FDA to treat bipolar disorder in children.

Anticonvulsant medications are commonly prescribed to treat seizures, but these medications can help stabilize moods too. They may be very helpful for difficult-to-treat bipolar episodes. For some children, anticonvulsants may work better than lithium. Not every child can take lithium.

Antidepressant medications are sometimes used to treat symptoms of depression in bipolar disorder. Doctors who prescribe antidepressants for bipolar disorder usually prescribe a mood stabilizer or anticonvulsant medication at the same time. If your child takes only an antidepressant, he or she may be at risk of switching to mania or hypomania. He or she may also be at risk of developing rapid cycling symptoms. Rapid cycling is when someone has four or more episodes of major depression, mania, hypomania, or mixed symptoms within a year.

Side effects: Before your child starts taking a new medication, talk with the doctor or pharmacist about possible risks and benefits of taking that medication.

The doctor or pharmacist can also answer questions about side effects. Over the last decade, treatments have improved, and some medications now have fewer or more tolerable side effects than past treatments. However, everyone responds differently to medications, and in some cases, side effects may not appear until a person has taken a medication for some time.

If your child develops any severe side effects from a medication, talk to the doctor who prescribed it as soon as possible. The doctor may change the dose or prescribe a different medication. Children and teens being treated for bipolar disorder should not stop taking a medication without talking to a doctor first. Suddenly stopping a medication may lead to "rebound," or worsening of bipolar disorder symptoms or other uncomfortable or potentially dangerous withdrawal effects.

Psychotherapy

In addition to medication, psychotherapy ("talk" therapy) can be an effective treatment for bipolar disorder. Studies in adults show that it can provide support, education, and guidance to people with bipolar disorder and their families. Psychotherapy may also help children keep taking their medications to stay healthy and prevent relapse.

Children and teens may also benefit from therapies that address problems at school, work, or in the community.

Some psychotherapy treatments used for bipolar disorder include the following:

- Cognitive behavioral therapy helps young people with bipolar disorder learn to change harmful or negative thought patterns and behaviors.

- Family-focused therapy includes a child's family members. It helps enhance family coping strategies, such as recognizing new episodes early and helping their child. This therapy also improves communication and problem solving.

- Interpersonal and social rhythm therapy helps children and teens with bipolar disorder improve their relationships with others and manage their daily routines. Regular daily routines and sleep schedules may help protect against manic episodes.

- Psychoeducation teaches young people with bipolar disorder about the illness and its treatment. This treatment helps people recognize signs of relapse so they can seek treatment early, before a full-blown episode occurs. Psychoeducation also may be helpful for family members and caregivers.

Help for Families

As with other serious illnesses, taking care of a child with bipolar disorder is incredibly hard on the parents, family, and other caregivers.

Caregivers often must tend to the medical needs of their child while dealing with how it affects their own health. The stress that caregivers are under may lead to missed work or lost free time. It can strain relationships with people who do not understand the situation and lead to physical and mental exhaustion.

It is important to take care of your own physical and mental health. You may also find it helpful to join a local support group. If your child's illness prevents you from attending a local support group, try an online support group. If you are unsure where to go for help, ask your family doctor.

If You Think Your Child Is in Crisis

- Call your doctor.

- Call 911 or go to a hospital emergency room to get immediate help or ask a friend or family member to help you do these things.

- Call the toll-free, 24-hour hotline of the National Suicide Prevention Lifeline at 800-273-TALK (800-273-8255); TTY 800-799-4TTY (800-799-4889) to talk to a trained counselor

- Make sure your child is not left alone.

Section 35.3

Depression

What Is Depression?

Depression is a medical disorder that causes a person to feel persistently sad, low, or disinterested in daily activities. While everyone may have occasional moments of feeling sad or "blue," or a temporary period of sadness in response to a major loss, a depressive disorder causes those feelings to continue for an extended period. The tendency to develop depression involves complex genetic and environmental factors.

Depression in a child or adolescent is usually in the form of a major depressive disorder, in which multiple, significant symptoms of depression persist nearly every day for at least two weeks. Major depressive disorder affects about 2% of children and about 5% of adolescents. It can develop in response to a stressful situation or it may develop on its own.

Many children have symptoms of a milder depression, known as dysthymic disorder, that last for at least one year and impair their functioning at home and at school. Another type of depressive disorder is seasonal affective disorder or seasonal depression, which is diagnosed when the depression is triggered each year by the change of seasons (most often, during fall or winter). Symptoms or episodes of depression can also be seen in children or adolescents with bipolar disorder.

What Does Depression Look Like in Children and Adolescents?

Depression in young people often looks different than it does in adults. In some cases, children or adolescents with depression may look sad or tearful more frequently than they had previously. In other cases, they may be constantly irritable, or they may be tired, listless, or uninterested in favorite activities. In general, depression is an episodic condition in which a child has symptoms for several weeks or months, which may then gradually resolve. A child or adolescent may have recurring depression or a single episode.

Treatment for depression usually speeds the process of reducing symptoms, reduces recurrence, and diminishes the time the child may be at risk for suicide or other consequences of the depressive episodes (such as school failure, loss of friends, or family conflict). Variations in the course and presentation of depressive episodes can make diagnosing depression a challenge. A trained clinician (such as a child psychiatrist, child psychologist, or pediatric neurologist) should integrate information from home, school, and the clinical visit to make a diagnosis.

At Home

At home, children with depression may have a combination of the symptoms listed here.

- Persistent sadness, downcast expression, or low mood, which may include tearfulness

- Persistently decreased interest in activities they previously enjoyed (hobbies, sports, friends, family outings, foods, etc.)

- Sleep disturbances, including difficulty falling asleep, restlessness, early awakening, excessive sleeping, taking more naps, wanting to go to bed after school, or going to sleep earlier at night

- Appetite disturbance, either eating much more or much less than typically; a change in weight may occur

- Increased fatigue or difficulty having enough energy to get through the day

- Increased irritability, such as more frequent tantrums and arguments or greater frustration over small disappointments

- Increased physical complaints such as headaches and stomach aches

- Feelings of worthlessness or low self-esteem, often revealed by repetitive comments such as "I'm no good," "I can't do it," and by refusal to even try activities or to complete chores

- Suicide risk, self-harm behaviors, preoccupation with death, or thoughts about hurting oneself or others may accompany depressed moods; children and adolescents may make comments about not caring whether they live or die, may give possessions away, or talk about how life would be different if they were no longer alive

- Irrational worries or fears of being watched or listened to by others, or unusual worries of having thoughts or internal voices controlled by others

- Experimentation with alcohol or drugs as a way to reduce suffering; drugs and alcohol can themselves produce or worsen depressive symptoms

At School

At school, a child with depression may have a combination of the symptoms listed here.

- Difficulty concentrating and/or forgetfulness, which may affect many aspects of school activities, from following directions and completing assignments to paying attention in class

- Impaired ability to plan, organize, concentrate, and use abstract reasoning; this can affect behavior and academic performance

- Social isolation or withdrawal from interactions with peers

- Problem behaviors at school, such as increased fights, arguments, or unusual behaviors

- Heightened sensitivity to perceived criticism

- Other conditions, such as attention deficit/hyperactivity disorder (ADHD), which may also be present, compounding any learning challenges; having one mental health condition does not "inoculate" the child from having other conditions as well

- Anxiety disorders which may lead to difficulty separating from parents, trouble transitioning from home to school, reluctance to attend school, or avoidance of play time with peers

- Learning disorders, particularly if undiagnosed or untreated, because the stress of coping with a learning disorder can trigger depression (A child's difficulties or frustrations in school should not be presumed to be due entirely to the depression. If the child still has academic difficulty after depression is treated, an educational evaluation for a learning disorder should be considered. A child's repeated reluctance to attend school may be an indicator of an undiagnosed learning disability.)

At the Doctor's Office

Depression can be difficult to diagnose, and a clinician may need to see a child over time to determine the appropriate diagnosis. A trained clinician (such as a child psychiatrist, child psychologist, or pediatric neurologist) should integrate information from home, school, and the clinical visit to make a diagnosis of depression. Diagnosing and treating children with depression may involve some of the following challenges.

- Symptoms may vary over time, and the appearance of depression may change as a child grows.

- Other conditions may look like depression (for example, bipolar disorder, learning disorders, developmental disorders, and certain medical conditions).

- Symptoms may be attributed to other factors such as conduct problems, oppositionality, disinterest in school, family stresses, or substance abuse.

- Young people with symptoms of depression may not feel comfortable about their own feelings and may not volunteer information. Phrasing questions with particular sensitivity and compassion may allow a more complete picture of symptoms to emerge.

- Children may be unaware, or unwilling to admit, that their behavior may indicate symptoms of a disorder.

- Families may need to be coached about what they can reasonably expect from their child. Children who suffer from depression will benefit if their family understands that therapy and medicines may reduce, but may not cure, symptoms.

- Symptoms may return during periods of high stress.

How Is Depression Treated?

Determining the correct underlying diagnosis will allow the clinician to select the appropriate treatment recommendations. Depression is treatable through ongoing interventions provided by a child's medical practitioners, therapists, school staff, and family. These treatments include psychological interventions (counseling), biological interventions (medicines), and accommodations at home and school that reduce sources of stress for the child. Open, collaborative communication between a child's family, school, and clinicians optimizes the care and quality of life for the child with depression.

Psychological Interventions (Counseling)

Counseling can help children with depression, and everyone around them, to understand that symptoms of depression are caused by an illness with complex genetic and environmental origins—not by flawed attitude or personality. Counseling also can reduce the impact of symptoms on daily life. A variety of psychological interventions can be helpful, and parents should discuss their child's particular needs with their clinician to determine which psychological treatments could be most beneficial for their child.

- Individual psychotherapy is generally recommended as the first line of treatment for children and adolescents with mild to moderate depression. Psychotherapy is also helpful when ongoing stressors exacerbate the symptoms. Depressed children or adolescents may carry a sense of failure, as if the illness was their fault. Individual psychotherapy can help reduce symptoms, and can help young people to become aware of, and address, their feelings of failure and self-blame.

- Cognitive behavior therapy (CBT) can teach a child new skills to reduce some symptoms of depression, particularly the negative thoughts or feelings accompanying depression. In CBT, a child or adolescent is helped to become aware of, and to describe, his or her negative thoughts or feelings. A trained clinician guides the child to think of new, more positive alternatives. The young person is then given a chance to practice new ways of thinking and feeling outside the clinical visit, and to discuss his or her experiences with the clinician afterwards. These methods are based upon well-researched practices that have helped many children and adolescents.

- Parent guidance sessions can help parents to manage their child's illness, identify effective parenting skills, learn how to function as a family despite the illness, and to address complex feelings that can arise when raising a child with a psychiatric disorder. Family therapy may be beneficial when issues are affecting the family as a whole.

- Group psychotherapy can be valuable to a child by providing a safe place to talk with other children who face adversity or allowing a child to practice social skills or symptom-combating skills in a carefully structured setting.

- School-based counseling can be effective in helping a child with depression navigate the social, behavioral, and academic demands of the school setting.

Biological Interventions (Medicines)

While psychotherapy may be sufficient to treat some children with depression, other children's symptoms do not improve significantly with psychotherapy alone. These children may benefit from medications.

The FDA has approved one antidepressant medication, Prozac (fluoxetine), for treating children and adolescents with depression. Medications approved by the FDA for other uses and age groups are also prescribed for young people with depression. The FDA allows doctors to use their best judgment to prescribe medication for conditions for which the medication has not specifically been approved.

The following medications are commonly prescribed for children and adolescents with depression:

- **Antidepressants:** The most commonly prescribed antidepressants, including Celexa, Lexapro, Luvox, Paxil, Prozac, and Zoloft, belong to a group of medications called selective serotonin reuptake inhibitors, or SSRIs. Other commonly prescribed antidepressants include Effexor, Remeron, and Wellbutrin.

- **Antipsychotic medications:** These medications (also called neuroleptics) may be prescribed if persistent and unusual worries develop, such as the fear of being harmed by others, or if the sensation develops of hearing or seeing things that are not really present. Examples of these drugs are Abilify, Geodon, Risperdal, Seroquel, and Zyprexa.

In most cases these medicines begin to be effective in reducing symptoms after the child or adolescent has taken them for at least 2–4 weeks. Fully 12 weeks may be required in order to determine whether the medication is going to be effective for a particular individual. Medications should only be started, stopped, or adjusted under the direct supervision of a trained clinician.

There is no "best" medicine to treat depression, and it is important to remember that medicines usually reduce rather than eliminate symptoms. Different medicines or dosages may be needed at different times in a child's life or to address the emergence of particular symptoms. Successful treatment requires taking medicine daily as prescribed, allowing time for the medicine to work, and monitoring for both effectiveness and side effects. The family, clinician, and school should maintain frequent communication to ensure that medications are working as intended and to monitor and manage side effects.

The following cautions should be observed when any child or adolescent is treated with antidepressants.

- Benefits and risks should be evaluated. Questions have arisen about whether antidepressants can cause some children or adolescents to have suicidal thoughts. The evidence to date shows that antidepressants, when carefully monitored, have safely helped many children and adolescents. The latest reports on this issue from the U.S. Food and Drug Administration can be found on its website at www.fda.gov. Consideration of any medicine deserves a discussion with the prescribing clinician about its risks and benefits.

- Careful monitoring is recommended for any child receiving medication. Though most side effects occur soon after starting a medicine, adverse reactions can occur months after medicines are introduced. Agitation, restlessness, increased irritability, or comments about self-harm should be addressed immediately with the clinician if any of these symptoms emerge after the child starts an antidepressant. Frequent follow-up (weekly for the first month) is now advocated by the FDA for children starting an antidepressant.

- Some children who appear depressed have bipolar disorder, which may need to be treated differently than depression. In some individuals with bipolar disorder, antidepressants may initially improve depressive symptoms but can sometimes worsen manic symptoms. While antidepressants do not "cause" bipolar disorder, they can unmask or worsen manic symptoms. For individuals with bipolar disorder, doctors commonly prescribe a mood stabilizer together with an antidepressant in order to minimize the risk that manic symptoms will be worsened by the antidepressant.

Helpful information about specific medications can be found at www.medlineplus.gov (click on "Drug Information") and in the book *Straight Talk about Psychiatric Medications for Kids (Revised Edition)* by Timothy E. Wilens, MD.

Interventions at Home

At home, as well as at school, interventions may be helpful to aid a child or adolescent.

- Adjust expectations until symptoms improve. Helping a child make more attainable goals during a depressive episode is important, so that the child can have the positive experience of success. Once symptoms improve and depression lifts, expectations can increase.

- Simplify home life. While the child is depressed, a busy after-school schedule or long list of household chores will likely add to feelings of being burdened. The number of commitments should be adjusted to the child's ability to be successful.

- Listen to the child's feelings. Isolation often perpetuates depression. The simple experience of being listened to sympathetically, without receiving advice, may have a powerful and helpful effect. Parents should not let their own worries prevent them from talking with their child at a time when their support is most needed.

- Small steps can make a difference. Keep a positive attitude about whatever successes occur during this time. At the same time, it is important to validate the child's feelings of frustration when his or her efforts fail ("Okay, you didn't score 100 on this test, but you did get all of the items done this time—let's see where you started missing items.").

- Address comments about suicide. If a child makes a remark about wanting to die, talk to the child about it without delay. Talking about suicide does not encourage self-harm acts. It may help clarify what the child meant by the remark, or help the child determine what might be changed in order to make that feeling go away.

- Talk as a family about what to say to people outside of the family. Determine what feels comfortable for the child (for example, "I was sick and got some help, and now I'm better."). Even if the decision is made not to discuss this medical condition with others, having an agreed-on plan will make it easier to handle unexpected questions and minimize family conflicts about this.

- Help prevent relapse. Assuring that a child takes medicine daily for as long as prescribed, watching for symptoms of another episode, and reducing stressors may all help prevent or postpone another episode of depression. If symptoms do return, it is important to know it is not anyone's fault but, rather, the nature of the illness.

Interventions at School

There are many ways that schools can help a child with depression succeed in the classroom. Parents and school staff, including teachers, guidance counselors, and nurses, should collaborate to develop helpful school structure for the child. The child may need particular changes (accommodations/modifications) within a classroom.

Examples of some accommodations, modifications, and school strategies include the following:

- Schedule check-ins on arrival to see if the child can succeed in certain classes that day. Check-ins also provide an opportunity to share an encouraging word or to identify worries the child has for the day. Note that some children may want less attention, so finding the right balance of attention will be helpful.

- Provide more time to complete certain types of assignments.

- Adjust homework load to prevent the child from becoming overwhelmed. Academic stressors, along with other stresses, are difficult for children to manage during a depressive episode.

- Anticipate issues such as school avoidance if there are unresolved social and/or academic problems.

- Be aware that some situations may be particularly difficult for the child. When a child with depression refuses to follow directions, for example, the reason may be anxiety, rather than intentional oppositionality.

- Encourage the child to help develop interventions. Enlisting the child in the task will lead to more successful strategies and will foster the child's ability to problem-solve.

Flexibility and a supportive environment are essential for a student with depression to achieve success in school. School faculty and parents together may be able to identify difficult areas and develop remedies to reduce a child's challenges at these times.

Section 35.4

Obsessive-Compulsive Disorder

This section excerpted from "Obsessive-Compulsive Disorder: When Unwanted Thoughts Take Over," National Institute of Mental Health (www .nimh.nih.gov), 2010. Additional information from International OCD Foundation is cited separately within the section.

What is obsessive-compulsive disorder (OCD)?

Everyone double checks things sometimes. For example, you might double check to make sure the stove or iron is turned off before leaving the house. But people with OCD feel the need to check things repeatedly, or have certain thoughts or perform routines and rituals over and over. The thoughts and rituals associated with OCD cause distress and get in the way of daily life.

The frequent upsetting thoughts are called obsessions. To try to control them, a person will feel an overwhelming urge to repeat certain rituals or behaviors called compulsions. People with OCD can't control these obsessions and compulsions.

For many people, OCD starts during childhood or the teen years. Most people are diagnosed by about age 19. Symptoms of OCD may come and go and be better or worse at different times.

What are the signs and symptoms of OCD?

People with OCD generally show these symptoms:

- Have repeated thoughts or images about many different things, such as fear of germs, dirt, or intruders; acts of violence; hurting loved ones; sexual acts; conflicts with religious beliefs; or being overly tidy

- Do the same rituals over and over such as washing hands, locking and unlocking doors, counting, keeping unneeded items, or repeating the same steps again and again

- Can't control the unwanted thoughts and behaviors

- Don't get pleasure when performing the behaviors or rituals, but get brief relief from the anxiety the thoughts cause

- Spend at least one hour a day on the thoughts and rituals, which cause distress and get in the way of daily life

What causes OCD?

OCD sometimes runs in families, but no one knows for sure why some people have it, while others don't. Researchers have found that several parts of the brain are involved in fear and anxiety. Researchers are also looking for ways in which stress and environmental factors may play a role.

How is OCD treated?

First, talk to your doctor about your symptoms. Your doctor should do an exam to make sure that another physical problem isn't causing the symptoms. The doctor may refer you to a mental health specialist.

OCD is generally treated with psychotherapy, medication, or both.

A type of psychotherapy called cognitive behavior therapy is especially useful for treating OCD. It teaches a person different ways of thinking, behaving, and reacting to situations that help him or her feel less anxious or fearful without having obsessive thoughts or acting compulsively.

Doctors also may prescribe medication to help treat OCD. The most commonly prescribed medications for OCD are anti-anxiety medications and antidepressants. Anti-anxiety medications are powerful and there are different types.

Antidepressants are used to treat depression, but they are also particularly helpful for OCD, probably more so than anti-anxiety medications. They may take several weeks—10 to 12 weeks for some—to start working.

It's important to know that although antidepressants can be safe and effective for many people, they may be risky for some, especially children, teens, and young adults. Anyone taking antidepressants should be monitored closely, especially when they first start treatment with medications.

OCD in Children and Teens

"What Is Life Like for Children and Teens Who Have OCD?" by S. Evelyn Stewart, M.D. © 2012 International OCD Foundation (www.ocfoundation .org). Reprinted with permission.

At least 1 in 200 children and teens in the United States have OCD. Understanding the special impact that the disorder has on their lives is important in helping them get the right treatment. Some common issues with OCD in children and teens follow:

Disrupted routines: OCD can make daily life very difficult and stressful for kids and teens. In the morning, they feel they must do their rituals right, or the rest of the day will not go well. In the evenings, they must finish all of their compulsive rituals before they go to bed. Some kids and teens even stay up late because of their OCD, and are often exhausted the following day.

Problems at school: OCD can affect homework, attention in class, and school attendance. If this happens, you need to be an advocate for your child. It is your right under the Disabilities Education Act (IDEA) to ask for changes from the school that will help your child succeed.

Physical complaints: Stress, poor nutrition, and/or the loss of sleep can make children physically ill.

Social relationships: The stress of hiding their rituals from peers, times spent with obsessions and compulsions, and how their friends react to their OCD-related behaviors can all affect friendships.

Problems with self-esteem: Kids and teens worry that they are "crazy" because their thinking is different than their friends and family. Their self-esteem can be negatively affected because the OCD has led to embarrassment or has made them feel "bizarre" or "out of control."

Anger management problems: This is because the parents have become unwilling (or are unable!) to comply with the child's OCD-related demands. Even when parents set reasonable limits, kids and teens with OCD can become anxious and angry.

Additional mental health problems: Kids and teens with OCD are more likely to have additional mental health problems than those who do not have the disorder. Sometimes these other disorders can be treated with the same medicine prescribed to treat the OCD. Depression, anxiety disorders, and trichotillomania (compulsive hair or skin picking) may improve when a child takes anti-OCD medicine. On the other hand, attention-deficit hyperactivity disorder (ADHD), tic disorders, and disruptive behavior disorders usually require additional treatments, including medicines that are not specific to OCD.

Part Five

Additional Help and Information

Chapter 36

Glossary of Terms Related to Childhood Diseases and Disorders

Active immunity: The production of antibodies against a specific disease by the immune system. Active immunity can be acquired in two ways, either by contracting the disease or through vaccination. Active immunity is usually permanent, meaning an individual is protected from the disease for the duration of their lives.[1]

Adenovirus: A member of a family of viruses that can cause infections in the respiratory tract, eye, and gastrointestinal tract. Forms of adenoviruses that do not cause disease are used in gene therapy. They carry genes that may fix defects in cells or kill cancer cells.[2]

Adrenal gland: A small gland that makes steroid hormones, adrenaline, and noradrenaline. These hormones help control heart rate, blood pressure, and other important body functions. There are two adrenal glands, one on top of each kidney. Also called suprarenal gland.[2]

Allergy: A condition in which the body has an exaggerated response to a substance (e.g. food or drug). Also known as hypersensitivity.[1]

Antibody: A protein found in the blood that is produced in response to foreign substances (e.g., bacteria or viruses) invading the body. Antibodies protect the body from disease by binding to these organisms and destroying them.[1]

The terms in this glossary were excerpted from "Vaccines & Immunizations Glossary," Centers for Disease Control and Prevention (www.cdc.gov) [marked 1] and "Dictionary of Cancer Terms," National Cancer Institute (www.cancer.gov) [marked 2].

Arthritis: A disease that causes inflammation and pain in the joints.[2]

Asthma: A chronic medical condition where the bronchial tubes (in the lungs) become easily irritated. This leads to constriction of the airways resulting in wheezing, coughing, difficulty breathing, and production of thick mucus. The cause of asthma is not yet known but environmental triggers, drugs, food allergies, exercise, infection, and stress have all been implicated.[1]

Autism: A chronic developmental disorder usually diagnosed between 18 and 30 months of age. Symptoms include problems with social interaction and communication as well as repetitive interests and activities. At this time, the cause of autism is not known although many experts believe it to be a genetically based disorder that occurs before birth.[1]

Bacteria: Tiny one-celled organisms present throughout the environment that require a microscope to be seen. While not all bacteria are harmful, some cause disease. Examples of bacterial disease include diphtheria, pertussis, tetanus, *Haemophilus influenzae*, and pneumococcal.[1]

Biopsy: The removal of cells or tissues for examination by a pathologist. The pathologist may study the tissue under a microscope or perform other tests on the cells or tissue. There are many different types of biopsy procedures. The most common types include: (1) incisional biopsy, in which only a sample of tissue is removed; (2) excisional biopsy, in which an entire lump or suspicious area is removed; and (3) needle biopsy, in which a sample of tissue or fluid is removed with a needle.[2]

Carrier: A person who has a mutated (changed) copy of a gene. This change may cause a disease in that person or in his or her children.[2]

Chromosome: Part of a cell that contains genetic information. Except for sperm and eggs, all human cells contain 46 chromosomes.[2]

Crohn disease: A chronic medical condition characterized by inflammation of the bowel. Symptoms include abdominal pain, diarrhea, fever, loss of appetite, and weight loss. The cause of Crohn disease is not yet known, but genetic, dietary, and infectious factors may play a part.[1]

CT scan: A series of detailed pictures of areas inside the body taken from different angles. The pictures are created by a computer linked to an X-ray machine. Also called CAT scan, computed tomography scan, computerized axial tomography scan, and computerized tomography.[2]

Cystic fibrosis: A common hereditary disease in which exocrine (secretory) glands produce abnormally thick mucus. This mucus can cause problems in digestion, breathing, and body cooling.[2]

Diabetes: A chronic health condition where the body is unable to produce insulin and properly break down sugar (glucose) in the blood. Symptoms include hunger, thirst, excessive urination, dehydration, and weight loss. The treatment of diabetes requires daily insulin injections, proper nutrition, and regular exercise. Complications can include heart disease, stroke, neuropathy, poor circulation leading to loss of limbs, hearing impairment, vision problems, and death.[1]

Encephalopathy: A general term describing brain dysfunction. Examples include encephalitis, meningitis, seizures, and head trauma.[1]

Endocrine system: A system of glands and cells that make hormones that are released directly into the blood and travel to tissues and organs all over the body. The endocrine system controls growth, sexual development, sleep, hunger, and the way the body uses food.[2]

Epilepsy: A group of disorders marked by problems in the normal functioning of the brain. These problems can produce seizures, unusual body movements, a loss of consciousness or changes in consciousness, as well as mental problems or problems with the senses.[2]

Exposure: Contact with infectious agents (bacteria or viruses) in a manner that promotes transmission and increases the likelihood of disease.[1]

Fever: An increase in body temperature above normal (98.6° F), usually caused by disease.[2]

Gastric reflux: The backward flow of stomach acid contents into the esophagus (the tube that connects the mouth to the stomach). Also called esophageal reflux and gastroesophageal reflux.[2]

Genetic counseling: A communication process between a specially trained health professional and a person concerned about the genetic risk of disease. The person's family and personal medical history may be discussed, and counseling may lead to genetic testing.[2]

***Haemophilus influenzae* type b (Hib):** A bacterial infection that may result in severe respiratory infections, including pneumonia, and other diseases such as meningitis.[1]

Hepatitis: Disease of the liver causing inflammation. Symptoms include an enlarged liver, fever, nausea, vomiting, abdominal pain, and dark urine.[2]

Hereditary: Transmitted from parent to child by information contained in the genes.[2]

Immune system: The complex system in the body responsible for fighting disease. Its primary function is to identify foreign substances in the body (bacteria, viruses, fungi, or parasites) and develop a defense against them. This defense is known as the immune response. It involves production of protein molecules called antibodies to eliminate foreign organisms that invade the body.[1]

Incubation period: The time from contact with infectious agents (bacteria or viruses) to onset of disease.[1]

Infection: Invasion and multiplication of germs in the body. Infections can occur in any part of the body and can spread throughout the body. The germs may be bacteria, viruses, yeast, or fungi. They can cause a fever and other problems, depending on where the infection occurs. When the body's natural defense system is strong, it can often fight the germs and prevent infection. Some cancer treatments can weaken the natural defense system.[2]

Inflammatory bowel disease (IBD): A general term for any disease characterized by inflammation of the bowel. Examples include colitis and Crohn disease. Symptoms include abdominal pain, diarrhea, fever, loss of appetite, and weight loss.[1]

Influenza: A highly contagious viral infection characterized by sudden onset of fever, severe aches and pains, and inflammation of the mucous membrane.[1]

MRI: A procedure in which radio waves and a powerful magnet linked to a computer are used to create detailed pictures of areas inside the body. These pictures can show the difference between normal and diseased tissue. MRI makes better images of organs and soft tissue than other scanning techniques, such as computed tomography (CT) or X-ray. MRI is especially useful for imaging the brain, the spine, the soft tissue of joints, and the inside of bones. Also called magnetic resonance imaging, NMRI, and nuclear magnetic resonance imaging.[2]

Otitis media: A viral or bacterial infection that leads to inflammation of the middle ear. This condition usually occurs along with an upper respiratory infection. Symptoms include earache, high fever, nausea, vomiting, and diarrhea. In addition, hearing loss, facial paralysis, and meningitis may result.[1]

Parasitic: Having to do with or being a parasite (an animal or plant that gets nutrients by living on or in an organism of another species).[2]

Pathogens: Organisms (e.g. bacteria, viruses, parasites, and fungi) that cause disease in human beings.[1]

Pertussis (whooping cough): Bacterial infectious disease marked by a convulsive spasmodic cough, sometimes followed by a crowing intake of breath.[1]

Pinkeye: A condition in which the conjunctiva (membranes lining the eyelids and covering the white part of the eye) become inflamed or infected. Also called conjunctivitis.[2]

Pneumonia: Inflammation of the lungs characterized by fever, chills, muscle stiffness, chest pain, cough, shortness of breath, rapid heart rate, and difficulty breathing.[1]

Reye syndrome: Encephalopathy (general brain disorder) in children following an acute illness such as influenza or chickenpox. Symptoms include vomiting, agitation, and lethargy. This condition may result in coma or death.[1]

Sarcoma: A cancer of the bone, cartilage, fat, muscle, blood vessels, or other connective or supportive tissue.[2]

Seizure: Sudden, uncontrolled body movements and changes in behavior that occur because of abnormal electrical activity in the brain. Symptoms include loss of awareness, changes in emotion, loss of muscle control, and shaking. Seizures may be caused by drugs, high fevers, head injuries, and certain diseases, such as epilepsy.[2]

Tumor: An abnormal mass of tissue that results when cells divide more than they should or do not die when they should. Tumors may be benign (not cancer) or malignant (cancer). Also called neoplasm.[2]

Ultrasound: A procedure in which high-energy sound waves are bounced off internal tissues or organs and make echoes. The echo patterns are shown on the screen of an ultrasound machine, forming a picture of body tissues called a sonogram. Also called ultrasonography.[2]

Vaccine: A product that produces immunity therefore protecting the body from the disease. Vaccines are administered through needle injections, by mouth, and by aerosol.[1]

Virus: A tiny organism that multiplies within cells and causes disease such as chickenpox, measles, mumps, rubella, pertussis, and hepatitis. Viruses are not affected by antibiotics, the drugs used to kill bacteria.[1]

Chapter 37

Resource List for Parents and Caregivers

General Health Organizations

American Academy of Pediatrics
National Headquarters
141 Northwest Point Boulevard
Elk Grove Village, IL 60007-1098
Phone: 847-434-4000
Fax: 847-434-8000
Website: http://www.aap.org
E-mail: csc@aap.org

Centers for Disease Control and Prevention (CDC)
1600 Clifton Road
Atlanta, GA 30333
Toll-Free: 800-CDC-INFO
(800-232-4636)
Website: http://www.cdc.gov
E-mail: cdcinfo@cdc.gov

Cleveland Clinic
9500 Euclid Avenue
Cleveland, OH 44195
Toll-Free: 800-223-2273
Phone: 216-444-2200
TTY: 216-444-0261
Website:
http://www.clevelandclinic.org

The information in this chapter was compiled from various sources deemed accurate. All contact information was verified and updated in March 2012. Inclusion does not imply endorsement. This list is not comprehensive.

Eunice Kennedy Shriver National Institute of Child Health and Development (NICHD) Information Resource Center
P.O. Box 3006
Rockville, MD 20847
Toll-Free: 800-370-2943
Toll-Free TTY: 888-320-6942
Toll-Free Fax: 866-760-5947
Website:
http://www.nichd.nih.gov
E-mail: NICHDInformation
ResourceCenter@ mail.nih.gov

Kidshealth.org
Nemours Foundation
10140 Centurion Parkway
Jacksonville, FL 32256
Phone: 904-697-4100
Fax: 904-697-4220
Website:
http://www.kidshealth.org

National Heart, Lung, and Blood Institute (NHLBI)
NHLBI Health Information Center
P.O. Box 30105
Bethesda, MD 20824-0105
Phone: 301-592-8573
TTY: 240-629-3255
Fax: 240-629-3246
Website:
http://www.nhlbi.nih.gov
E-mail:
nhlbiinfo@nhlbi.nih.gov

National Institute of Allergy and Infectious Diseases (NIAID)
Office of Communications
and Government Relations
6610 Rockledge Drive
MSC 6612
Bethesda, MD 20892-6612
Toll-Free: 866-284-4107
Toll-Free TDD: 800-877-8339
Phone: 301-496-5717
Toll-Free TDD: 800-877-8339
Fax: 301-402-3573
Website: http://www.niaid.nih.gov
E-mail: ocpostoffice@niaid.nih.gov

National Institute of Diabetes and Digestive and Kidney Diseases (NIDDK)
Office of Communications and Public Liaison
NIDDK, NIH
Building 31, Room 9A06
31 Center Drive, MSC 2560
Bethesda, MD 20892-2560
Phone: 301-496-3583
Website:
http://www.niddk.nih.gov

National Organization for Rare Disorders (NORD)
55 Kenosia Avenue
P.O. Box 1968
Danbury, CT 06813-1968
Toll-Free: 800-999-6673
Phone: 203-744-0100
TDD: 203-797-9590
Fax: 203-798-2291
Website:
http://www.rarediseases.org
E-mail: orphan@rarediseases.org
or RN@rarediseases.org

U.S. Department of Health and Human Services
200 Independence Avenue SW
Washington, DC 20201
Toll-Free: 877-696-6775
Website: http://www.hhs.gov

U.S. Environmental Protection Agency
Ariel Rios Building
1200 Pennsylvania Avenue NW
Washington, DC 20460
Phone: 202-272-0167
TTY: 202-272-0165
Website: http://www.epa.gov

U.S. Food and Drug Administration
10903 New Hampshire Avenue
Silver Spring, MD 20993
Toll-Free: 888-INFO-FDA
(888-463-6332)
Website: http://www.fda.gov

Weight-Control Information Network (WIN)
1 WIN Way
Bethesda, MD 20892-3665
Toll-Free: 877-946-4627
Phone: 202-828-1025
Fax: 202-828-1028
Website: http://www.win.niddk.nih.gov
E-mail: win@info.niddk.nih.gov

Allergies and Asthma

Asthma and Allergy Foundation of America
8201 Corporate Drive, Suite 1000
Landover, MD 20785
Toll-Free: 800-7-ASTHMA
(800-727-8462)
Website: http://www.aafa.org
E-mail: info@aafa.org

Arthritis and Musculoskeletal Diseases

American College of Rheumatology
2200 Lake Boulevard NE
Atlanta, GA 30319
Phone: 404-633-3777
Fax: 404-633-1870
Website: http://www.rheumatology.org
E-mail: acr@rheumatology.org

Arthritis Foundation
P.O. Box 7669
Atlanta, GA 30357-0669
Toll-Free: 800-283-7800
Website: http://www.arthritis.org

National Institute of Arthritis and Musculoskeletal and Skin Diseases (NIAMS)
1 AMS Circle
Bethesda, MD 20892-3675
Toll-Free: 877-22-NIAMS
(877-226-4267)
Phone: 301-495-4484
TYY: 301-565-2966
Fax: 312-718-6366
Website: http://www.niams.nih.gov
E-mail: NIAMSinfo@mail.nih.gov

Cancer

American Cancer Society
250 Williams Street NW
Atlanta, GA 30303
Toll-Free: 800-ACS-2345
(800-227-2345)
Toll-Free TTY: 866-228-4327
Website: http://www.cancer.org

Leukemia and Lymphoma Society
1311 Mamaroneck Ave., Suite 310
White Plains, NY 10605-5221
Toll-Free: 800-955-4LSA
(800-955-4572)
Phone: 914-949-5213
Fax: 914-949-6691
Website: http://www.lls.org
E-mail: infocenter@lls.org

National Cancer Institute (NCI)
NCI Public Inquiries Office
6116 Executive Blvd., Suite 300
Bethesda, MD 20892-8322
Toll-Free: 800-422-6237
(800-4-CANCER), Monday
through Friday 9:00 a.m. to 4:30
p.m., EST
Website: http://www.cancer.gov

National Children's Cancer Society
1 South Memorial Dr., Suite 800
St. Louis, MO 63102
Toll-Free: 800-5-FAMILY
(800-532-6459)
Phone: 314-241-1600
Fax: 314-241-1996
Website:
http://www.children-cancer.com

Pediatric Brain Tumor Foundation
302 Ridgefield Court
Asheville, NC 28806
Toll-Free: 800-253-6530
Phone: 828-665-6891
Fax: 828-665-6894
Website:
http://www.pbtfus.org
E-mail: info@pbtfus.org

Cardiovascular Disorders

American Heart Association
7272 Greenville Avenue
Dallas, TX 75231-4596
Toll-Free: 800-AHA-USA1
(800-242-8721)
Website:
http://www.americanheart.org

National Hemophilia Foundation
116 West 32nd Street
11th Floor
New York, NY 10001
Toll-Free: 800-42-HANDI
(800-424-2634)
Phone: 212-328-3700
Fax: 212-328-3777 or
212-328-3799
Website:
http://www.hemophilia.org
E-mail: handi@hemophilia.org

Developmental Disorders

Attention Deficit Disorder Association
P.O. Box 7557
Wilmington, DE 19803-9997
Toll-Free Phone/Fax:
800-939-1019
Website: http://www.add.org
E-mail: info@add.org

Autism Society of America
4340 East-West Highway
Suite 350
Bethesda, MD 20814
Toll-Free: 800-3-AUTISM
(800-328-8476)
Phone: 301-657-0881
Website:
http://www.autism-society.org

Autism Speaks
1 East 33rd Street, 4th Floor
New York, NY 10016
Phone: 212-252-8584
Fax: 212-252-8676
Website:
http://www.autismspeaks.org
E-mail:
contactus@autismspeaks.org

Learning Disabilities Association of America
4156 Library Road
Pittsburgh, PA 15234-1349
Phone: 412-341-1515
Fax: 412-344-0224
Website:
http://www.ldaamerica.org
E-mail:
info@ldaamerica.org

National Center for Learning Disabilities
381 Park Avenue South
Suite 1401
New York, NY 10016
Toll-Free: 888-575-7373
Phone: 212-545-7510
Fax: 212-545-9665
Website: http://www.ncld.org

Diabetes

American Diabetes Association
Attention: Center for Information
1701 North Beauregard Street
Alexandria, VA 22311
Toll-Free: 800-DIABETES
(342-2383)
Website: http://www.diabetes.org
E-mail: AskADA@diabetes.org

Juvenile Diabetes Research Foundation International (JDRF)
26 Broadway
New York, NY 10004
Toll-Free: 800-533-CURE
(800-533-2873)
Fax: 212-785-9595
Website: http://www.jdrf.org
E-mail: info@jdrf.org

National Diabetes Education Program (NDEP)
1 Diabetes Way
Bethesda, MD 20814-9692
Toll-Free: 888-693-NDEP
(888-693-6337 to order materials)
Phone: 301-496-3583
Website: http://www.ndep.nih.gov
E-mail: ndep@mail.nih.gov

National Diabetes Information Clearinghouse (NDIC)

1 Information Way
Bethesda, MD 20892-3560
Toll-Free: 800-860-8747
Toll-Free TTY: 866-569-1162
Fax: 703-738-4929
Website:
http://diabetes.niddk.nih.gov
E-mail: ndic@info.niddk.nih.gov

Foodborne Illnesses

Center for Food Safety and Applied Nutrition

5100 Paint Branch Parkway
College Park, MD 20740-3835
Food Information Line:
888-SAFEFOOD (888-723-3366)
Website: http://www.fda.gov/Food
E-mail: consumers@fda.gov

Partnership for Food Safety Education

2345 Crystal Drive, Suite 800
Arlington, VA 22202
Phone: 202-220-0651
Fax: 202-220-0873
Website: http://www.fightbac.org
E-mail: info@fightbac.org

U.S. Department of Agriculture

1400 Independence Avenue SW
Washington, DC 20250
Toll-Free: 888-674-6854
(Meat and Poultry Hotline)
Phone: 202-720-2791
(Information Hotline)
Website: http://www.usda.gov

Gastrointestinal and Digestive Disorders

Academy of Nutrition and Dietetics

120 South Riverside Plaza
Suite 2000
Chicago, IL 60606-6995
Toll-Free: 800-877-1600
Phone: 312-899-0040
Website: http://www.eatright.org
E-mail: knowledge@eatright.org

American Celiac Disease Alliance

2504 Duxbury Place
Alexandria, VA 22308
Phone: 703-622-3331
Website:
http://www.americanceliac.org
E-mail: info@americanceliac.org

American College of Gastroenterology

6400 Goldsboro Road
Suite 450
Bethesda, MD 20817
Phone: 301-263-9000
Website:
http://www.acg.gi.org
Fax: info@acg.gi.org

American Gastroenterological Association

4930 Del Ray Avenue
Bethesda, MD 20814
Phone: 301-654-2055
Fax: 301-654-5920
Website: http://www.gastro.org
E-mail: member@gastro.org

Celiac Disease Foundation
13251 Ventura Boulevard, Suite 1
Studio City, CA 91604
Phone: 818-990-2354
Fax: 818-990-2379
Website: http://www.celiac.org
E-mail: cdf@celiac.org

Celiac Sprue Association/ USA Inc.
P.O. Box 31700
Omaha, NE 68131-0700
Toll-Free: 877-CSA-4CSA
(877-272-4272)
Phone: 402-558-0600
Fax: 402-643-4108
Website:
http://www.csaceliacs.org
E-mail: celiacs@csaceliacs.org

Crohn's and Colitis Foundation of America (CCFA)
386 Park Avenue South
17th Floor
New York, NY 10016
Toll-Free: 800-932-2423
Phone: 212-685-3440
Fax: 212-779-4098
Website: http://www.ccfa.org
E-mail: info@ccfa.org

Cyclic Vomiting Syndrome Association (CVSA)
10520 West Bluemound Road
Suite 106
Milwaukee, WI 53226
Phone: 414-342-7880
Fax: 414-342-8980
Website: http://www.cvsaonline.org
E-mail: cvsa@cvsaonline.org

Digestive Disease National Coalition (DDNC)
507 Capitol Court NE, Suite 200
Washington, DC 20002
Phone: 202-544-7497
Fax: 202-546-7105
Website: http://www.ddnc.org
E-mail: ddnc@hmcw.org

Food Allergy and Anaphylaxis Network
11781 Lee Highway, Suite 160
Fairfax, VA 22033
Toll-Free: 800-929-4040
Fax: 703-691-2713
Website:
http://www.foodallergy.org
E-mail: faan@foodallergy.org

International Foundation for Functional Gastrointestinal Disorders
P.O. Box 170864
Milwaukee, WI 53217-8076
Toll-Free: 888-964-2001
Phone: 414-964-1799
Fax: 414-964-7176
Website: http://www.iffgd.org
E-mail: iffgd@iffgd.org

National Digestive Diseases Information Clearinghouse (NDDIC)
2 Information Way
Bethesda, MD 20892-3570
Toll-Free: 800-891-5389
Toll-Free TTY: 866-569-1162
Fax: 703-738-4929
Website: http://www.digestive
.niddk.nih.gov
E-mail: nddic@info.niddk.nih.gov

North American Society for Pediatric Gastroenterology, Hepatology, and Nutrition
NASPGHAN
P.O. Box 6
Flourtown, PA 19031
Phone: 215-233-0808
Fax: 215-233-3918
Website:
http://www.naspghan.org
E-mail: naspghan@naspghan.org

Pediatric/Adolescent Gastroesophageal Reflux Association (PAGER)
P.O. Box 7728
Silver Spring, MD 20907
Phone: 301-601-9541
Website: http://www.reflux.org
E-mail: gergroup@aol.com

Growth Disorders

Hormone Foundation
8401 Connecticut Ave., Suite 900
Chevy Chase, MD 20815-5817
Toll-Free: 800-HORMONE
(800-467-6663)
Fax: 301-941-0259
Website: http://www.hormone.org
E-mail:
hormone@endo-society.org

Human Growth Foundation
997 Glen Cove Avenue, Suite 5
Glen Head, NY 11545
Toll-Free: 800-451-6434
Fax: 516-671-4055
Website: http://www.hgfound.org
E-mail: hgf1@hgfound.org

MAGIC Foundation
6645 West North Avenue
Oak Park, IL 60302
Toll-Free: 800-3-MAGIC-3
(800-362-4423)
Phone: 708-383-0808
Website:
http://www.magicfoundation.org
E-mail:
ContactUs@magicfoundation.org

Hearing Disorders

National Institute on Deafness and Other Communication Disorders
NIDCD Information
Clearinghouse
31 Center Drive, MSC 2320
Bethesda, MD 20892-2320
Toll-Free: 800-241-1044
Toll-Free TTY: 800-241-1055
Fax: 301-770-8977
Website:
http://www.nidcd.nih.gov
E-mail: nidcdinfo@nidcd.nih.gov

Injury Prevention

Safe Kids Worldwide
1301 Pennsylvania Avenue NW
Suite 1000
Washington, DC 20004-1707
Phone: 202-662-0600
Fax: 202-393-2072
Website: http://www.safekids.org

Kidney and Urological Disorders

American Society of Pediatric Nephrology
3400 Research Forest Drive
Suite B-7
The Woodlands, TX 77381
Phone: 281-419-0052
Fax: 281-419-0082
Website: http://www.aspneph.com
E-mail: info@aspneph.com

American Urological Association Foundation
1000 Corporate Boulevard
Linthicum, MD 21090
Toll-Free: 800-828-7866
Phone: 410-689-3700
Fax: 410-689-3998
Website:
http://www.urologyhealth.org
E-mail: auafoundation@
auafoundation.org

National Association for Continence (NAFC)
P.O. Box 1019
Charleston, SC 29402-1019
Toll-Free: 800-BLADDER
(800-252-3337)
Phone: 843-377-0900
Fax: 843-377-0905
Website: http://www.nafc.org
E-mail:
memberservices@nafc.org

National Kidney Foundation
30 East 33rd Street
New York, NY 10016
Toll-Free: 800-622-9010
Phone: 212-889-2210
Fax: 212-689-9261
Website: http://www.kidney.org

Liver Disorders

Alpha-1 Foundation
2937 SW 27th Avenue, Suite 302
Miami, FL 33133
Toll-Free: 877-2-CURE-A1
(877-228-7321)
Phone: 305-567-9888
Fax: 305-567-1317
Website: http://www.alphaone.org
E-mail: info@alphaone.org

American Association for the Study of Liver Diseases
1001 North Fairfax St., Suite 400
Alexandria, VA 22314
Phone: 703-299-9766
Fax: 703-299-9622
Website: http://www.aasld.org
E-mail: aasld@aasld.org

American Liver Foundation
39 Broadway, Suite 2700
New York, New York 10006
Toll-Free: 800-GO-LIVER
(800-465-4837)
Phone: 212-668-1000
Fax: 212-483-8179
Website:
http://www.liverfoundation.org
E-mail: info@liverfoundation.org

Hepatitis Foundation International
504 Blick Drive
Silver Spring, MD 20904-2901
Toll-Free: 800-891-0707
Phone: 301-622-4200
Fax: 301-622-4702
Website: http://www.hepatitis
foundation.org
E-mail: info@
hepatitisfoundation.org

Mental Health

American Academy of Child and Adolescent Psychiatry
3615 Wisconsin Avenue NW
Washington, DC 20016-3007
Phone: 202-966-7300
Fax: 202-966-2891
Website: http://www.aacap.org
E-mail:
communications@aacap.org

American Psychological Association
750 First Street NE
Washington, DC 20002-4242
Toll-Free: 800-374-2721
Phone: 202-336-5500
TDD/TTY: 202-336-6123
Website: http://www.apa.org

Mental Health America
2000 North Beauregard Street
6th Floor
Alexandria, VA 22311
Toll-Free: 800-969-6642
Toll-Free Crisis Line:
800-273-TALK (800-273-8255)
Toll-Free TTY: 800-433-5959
Phone: 703-684-7722
Fax: 703-684-5968
Website: http://www.mental
healthamerica.net
E-mail:
info@mentalhealthamerica.net

National Association for Children's Behavioral Health
NACBH
1025 Connecticut Avenue NW
Suite 1012
Washington, DC 20036
Phone: 202-857-9735
Fax: 202-362-5145
Website: http://www.nacbh.org

National Federation of Families for Children's Mental Health
9605 Medical Center Drive
Suite 280
Rockville, MD 20850
Phone: 240-403-1901
Fax: 240-403-1909
Website: http://www.ffcmh.org
E-mail: ffcmh@ffcmh.org

National Institute of Mental Health

6001 Executive Boulevard
Room 8184, MSC 9663
Bethesda, MD 20892-9663
Toll-Free: 866-615-NIMH
(866-615-6464)
Toll-Free TTY: 866-415-8051
Phone: 301-443-4513
TTY: 301-443-8431
Fax: 301-443-4279
Website:
http://www.nimh.nih.gov
E-mail: nimhinfo@nih.gov

Substance Abuse and Mental Health Services Administration (SAMHSA)

SAMHSA's Health Information
Network
P.O. Box 2345
Rockville, MD 20847-2345
Toll-Free: 877-SAMHSA-7
(877-726-4727)
Toll-Free Suicide Prevention
Lifeline: 800-273-TALK
(800-273-8255)
Toll-Free 24/7 Treatment
Referral Line: 800-622-HELP
(800-622-4357)
Toll-Free TTY: 800-487-4889
Toll-Free TDD: 866-889-2647
Phone: 240-276-1310 (Center for
Mental Health Services)
Fax: 240-221-4295
Fax: 240-276-1320 (Center for
Mental Health Services)
Website: http://samhsa.gov
E-mail: SAMHSAInfo@samhsa
.hhs.gov

Muscular Dystrophy

Muscular Dystrophy Association (MDA)

National Headquarters
3300 East Sunrise Drive
Tucson, AZ 85718-3208
Toll-Free: 800-572-1717
Phone: 520-529-2000
Fax: 520-529-5300
Website: http://www.mda.org
E-mail: mda@mdausa.org

Neurological Disorders

Charlie Foundation to Help Cure Pediatric Epilepsy

515 Ocean Avenue, Suite 602N
Santa Monica, CA 90402
Phone: 310-393-2347
Website: http://www.charlie
foundation.org
E-mail: ketoman@aol.com

Children's Neurobiological Solutions (CNS) Foundation

1726 Franceschi Road
Santa Barbara, CA 93103-1870
Toll-Free: 866-CNS-5580
(866-267-5580)
Phone: 805-898-4442
Fax: 805-898-4448
Website: http://www.cns
foundation.org
E-mail: info@cnsfoundation.org

Epilepsy Foundation
8301 Professional Place
Landover, MD 20785-7223
Toll-Free: 800-EFA-1000
(800-332-1000)
Phone: 301-459-3400
Fax: 301-577-2684
Website: http://www.epilepsy
foundation.org
E-mail: ContactUs@efa.org

Scoliosis

National Scoliosis Foundation
5 Cabot Place
Stoughton, MA 02072
Toll-Free: 800-NSF-MYBACK
(800-673-6922)
Phone: 781-341-6333
Fax: 781-341-8333
Website: http://www.scoliosis.org
E-mail: nsf@scoliosis.org

Scoliosis Association, Inc.
P.O. Box 811705
Boca Raton, FL 33481-1705
Toll-Free: 800-800-0669
Phone: 561-994-4435
Fax: 561-994-2455
Website:
http://www.scoliosis-assoc.org
E-mail: scolioassn2@aol.com

Skin Disorders

American Academy of Dermatology
P.O. Box 4014
Schaumburg, IL 60618-4014
Toll-Free: 866-503-SKIN
(866-503-7546)
Phone: 847-240-1280
Fax: 847-240-1859
Website: http://www.aad.org
E-mail: MRC@aad.org

Sleep Disorders

National Sleep Foundation
1010 North Glebe Rd., Suite 310
Arlington, VA 22201
Phone: 703-243-1697
Website: http://www.sleep
foundation.org
E-mail: nsf@sleepfoundation.org

Vision Disorders

Lighthouse International
111 East 59th Street
New York, NY 10022-1202
Toll-Free: 800-829-0500
Phone: 212-821-9200
TTY: 212-821-9713
Fax: 212-821-9707
Website: http://lighthouse.org
E-mail: info@lighthouse.org

National Eye Institute
Information Office
31 Centers Drive, MSC 2510
Bethesda, MD 20892-2510
Phone: 301-496-5248
Website: http://nei.nih.gov
E-mail: 2020@nei.nih.gov

Index

Index

Page numbers followed by 'n' indicate a footnote. Page numbers in *italics* indicate a table or illustration.

679

Health Reference Series